Diabetes Meal Planning & Nutrition

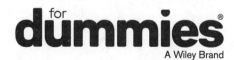

A Wiley Brand

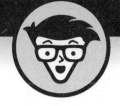

Diabetes Meal Planning & Nutrition

2nd Edition

By Dr. Simon Poole and Amy Riolo with Dr. Alan Rubin and Toby Smithson, RDN, CDE

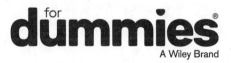

A Wiley Brand

Diabetes Meal Planning & Nutrition For Dummies®, 2nd Edition

Published by: **John Wiley & Sons, Inc.,** 111 River Street, Hoboken, NJ 07030-5774, www.wiley.com

Copyright © 2024 by John Wiley & Sons, Inc., Hoboken, New Jersey

Published simultaneously in Canada

No part of this publication may be reproduced, stored in a retrieval system or transmitted in any form or by any means, electronic, mechanical, photocopying, recording, scanning or otherwise, except as permitted under Sections 107 or 108 of the 1976 United States Copyright Act, without the prior written permission of the Publisher. Requests to the Publisher for permission should be addressed to the Permissions Department, John Wiley & Sons, Inc., 111 River Street, Hoboken, NJ 07030, (201) 748-6011, fax (201) 748-6008, or online at http://www.wiley.com/go/permissions.

Trademarks: Wiley, For Dummies, the Dummies Man logo, Dummies.com, Making Everything Easier, and related trade dress are trademarks or registered trademarks of John Wiley & Sons, Inc. and may not be used without written permission. All other trademarks are the property of their respective owners. John Wiley & Sons, Inc. is not associated with any product or vendor mentioned in this book.

LIMIT OF LIABILITY/DISCLAIMER OF WARRANTY: WHILE THE PUBLISHER AND AUTHORS HAVE USED THEIR BEST EFFORTS IN PREPARING THIS WORK, THEY MAKE NO REPRESENTATIONS OR WARRANTIES WITH RESPECT TO THE ACCURACY OR COMPLETENESS OF THE CONTENTS OF THIS WORK AND SPECIFICALLY DISCLAIM ALL WARRANTIES, INCLUDING WITHOUT LIMITATION ANY IMPLIED WARRANTIES OF MERCHANTABILITY OR FITNESS FOR A PARTICULAR PURPOSE. NO WARRANTY MAY BE CREATED OR EXTENDED BY SALES REPRESENTATIVES, WRITTEN SALES MATERIALS OR PROMOTIONAL STATEMENTS FOR THIS WORK. THE FACT THAT AN ORGANIZATION, WEBSITE, OR PRODUCT IS REFERRED TO IN THIS WORK AS A CITATION AND/OR POTENTIAL SOURCE OF FURTHER INFORMATION DOES NOT MEAN THAT THE PUBLISHER AND AUTHORS ENDORSE THE INFORMATION OR SERVICES THE ORGANIZATION, WEBSITE, OR PRODUCT MAY PROVIDE OR RECOMMENDATIONS IT MAY MAKE. THIS WORK IS SOLD WITH THE UNDERSTANDING THAT THE PUBLISHER IS NOT ENGAGED IN RENDERING PROFESSIONAL SERVICES. THE ADVICE AND STRATEGIES CONTAINED HEREIN MAY NOT BE SUITABLE FOR YOUR SITUATION. YOU SHOULD CONSULT WITH A SPECIALIST WHERE APPROPRIATE. FURTHER, READERS SHOULD BE AWARE THAT WEBSITES LISTED IN THIS WORK MAY HAVE CHANGED OR DISAPPEARED BETWEEN WHEN THIS WORK WAS WRITTEN AND WHEN IT IS READ. NEITHER THE PUBLISHER NOR AUTHORS SHALL BE LIABLE FOR ANY LOSS OF PROFIT OR ANY OTHER COMMERCIAL DAMAGES, INCLUDING BUT NOT LIMITED TO SPECIAL, INCIDENTAL, CONSEQUENTIAL, OR OTHER DAMAGES.

For general information on our other products and services, please contact our Customer Care Department within the U.S. at 877-762-2974, outside the U.S. at 317-572-3993, or fax 317-572-4002. For technical support, please visit https://hub.wiley.com/community/support/dummies.

Wiley publishes in a variety of print and electronic formats and by print-on-demand. Some material included with standard print versions of this book may not be included in e-books or in print-on-demand. If this book refers to media such as a CD or DVD that is not included in the version you purchased, you may download this material at http://booksupport.wiley.com. For more information about Wiley products, visit www.wiley.com.

Library of Congress Control Number: 2023946157

ISBN 978-1-394-20686-5 (pbk); ISBN 978-1-394-20688-9 (ebk); ISBN 978-1-394-20689-6 (ebk)

SKY10056017_092523

Contents at a Glance

Introduction 1

Part 1: Diabetes and Food: Culinary Therapy 7

CHAPTER 1: Eating Well with Diabetes 9

CHAPTER 2: Understanding Diabetes : A Holistic Approach 23

CHAPTER 3: Managing Diabetes and Blood Glucose 39

CHAPTER 4: Incorporating Easy Lifestyle Hacks 55

Part 2: Nutrition with Purpose 63

CHAPTER 5: Explaining Nutrition Requirements for Diabetes 65

CHAPTER 6: Meeting the Macronutrients: Carbohydrates, Fat, and Protein 81

CHAPTER 7: Making Micronutrients Work for You 105

CHAPTER 8: Eating a Rainbow: Bioactive Compounds and Polyphenols 125

CHAPTER 9: Equipping Yourself for Success 143

Part 3: Eating for Pleasure and Better Health 159

CHAPTER 10: Exposing Barriers to Healthy Eating 161

CHAPTER 11: Setting Priorities and Staying on Track 177

CHAPTER 12: Choosing the Best Food When Shopping 191

Part 4: Ready, Set, Plan 211

CHAPTER 13: Customizing Your Meals 213

CHAPTER 14: Analyzing Popular Diet Plans 237

CHAPTER 15: What's on the Menu: Having a Plan for Eating Out 259

CHAPTER 16: Choosing Sensible Beverages and Snacks 275

Part 5: Putting It All Together: Meals to Manage Your Diabetes 289

CHAPTER 17: Reviewing a Seven-Day Menu 291

CHAPTER 18: Creating Delicious and Nutritious Meals 301

Part 6: The Part of Tens 345

CHAPTER 19: Ten Diabetes "Power Foods" 347

CHAPTER 20: Ten Inexpensive Diabetes-Friendly Foods 355

CHAPTER 21: Ten Healthful Food Swaps for Losing Weight 361

Appendix A: Diabetes Exchange Lists 369

Appendix B: Glycemic Index and Glycemic Load Values 387

Appendix C: Examples of Bioactive Compounds in Foods 391

Index 397

Table of Contents

INTRODUCTION 1

About This Book 2

Foolish Assumptions 4

Icons Used in This Book 4

Beyond the Book 5

Where to Go from Here 6

PART 1: DIABETES AND FOOD: CULINARY THERAPY 7

CHAPTER 1: Eating Well with Diabetes 9

Balancing Glucose in the Body 10

Taking Your Place in Diabetes Management 11

Understanding Your Brain's Role in Eating 13

Making the mind-body connection 13

Exploring how emotion and eating are connected 14

Explaining impulsive eating 15

Deciding What to Eat and When 17

Helping your body manage blood glucose 18

Considering carbohydrates 18

Keeping your heart healthy 20

Making It Easy on Yourself 21

CHAPTER 2: Understanding Diabetes : A Holistic Approach 23

Defining Diabetes Mellitus 24

Explaining the role of glucose 25

Simplifying insulin 26

Exploring Type 1 Diabetes 27

Losing the capacity to produce insulin 27

Comparing LADA with type 1 29

Puzzling over the causes of type 1 29

Analyzing Type 2 and Gestational Diabetes 30

Prediabetes and the possible progression of type 2 30

Weighing the role of body mass 32

Considering ethnicity, genetics, and age 32

Developing diabetes during pregnancy 34

Summing Up the Potential Complications of Diabetes 34

Linking diabetes and inflammation 36

Exploring diabetes and immunity: COVID-19 and
other infections 38

CHAPTER 3: **Managing Diabetes and Blood Glucose** 39

Regulating Your Body's Blood Glucose Levels. 40
Understanding how insulin works 41
Storing glucose for later 42
Losing the Glucose Balance 43
Measuring Blood Glucose 44
Testing blood glucose at home 45
Getting the averages. 46
Ensuring the Best Diabetes Care. 47
Choosing your medical team. 47
Monitoring your medications 49
Explaining insulin therapy 51
Seeing a Registered Dietitian or Certified Nutrition Specialist 52
Achieving and maintaining a healthy body weight. 53
Reducing risk for a variety of complications 53
Getting to know quality carbohydrates .54

CHAPTER 4: **Incorporating Easy Lifestyle Hacks**. 55

Adopting a Healthful and Enjoyable Diabetes Lifestyle. 56
Enjoying physical activity 56
Transforming stress 59
Prioritizing Your Health 60
Making the commitment 61
Enjoying the community, fresh air, and pleasurable activities 61
Valuing prevention 62

PART 2: NUTRITION WITH PURPOSE 63

CHAPTER 5: **Explaining Nutrition Requirements
for Diabetes**. 65

Five Principles of Excellent Nutrition 66
Targeting Blood Glucose Control in Type 1 and Type 2 Diabetes 67
Matching medication and food. 67
Keeping A1C in range 69
Losing to Win: Weight Loss 70
Monitoring Cardiovascular Risks. 72
Normalizing high blood pressure 73
Lowering LDL cholesterol. 74
Looking at other risks 76
Being Aware of Special Circumstances 76
Children. 76
Elderly 77
Athletes. 78
Celiac and gluten sensitivity. 78

Gastroparesis. 79
Kidney failure 79

CHAPTER 6: **Meeting the Macronutrients: Carbohydrates, Fat, and Protein**. 81

Food Is More than Macronutrients. 82
Building a Complete Meal Is Important 83
Energizing with Quality Carbohydrates 84
Looking at sugar and diabetes 86
Not all carbs are created equal: Complex carbohydrates. 88
Evaluating glycemic index and glycemic load 88
Counting Carbs 91
Counting to 15 grams 91
Comparing carb choices. 92
Insulin bolus dosing 93
Putting Carbs on Your Plate. 94
Filling Fiber and How to Use It. 95
Embracing Healthful Fats. 96
Going beyond insulation 97
Highlighting unsaturated fat 97
Debating saturated fat and cholesterol. 99
Identifying the Best Quality Proteins 100
Recycling amino acids from food 101
Identifying the best animal sources of protein. 102
Using plants for protein 104

CHAPTER 7: **Making Micronutrients Work for You**. 105

Introducing Versatile Vitamins 106
Give me a "B" (vitamin or two). 106
A sunny day with vitamin D 108
Finding Marvelous Minerals. 110
Calcium: More than strong bones. 111
Chromium: From the Emerald City. 112
Magnesium: A crucial player 113
Potassium: Too much, or too little 114
Sodium: A little goes a long way 115
Insulin and zinc: Two peas in a pancreas. 117
Sorting Out Supplements. 117
The Gut Microbiome and Its Role in Diabetes. 120
Understanding the role of prebiotics. 122
Learning how probiotics can help. 122

CHAPTER 8: **Eating a Rainbow: Bioactive Compounds and Polyphenols**...................................125

Defining Bioactive Compounds.................................126
Understanding Bioactives and Their Role in Health.............127
Analyzing Oxidation and Antioxidants.........................129
Inflammation: The Good, the Bad, and the Ugly................130
    Chronic inflammation and disease.........................131
    The Dietary Inflammatory Index...........................132
Getting to Know Carotenoids, Glucosinolates, and Polyphenols....133
    Colorful carotenoids.....................................133
    Glucosinolates and garlic................................135
    Powerful polyphenols.....................................136
    Flavorful flavonoids.....................................136
    Non-flavonoid polyphenols................................137
Enjoying the Taste of Bioactives.............................140
How to Recognize Foods with Bioactives.......................141

CHAPTER 9: **Equipping Yourself for Success**.......................143

Stocking Your Kitchen..143
    Gathering tools and gadgets..............................144
    Planning a pantry..146
Understanding Nutrition Facts Labels.........................148
    Calories...150
    Grams and milligrams.....................................151
    Serving sizes..152
Calculating Food Choices.....................................152
    Sizing up your food: Portion sizes.......................153
    Estimating tricks..154
Referencing the Right Resources 155
    Searching websites and apps 155
    Collecting recipes.......................................156
    Converting recipes.......................................156
Considering Exchanges..156

PART 3: EATING FOR PLEASURE AND BETTER HEALTH..159

CHAPTER 10: **Exposing Barriers to Healthy Eating**................161

Tracing Changes in the Food Environment......................162
    Surviving scarcity.......................................163
    Being overwhelmed by food 164
Recognizing Emotional Attachments to Food....................166
    Identifying with a particular culture....................167
    Making the social connection 168
    Seeking the pleasure response............................168

Losing logic to impulse from stress 170
Uncovering the mindless subconscious. .171
Eating Healthier Forever. 173
Creating the right environment. 173
Asking for help when needed 175
Planning: Deciding what to eat in advance 175

CHAPTER 11: Setting Priorities and Staying on Track 177
Committing to Your Future 178
Adhering to a new philosophy. 178
Making time for healthy eating 179
Enjoying the process. 180
Learning new things 181
Standing your ground. 182
Adopting Better Habits. 182
Eating at home more often 183
Timing is everything 183
Staying on Track 185
Discovering delicious solutions 185
Embracing imperfection. 186
Ignoring fads and quick fixes. 187
Achieving Your Goals 188
Writing it all down 189
Using blood glucose readings 189

CHAPTER 12: Choosing the Best Food When Shopping 191
Starting Healthy Meal Planning. 192
Making Your Menus 192
Compiling a list. 193
Stretching your money 194
Avoiding temptation 195
Assessing the Quality of Your Food 195
Unraveling Food Terminology. 196
Prepackaged food 196
Processed foods 198
Frozen and canned foods. 199
Organic foods. 200
Choosing the Best Foods 201
Picking produce: The colorful base of your diet 201
Incorporating whole grains 202
Adding beans and legumes 203
Enjoying nuts and seeds. 204
Increasing flavor with spices, herbs, and alums 204
Dressing dishes with extra-virgin olive oil 204

Considering fats and oils 205
Selecting condiments 207
Consuming yogurt, eggs, and dairy 207
Choosing fish and seafood. 208
Looking at poultry 209
What you need to know about red meat. 209

PART 4: READY, SET, PLAN. 211

CHAPTER 13: **Customizing Your Meals**. 213
Laying the Foundation 214
Knowing your personal meal plan 215
Making MyPlate into YourPlate 217
Understanding carb portions 219
Starting simple. 221
Picking a perfect protein. 222
Isolating carbohydrates 223
Filling up on vegetables 224
Moving Beyond Simple. 226
Knowing the sneaky foods. 226
Estimating mixed dishes and casseroles 227
Knowing basic recipe formulas 229
Pairing complete meals 230
Planning breakfast and lunch 231
Swapping out popular condiments. 232
Adding in snacks 234
Salvaging Heirloom Recipes. 234

CHAPTER 14: **Analyzing Popular Diet Plans**. 237
Basking in the Mediterranean. 238
Balancing grains, legumes, and fruit 240
Swapping meat for fish and extra-virgin olive oil 241
Understanding Heritage Diets. 243
Dining with DASH 244
Controlling high blood pressure with diet. 245
Considering grains, fruit, and dairy. 245
Finding potassium, magnesium, and calcium. 247
Losing sodium is even better. 247
Preferring Plants: Vegetarian Diets. 248
Adopting the ovo-lacto view. 249
Being vegan 250
Thinking About Low-Carb Diets. 251
Atkins diet. 252
Keto diet 253
Paleo diet 253

Counting Points: Weight Watchers 253
Food By Mail. 255
   Nutrisystem 255
   Noom. 256
   Hello Fresh 256
   BistroMD. 256
Resisting Fads. 257
   Promising the quick fix 257
   Trumpeting miracle weight-loss foods. .258

CHAPTER 15: What's on the Menu: Having a Plan for Eating Out 259
Making Decisions First 260
   Remembering your meal plan. 261
   Checking ahead 262
   Sticking to a plan 263
Dining Out 264
   Analyzing the menu. 264
   Asking the right people. 266
   Bringing your own. 267
   Taking some home 267
Keeping It Honest 268
   Drinks and bar snacks. 269
   Hors d'oeuvres, appetizers, bread, and dessert 270
   Salad bar foolers 271
   Buffets: Wanting it all 272

CHAPTER 16: Choosing Sensible Beverages and Snacks 275
Beverages. 276
   Water. 276
   Alcohol. 276
   Coffee and tea 279
   Soft drinks and flavored waters 280
   Sports and energy drinks. 281
Snacks. 282
   Nuts and seeds 282
   Yogurt 283
   Fruit. 284
   Veggies and dips 284
   Dark chocolate. 284
Low-Carb Healthy Snacks. 285
   15-gram snacks 286
   30-gram snacks 286
Alternative Sweeteners. 287

PART 5: PUTTING IT ALL TOGETHER: MEALS TO MANAGE YOUR DIABETES 289

CHAPTER 17: **Reviewing a Seven-Day Menu** 291

    Day 1 293
    Day 2 294
    Day 3 294
    Day 4 295
    Day 5 296
    Day 6 297
    Day 7 298
    Snacks 299

CHAPTER 18: **Creating Delicious and Nutritious Meals** 301

    Bountiful Breakfasts 302
        Poached Egg and Avocado Toast with Warm Cherry Tomatoes and Sea Salt 303
        Blueberry-Almond Yogurt Bowls with Honey, Cinnamon, and Chia Seeds 305
        Fresh Fruit Salad with Homemade Vanilla and Flaxseed Granola.......................................306
        Warm Raspberry and Cocoa Quinoa with Almond Milk and Sesame Seeds 307
        Middle Eastern–Style Breakfast Platter 308
        Egyptian Fuul Medammes with Extra-Virgin Olive Oil, Tomato, and Eggs 309
        Cardamom-Scented Kefir, Pineapple, and Kiwi Smoothie.......310
    Looking Forward to Lunch 311
        Homemade Hummus and Whole Wheat Pita with Fresh Vegetables 312
        Moroccan Rice, Lamb, Vegetable, and Lentil Soup 313
        Roasted Sweet Potato, Avocado, and Quinoa Bowls with Honey-Lime Dressing and Cashews....................314
        Lebanese Fattoush Salad with Citrus-Infused Chicken 315
        Asian Noodle and Seven-Vegetable Salad with Sweet and Tangy Ginger Sauce 316
        Broccoli and Pecorino Cheese Soup with Stuffed Baby Portobello Mushrooms.....................................317
        Hearty Farro and Five-Vegetable Minestrone 319
        Cucumber and Smoked Salmon Pinwheels with Mixed Green Salad 320
        Baba Ghanouj with Crudités and Roasted Chickpeas 321
    Delicious Dinners..323
        Citrus-Marinated Salmon with Fiery Potatoes and Kale 324
        Red Lentil Croquettes over Baby Spinach with Tzatziki Sauce ...325

Chicken Simmered in Tomatoes, Olives, and
Capers with Sautéed Dandelion Greens and Salad 327

Turkish-Style Eggplant and Chickpea Stew with
Brown Basmati Rice Pilaf 328

Fresh Herb and Parmigiano Crusted Fish with
Apple, Beet, and Carrot Salad with Citrus Vinaigrette 330

Pasta with Pistachio Pesto, Fresh Tuna, and
Yellow Tomato Sauce 331

Sizzling Rosemary Shrimp over Cannellini Bean
Puree and Sautéed Greens with Mixed Peppers 332

Assorted Seafood Tartines with Microgreen,
Red Cabbage, Carrot, and Corn Slaw 334

Asparagus, Red Pepper, and Tempeh Stir-Fry
with Soba Noodles and Sesame Seeds .335

Must-Have Base Recipes 336

Dried Beans 337

Lentils 338

Homemade Vegetable Stock 339

Homemade Seafood Stock 340

Homemade Chicken Stock 341

Fresh Bread Crumbs 342

Fresh Tomato Sauce 343

PART 6: THE PART OF TENS 345

CHAPTER 19: **Ten Diabetes "Power Foods"** 347

Extra-Virgin Olive Oil 348

Beans 349

Salmon and Tuna 349

Nuts 350

Oranges and Lemons 350

Kale (and Other Leafy Greens) 351

Dark Chocolate 351

Soybeans 352

Full-Fat Greek-Style Plain Yogurt 353

Whole Grains: Oats and Barley 353

Oats 354

Barley 354

CHAPTER 20: **Ten Inexpensive Diabetes-Friendly Foods** 355

Beans 356

Lentils 356

Apples 357

Yogurt 357

Potatoes 358

Bananas 358

Carrots 358
Eggs 359
Beets 359
Peanut Butter. 360

CHAPTER 21: **Ten Healthful Food Swaps for Losing Weight**. 361
Swap Bottled Dressings for Extra-Virgin Olive Oil
and Vinegar or Lemon Juice. 362
Make Your Own Fresh Tomato Sauce 362
Skip Sour Cream and Go Greek Instead. 363
Flavor Your Foods with Aromatics 364
Use Raw Vegetables for Dipping. 365
Spice It Up. 366
Reach for a Healthier Chocolate Fix .366
Choose Fresh or Frozen over Canned and Jarred. 367
Opt For Nutrient-Dense Foods over Processed and
Packaged Foods. 368
Eat Fresh Fish or Legumes over Red Meat. 368

APPENDIX A: DIABETES EXCHANGE LISTS 369

APPENDIX B: GLYCEMIC INDEX AND GLYCEMIC
LOAD VALUES 387

APPENDIX C: EXAMPLES OF BIOACTIVE
COMPOUNDS IN FOODS 391

INDEX. 397

Introduction

This book was written to give you the nutritional and culinary knowledge necessary to prevent, treat, and even reverse diabetes. Armed with simple strategies and sound advice, *Diabetes Meal Planning & Nutrition For Dummies* enables you to take control of diabetes. Whether you purchased this book for yourself or for a loved one and use it to prevent, treat, or reverse a diabetes diagnosis, you will find the answers you need all in one place.

There should be no such thing as a "diabetic diet." A person with diabetes should not need to choose from a different restaurant menu or be limited to looking for specifically labeled products that have sugar substituted by an artificial sweetener. With the number of people worldwide estimated to have diabetes projected to rise to 642 million by 2040, there is a compelling case for looking at nutrition for managing type 2 diabetes not only when it occurs but also as a strategy to prevent it from developing.

More than half of the population of many countries is now defined as being overweight and at risk of having established type 2 diabetes, undiagnosed type 2 diabetes, or its precursor, prediabetes. The reasons for the dramatic rise in type 2 diabetes and prediabetes are almost certainly related to the move away from traditional healthy lifestyles to our current so-called "Western" processed diets with refined sugars and additives and sedentary patterns of behavior. It is also clear that the complications of poorly controlled diabetes such as heart disease, stroke, dementia, and kidney disease are conditions that can also cause chronic illnesses in people, especially those with poor diets who do not have diabetes.

The dietary advice we give in this book aims to help you achieve excellent blood glucose control, optimum weight maintenance, and better overall health — things that can benefit the majority of people with or without diabetes. The best nutritional advice for people with or without diabetes is to enjoy a diet of foods and nutrients that reduce the likelihood of many of these chronic illnesses. This makes diabetes, its prevention, possible reversal and management, and reduction in its complications everybody's business.

Best of all, this book exemplifies how you don't need to give up good-tasting food in order to maintain a diabetes-friendly lifestyle! On the contrary, it shows how to pair ingredients together for maximum flavor and nutritional benefits. You'll fall in love with culinary therapy techniques that have the power to transform your life. Food is the simplest, least expensive, most available, and most immediate treatment option for diabetes health and overall wellbeing.

Luckily, the foods used in this book are readily available and offer options for a wide variety of tastes. Many of the simple foods that we take for granted are the most beneficial to our diets, and this book shows you how to unleash their power, all while keeping an eye on the clock and the budget. Many people with diabetes struggle to adopt healthier eating habits, many to the point of giving up. This book, however, was built to inspire with enjoyable practices that will enrich your life as well as your meals.

If the word *planning* in the title seems like the least important (even least interesting) subject in the pages ahead, you are in for an amazing surprise — maybe even an epiphany. See, the struggle with healthy eating doesn't come from your stomach, your pancreas, or an uncontrollable hand that sneaks unhealthy food into your mouth when you're not looking. Your struggle with healthy eating is a struggle between your incredible brain and your primitive survival chemistry, and when it comes to food, chemistry often wins. You're about to learn how planning can tip the balance, and make healthier eating your newest accomplishment. Adopting the advice in this book can provide a way to establish a balanced, satisfying, and truly enjoyable relationship with food.

About This Book

Diabetes Meal Planning & Nutrition For Dummies zeroes in on the important relationship between diabetes and food, and helps you make choices that benefit your long-term health and satisfy your eating preferences. The book's focus is on which foods you can, and should, eat to improve your health with diabetes, and not on what you shouldn't eat. There is no doubt, by the way, that how you choose to eat when you have diabetes can have a remarkable effect on your health — this book helps ensure that effect is a positive one. And it is not just about considering the nutrients we eat in the greatest quantity — for diabetes the all-important carbohydrates, fats, and proteins — but also to understand the vital role of micronutrients such as vitamins and minerals, as well as the new science of our gut microbiome and food constituents called bioactive compounds that can have profound antioxidant and anti-inflammatory effects.

The book acknowledges and explains some of the barriers you may have experienced to adopting healthier eating habits, and how your best intentions can be sabotaged. And, you see how the power of making eating decisions in advance — planning — can get you beyond those barriers and keep you there. More than 80 percent of people with type 2 diabetes are overweight or obese, and many have made attempts to change eating habits without success. This discussion on planning may be just the advice you need.

The target audience is people already diagnosed with type 1 or type 2 diabetes, but the concepts and practical advice for managing diabetes with diet apply to gestational diabetes, to those with prediabetes, and even to people who feel they may be at risk of diabetes. This book doesn't substitute for medical nutrition therapy from a registered dietitian, but should help you put your personalized diabetes meal plan into action.

TIP

Diabetes Meal Planning & Nutrition For Dummies does discuss diabetes as a disease, but if you're new to diabetes you may want to grab one of Dr. Poole's and Amy Riolo's other books, such as *Diabetes For Dummies,* for a more detailed discussion. Food is an important part of managing diabetes over the long term, but there's a lot more you need to know.

Diabetes often occurs with medical conditions, like celiac disease or lactose intolerance, that limit food choices. And, diabetes can promote health conditions, like kidney failure, that trigger very specific dietary requirements that are significantly different than general recommendations for a diabetes meal plan. Your doctor and a registered dietitian can advise you in these cases, but advice in this book may not always apply.

REMEMBER

You should know that you don't have to read this book from front to back. All *For Dummies* books are written so that each chapter will make sense on its own. It's not necessary that you remember anything either — a detailed table of contents helps you find what you need whenever you need it. This book is meant to be a reference; there will be no final exam to test your memorization skills.

Here are a few other tidbits that may answer your questions before you have to ask:

» Blood glucose is often casually called *blood sugar*. Blood glucose is the correct terminology and is used exclusively in the book. In common usage, the terms mean the same.

» Blood glucose is measured in milligrams per deciliter (mg/dl) in the United States, but many countries use the International System of Units measure of millimoles per liter (mmol/l). The same is true for cholesterol and triglycerides.

» Healthy eating is no less important for people with type 1 diabetes, but insulin does provide a more direct way to control blood glucose. Some discussion about managing food amount and timing may be less relevant to people with type 1 diabetes when rapid acting insulin is used.

>> The term *diabetic* is not used to refer to a person with diabetes. Diabetes is not who you are; it's a condition you have.

>> This book does not spend much time addressing the particulars of insulin dosing, insulin-carbohydrate ratios, or insulin correction factors. These are very individualized and must be worked out with your doctor or diabetes educator.

Foolish Assumptions

Your authors have some preconceived notions about you, and thought you might be interested in knowing what those are. This book assumes the following:

>> You have diabetes, or have an interest in someone who has diabetes. It's okay if neither is true, by the way.

>> You realize that effectively managing diabetes for better health includes managing what and how you eat. Maybe you've been advised about the importance of diet, or maybe you learned from previous experience with diabetes.

>> You are not expecting a miracle answer that requires no further thinking or effort from you.

>> Even though you are not expecting a miracle, you appreciate advice that makes healthy eating for diabetes easier.

Icons Used in This Book

Throughout *For Dummies* books you find icons that call your attention to something especially important, or something technical. This book includes the following icons:

TIP

A Tip icon often suggests you try something or check something out, and it usually points to something surprising about food or nutrition.

WARNING

A Warning icon does exactly what it sounds like. It warns against potential problems.

REMEMBER

The Remember icon might re-emphasize something discussed earlier in the section, or it may be a reminder to follow specific advice when you put what you've learned in practice.

TECHNICAL STUFF

The Technical Stuff icon highlights information that is beyond what's key to the book's message, but something some curious readers might find interesting.

ASK THE DOCTOR

This icon points out where Dr. Simon Poole added special insight from his medical expertise and practice.

FROM THE AUTHORS

This icon designates instances where Dr. Simon Poole and Chef Amy Riolo describe anecdotes and special tips from their experience.

Beyond the Book

There is much more information available from your authors and from the *For Dummies* brand for your learning pleasure. Check out these resources to learn more about diabetes and nutrition or to find some great recipes:

>> Check out this book's online Cheat Sheet for more help and information. Just go to www.dummies.com and search for "Diabetes Meal Planning & Nutrition For Dummies Cheat Sheet."

>> You can meet your authors face to face, literally, on their respective websites so that you can get an idea of who's giving you the wonderful advice in this book. You can find Dr. Poole at www.drsimonpoole.com and Amy Riolo at www.amyriolo.com.

>> And, although this book includes 25 diabetes-friendly complete meal recipes so that you don't have to worry about covering nutritional requirements and glucose managing in your meals, you can use what you learn about choosing diabetes-friendly dishes from other resources, too. An excellent place to start is *Diabetes For Dummies*, 6th Edition, published by Wiley.

Where to Go from Here

You can start anywhere with *For Dummies* books, but there's a logic to beginning at the beginning. If that's not in your personality, consider starting with Chapter 10 to see why healthy eating — diabetes or not — is so difficult in this society. Chapter 14 reviews how some popular diet plans will fit with effective diabetes self-management, and if you're not sure what diabetes self-management means, try Chapter 3.

Chapter 11 addresses how you can stay motivated and offers simple tricks that usually bring big rewards. If you're heading straight to the buffet or restaurant, check Chapter 15; the grocery can be found in Chapter 12.

Some final advice is don't get in such a rush. Diabetes will still be there, and changes often come slowly. Take your time, try different approaches to eating healthier, and be patient about seeing real improvements in your lab work. We find that lasting change is best achieved when done gradually. Little changes add up and are more easily sustained than drastic life changes. Start wherever you are with good intentions, knowing that you will eventually reach your objectives. In addition, if you have been living an unhealthy lifestyle or suffering from diabetes symptoms without any treatment at all, once you start making positive changes you will begin feeling better than before, and that is the best motivator of all.

TIP

Don't forget the famous speech Dr. Martin Luther King Jr. delivered at Spelman College in 1960: "If you can't fly then run, if you can't run then walk, if you can't walk then crawl, but whatever you do you have to keep moving forward."

1
Diabetes and Food: Culinary Therapy

Find out how to eat well with diabetes so that you can enjoy food while improving your health and balancing blood glucose levels.

Understand how the concept of culinary therapy can help you look and feel your best while enjoying yourself in the process.

Understand the difference between prediabetes, type 1, and type 2.

Know how to test your blood glucose levels at home, especially with type 1 diabetes. With so many different ways to test, you no longer have to guess your blood glucose level.

Be inspired to incorporate easy lifestyle hacks to take charge of your health and happiness.

Chapter 1

Eating Well with Diabetes

Hippocrates, sometimes called the father of modern medicine, once said "let food be thy medicine, and medicine be thy food." When it comes to diabetes, Hippocrates was absolutely correct. It would be difficult to think of another serious medical condition that's so intimately and immediately connected to food. Yes, there are drugs for diabetes — eight different classes of diabetes drugs, numerous formulations of insulin, drugs that help other drugs work better, and a few drugs that seem to benefit diabetes by accident — and diabetes drugs are extremely important. Without insulin, people with type 1 diabetes cannot live. However, putting your confidence in drugs alone is insufficient to keep diabetes from affecting your long-term health, and you don't have to rely on advice that's more than 2,300 years old to believe that.

Making healthy lifestyle choices that include eating the best foods and getting regular exercise dramatically improves diabetes control and may also prevent and even reverse type 2 diabetes. An excellent diet can protect us from many of the chronic diseases, including heart disease and stroke, that are common complications of type 1 and type 2 diabetes and that also frequently affect people without diabetes. A healthy and sustainable dietary pattern is one that will support achieving and maintaining an optimum weight.

Chances are you already have at least a vague idea that what you eat is important to diabetes. With or without diabetes, our food choices can contribute to a happy and heathy life. This book gives you the whole story on just how the food choices you make can work to add healthy and active years to your life — without sacrificing delicious foods and flavors. To start, this chapter explains how food is effective medicine for prediabetes, as well as type 1 and type 2. In the pages ahead you explore your role in preserving your health, how to make your brain work for you, and how to choose the most nutrient-boosting foods.

Balancing Glucose in the Body

Whether you have type 1 diabetes or type 2 diabetes, you share one crucial responsibility from your diagnosis going forward — doing your part. In simple terms, you must now become an active helper in your body's metabolism, and the better helper you become, the less likely you are to experience the damage that diabetes can do to your body.

Type 1 diabetes results when your capacity to produce insulin is lost. Type 2 diabetes is related more to your natural insulin being unable to do its job effectively. If you were a car and insulin was gasoline, type 1 diabetes is having an empty tank, and type 2 diabetes is more like lost efficiency from clogged fuel injectors. Managing type 1 diabetes requires constantly adding gasoline; type 2 diabetes requires that you get your fuel injectors to work better. The real story is a little more complicated.

Your body needs to keep a certain concentration of glucose circulating in your blood — a normal blood glucose level. Glucose is the favorite fuel of your trillions of cells, and some really important cells — your brain cells — can't get their energy from anything else. Glucose in your bloodstream is all about energy — it's delivered right to the doorstep of every cell that needs it.

Because glucose enters your blood after you eat carbohydrate foods, causing your blood glucose levels to rise, your body has a way to return those levels back to normal by storing the excess for later. The stored glucose can be released back into the blood when glucose levels drop between meals, keeping a constant supply available for your brain. This kind of balance in a biological system is called *homeostasis*.

The hormone responsible for escorting glucose into storage is insulin, and insulin is automatically released from special cells on your pancreas when blood glucose levels are going higher after eating. If insulin isn't available or isn't working properly, blood glucose can't be stored, and blood glucose levels remain high. High blood glucose levels not only upset glucose homeostasis, but begin to damage cells and tissue.

REMEMBER

Chronic high blood glucose levels is diabetes — literally. It's important that you understand diabetes, and Chapters 2 and 3 include a more in-depth explanation. In the simplest terms, having diabetes means your blood glucose levels go up after eating and don't come down to normal levels in a normal amount of time.

Type 1 diabetes results when insulin production capacity is destroyed, and no insulin is available to facilitate glucose homeostasis. Type 2 diabetes begins when the cells that normally store excess glucose stop responding to insulin. So, even though insulin may be available, blood glucose levels remain high. The long-term damage caused by high blood glucose, in either case, can progress to very serious consequences like heart attack, stroke, vision loss, nerve damage, kidney failure, and more. These secondary conditions are called *complications of diabetes,* and avoiding these outcomes is one reason that lowering blood glucose levels is so important.

High glucose levels not only mean that excess glucose can't get into cells to be stockpiled, but also that glucose can't get into cells to properly fuel energy needs. That means your microscopic cells, like the muscle cells you need to move, don't have access to their favored fuel and must turn to plan B or plan C for generating energy. Plans B and C are ordinarily temporary plans for times of shortage — generating energy without glucose is inefficient, and even produces toxic waste products. Diabetes upsets your entire energy balance.

Taking Your Place in Diabetes Management

Treating diabetes is not like treating an infected cut, where the problem goes away after a week or two. In fact, diabetes treatment is called *diabetes management,* hinting at a responsibility that requires continuous oversight. And, that's exactly what diabetes management is — continuous oversight. Managing diabetes is like managing a company, or a sports team, or a lawn, or anything else where the goal is to achieve and sustain a certain level of performance. The manager works to provide the best environment and materials for success, looks at performance indicators, sets priorities, makes adjustments to improve efficiency, tries to avoid disruptions, and always keeps a focus on surviving and prospering over the long term.

Effective management is a key to success in business, sports, lawn care, and diabetes. But, while the management responsibilities for businesses, sports teams, and even lawn care can be delegated to professional experts, the extraordinarily important job of managing your diabetes has suddenly fallen on you — diabetes self-management. Not only that, you've inherited responsibility for the equivalent of a business that's experiencing challenges, a sports team with some of its stars on injured reserve, and a lawn that's been overcome by weeds — and the stake is your long-term health.

Fortunately, if you're willing to take this responsibility seriously, there is a proven plan that can turn you into a successful manager of your body's metabolism. And, as daunting as this might sound, with some dedication and practice you'll be managing your metabolism like a pro and enjoying the rest of your life's activities even more than before. How's that? Well, like any good manager, success is a little bit of participating, but a whole lot of setting up a system where success is possible. You will also have professional advice as well as help from your team of supporters to guide you on your journey.

REMEMBER

You may not be able to permanently fix your glucose metabolism. You can, however, provide the best environment and materials for success, look at performance indicators, set priorities, make adjustments to improve efficiency, try to avoid disruptions, and always keep a focus on flourishing and prospering over the long term. That sort of management strategy lets your natural metabolism work as well as it possibly can, and that's effective diabetes self-management at its best. And, you can do it.

LEARNING TO MANAGE AND REVERSE DIABETES

The aim of eating well for diabetes is to optimize blood glucose control and to minimize the risks of complications, but it is also possible to prevent diabetes in someone who has *prediabetes* where measurements are suggesting signs of long-term blood glucose levels progressing toward the range of a type 2 diabetes diagnosis. Even when a person has been diagnosed with type 2 diabetes, it is possible to reverse the diagnosis and to remain in a range of blood glucose that is considered normal as long as dietary patterns and lifestyle changes can be sustained.

Understanding Your Brain's Role in Eating

Right between your ears is your incredible and mysterious brain, and your brain plays essential roles in managing diabetes. But, the different roles your brain plays in diabetes management aren't always in your best interests, and more often than you might imagine messages from your brain make managing diabetes more difficult.

On the surface, literally and anatomically, it's obvious that your brain helps you to understand diabetes, to remember what your healthcare team has advised you to do, to schedule your time, to decide what you're going to eat, and to comprehend what you read in this book. The part of your brain doing your thinking, the outer cerebral cortex layer, is an amazing problem-solver that has never been duplicated biologically or electronically. Your thinking brain can evaluate hundreds of variables, look at issues from every direction, factor in previous experience, apply concepts that are only abstract, project future outcomes, and come to solidly logical conclusions. When your thinking brain is in charge, it's hard to go wrong. And, if things do go wrong, your thinking brain will figure out exactly why and make sure the same thing doesn't go wrong again.

But, guess what? Your thinking brain isn't always in charge. At times, the well-thought recommendations from your marvelous thinking brain get outvoted. At other times, your thinking brain takes too long to make decisions, allowing another part of your brain to beat it to the punch. There's nothing abnormal about this. In fact, some completely illogical behaviors, like risking personal safety to assist another person, make humans human. But recognizing how your thinking brain can be nullified in diabetes management can lead to more success — you can change the circumstances and give power back to that part of your brain best suited for management.

Making the mind-body connection

Modern societies are only now beginning to appreciate the positive ways in which our mind influences our bodies. The old Italian adage, *mente sana, corpo sano* means "healthy mind, healthy body." For that reason, if we want to truly perform at our best, we need to make sure our minds are performing optimally.

In the United States and in some other cultures, the word "emotions" is often used with a negative connotation. "Emotional eating," "too emotional," "put your emotions aside," and "leave your emotions out of it" are phrases we hear repeatedly in the English language. Yet without our positive emotions like love, gratitude, joy, passion, and affection, the world would be a horrible place. It is through positive emotions that we can transform negative situations into blessings, sickness into health, and enjoy our lives.

THE MIND-BODY CONNECTION IN ACTION

FROM THE AUTHORS

Years ago, Amy was suffering from what she believed to be an incurable disease. She did everything her teams of doctors told her to do, as well as additional complimentary therapies, but she was legally disabled and progressing slowly. She remembers the day her doctor suggested she see a mind-body therapist. She was so offended by this because she thought her doctor thought she had mental problems. When she expressed her concerns, he said, "Amy, anyone with as many medical symptoms and pain as you have should talk to someone, if for nothing else than just to have a confidant who understands what you're going through." Amy followed his advice, and meeting her therapist eventually saved her life and led her to a new career. If she had known then what she knows now, she would never have thought twice about exploring the emotional factors she was dealing with. In fact, she would have gone sooner.

A modern discipline of healthcare based on ancient principles called *mind-body therapy* teaches people how to listen to their bodies to identify old patterns of thought that are keeping them stuck in undesirable situations and clear them out so that they can move forward in healing physically and mentally. It is worth exploring any thoughts and feelings that you think and feel in order to see if they might be contributing to your diabetes diagnosis. Conversely, if you have been suffering from any physical disease, this, as well as other types of therapy, can be helpful in coping with what you've experienced.

Exploring how emotion and eating are connected

It's easy to see how your thinking brain gets overruled if you think about emotions. Everyone makes emotional decisions, sometimes to feel a positive emotion, and sometimes to avoid a negative one. Emotional decisions are often completely conscious — you know the decision may not be completely logical, but you're willing to accept that. There's really no way to avoid some emotional decisions, and seeking or avoiding an emotion in a specific circumstance has an emotional benefit. An illogical decision now and then about diabetes is unavoidable.

It's when a particular pattern of emotional decision-making becomes a way of life that problems can arise, and when diabetes is involved, illogical emotional behavior can be dangerous. Chapter 10 gives you some important insight of how emotion and eating are tied together, but here are some common emotional patterns that really interfere with self-care:

>> **You are unable to digest the "sweetness of life."** Anger and resentment are common, and completely understandable, among people with type 1 diabetes. Type 1 diabetes is a virtually random and completely life-changing event that happens suddenly, mostly to young and otherwise healthy individuals. And, the management responsibilities are more complex than with type 2 diabetes and are unending. But, when natural anger and resentment at fate turns into a defiant refusal to give in to the management responsibilities of type 1 diabetes, serious consequences can result.

>> **You feel guilty.** Guilt can play a similar role in type 2 diabetes because type 2 diabetes usually develops slowly, and in many cases could have been pre-vented. Guilt is anger, but directed at oneself rather than at fate. Guilt about type 2 diabetes can lead to thinking you deserve the worst diabetes can offer, and that emotion is incompatible with managing diabetes to preserve your health.

>> **You view your illness as a personal weakness.** Viewing illness as a personal weakness keeps people from even acknowledging diabetes, or has them looking to challenge diabetes to a strength contest. Ironically, the greatest strength is acknowledging the reality of diabetes and taking self-management responsibilities seriously.

>> **You put your needs second.** Misplaced selflessness is an emotional reaction that can also be unhelpful. Managing diabetes effectively does require prioritiz-ing your own health, and taking time for exercise or changing a family's eating patterns can take a back seat to what's perceived as caring for others.

These emotional patterns usually impact the whole range of diabetes manage-ment, not just eating. With some self-analysis, maybe helped by counseling and easy-to-implement daily practices such as breathwork, meditation, and positive visioning, misdirected emotional responses to diabetes can be changed for the better.

Explaining impulsive eating

If you're like most people, you probably have a mobile phone full of photographs. To you, these photos are colorful and represent pleasant memories. But in com-puter language, your photos are just a series of black and white ones and zeros — it's a secret language, but looking at millions of ones and zeros won't stimulate any pleasant memories for you. Your body has a secret language, too — a chemical language. Although you don't consciously understand this chemical language any more than the ones and zeros on your computer, this chemical language stores vivid memories, especially about food, and you can understand those memories very, very well.

It's an amazing system that has helped humans survive the toughest times. For an overly simplistic explanation, consider that the part of your brain responsible for survival doesn't trust your thinking brain with some very important responsibilities. Your thinking brain can be so wrapped up evaluating something logically that it might forget to eat when food is available. And, in tough times, you have to grab food whenever you can. So this part of your brain gives you a chemical reward when you remember to eat — a chemical that brings a comforting feeling of wellbeing. It's a reward that's so satisfying that you'll remember to eat no matter what your thinking brain is preoccupied with. And to make doubly sure you won't miss an eating opportunity, your brain gives you a little boost even if you think about food, or see a picture of food. Eventually, impulsive eating when food is available is second nature and completely unconscious. Most important, in the contest between your impulse to eat and your thinking brain, impulse usually wins.

However, this amazing biological system is obsolete in a society where food is constantly available, and it runs on overload when images of unhealthful food surround you everywhere you look. It does not, however, have an off switch. Chapter 10 explains how being surrounded by food and food images doesn't need to trigger unhealthy impulses; in fact, it can actually do the opposite.

REMEMBER

Impulsive eating has a negative connotation in the modern world, but it doesn't have to. Hunger is our body's way of encouraging us to nourish ourselves. Even cravings for certain foods, which are often viewed as problematic, can deliver great clues into what your body needs. A strong urge to eat chocolate can be as a result of a zinc deficiency, for example, while craving leafy greens might be a sign that the body is fighting off an infection.

With industrialization, advertising propaganda, and the invention of fast and junk food, however, many people are no longer in control of their cravings. A late night TV ad may stir desires for a double cheeseburger with bacon, and a billboard will make a candy bar look like something you can't live without. When coupled with subliminal messages that these items provide "a break," "a complete meal," or "a sinful delight," it can be easy to get into temptation.

Many times we crave certain food styles when we are truly craving an emotional state. It is said that those who crave salty foods most (if their cortisol levels are not unbalanced) are truly craving adventure. Those who love comforting pastas and carbohydrate-rich products are truly in need of comfort. Craving sugary snacks and sweet treats most often is because of a lack of perceived sweetness in life. If any of these scenarios sound like you, it's worth exploring whether you are truly craving the emotion associated with that type of food.

Because our lives change, so do our cravings. You may have a particular craving for sweets more than normal while in a particular stressful period of life. When things get hard, you might find yourself craving more comforting foods.

TIP

It's worth taking a few minutes to pause each time you have strong cravings for certain foods. Try sitting with your feet flat on the floor. Put one hand on your heart and the other on your belly and breathe in and out very slowly three times. Ask yourself:

» Why am I craving this food?

» What is it that I'm truly craving?

» If I had a magic wand and could be doing anything right now, what would I rather be doing?

Then take a deep breath and write down your answers. Reminding yourself that your health is your first priority, ask yourself whether you can achieve the desired emotion (comfort, love, sweetness) another way. Calling a friend, going for a walk, watching a comedy, and eating more healthful versions of the foods you're craving can help a great deal in breaking negative habits.

Deciding What to Eat and When

A significant portion of this book is dedicated to giving you the nutrition facts you need to make the most out of your meals. Contrary to popular belief, eating well with diabetes doesn't have to be difficult or boring. With a little effort and consideration, you may be surprised to find yourself eating better-tasting meals than before. In addition, your body will respond favorably once you give it the super-charged fuel it needs.

That's where meal planning comes in because it enables you to eat with both pleasure and health in mind. Planning ahead puts your thinking brain in charge, and it's your thinking brain that understands how important what you eat today and tomorrow can be to your health ten years from now. Your thinking brain may not be good for making spur-of-the-moment decisions, but when you give it time, without standing in front of an open refrigerator or watching a waiter deliver food to the next table, you win.

REMEMBER

That is precisely what makes diabetes meal planning so crucial. Taking emotion and impulse out of your eating decisions means better decisions, and better decisions about food can have a direct and immediate benefit to your health.

Helping your body manage blood glucose

"Diabetic diet" is a phrase you'll hear constantly, and what is more discouraging than to imagine yourself sentenced to an eating plan that's so restrictive that only people with diabetes have to subject themselves to it? The truth is almost the complete opposite. An eating plan that works for diabetes is an appropriate eating plan for nearly anyone. It's a balanced eating plan with five clear objectives:

>> Help your body manage blood glucose levels as effectively as possible

>> Provide adequate nutrition with a focus on reducing recognized risks for chronic diseases, especially those associated as potential complications of diabetes

>> Be an enjoyable diet that can be maintained in the long term

>> Optimize weight and body fat

>> Be ethical and sustainable for the environment and planet

Other medical conditions, including common comorbidities like celiac disease or complications caused by long-term poorly controlled diabetes, may lead to adding an emphasis to other dietary concerns, too. Without any pressing health issues other than diabetes, however, the story is pretty simple.

The specific focus for accomplishing those two objectives is managing carbohydrates and managing dietary fat. Be assured, however, that managing does not mean eliminating. An effective diabetes eating plan commonly recommends that 50 percent of daily calories come from carbohydrates, and 30 percent of daily calories come from fat. It won't shock you to learn that whole-grain pasta primavera with a little olive oil is a better option to satisfy this calorie distribution than a frosted donut. It may shock you to learn that pasta is allowed at all.

Considering carbohydrates

Earlier in this chapter you read a short discussion of glucose homeostasis — glucose balance. Glucose is a sugar, and carbohydrates are made of glucose molecules bound together in chains. That is an oversimplification — other sugars join glucose to form some carbohydrates, too, but glucose is the most prominent, and the most relevant, to diabetes.

Carbohydrates have a prominent role in this book, and Chapter 6 is devoted to understanding carbohydrates in your diet. Carbohydrates are sugars, starches, and fiber, and if you can digest them (some fiber you can't), glucose molecules are unchained and absorbed directly into your blood. The glucose in table sugar is indistinguishable from the glucose in potatoes or milk or an orange. That does not mean these foods are equivalent, but only that a glucose molecule is a glucose molecule.

TECHNICAL STUFF

Glucose is your body's favorite fuel and the only fuel your brain can use. When you eat carbohydrates, your blood glucose levels go higher, whether you have diabetes or not. High blood glucose levels stimulate insulin secretion; low blood glucose levels stimulate another hormone, *glucagon*. Insulin and glucagon work together to lower, or to raise, blood glucose so a normal level is maintained.

Insulin reduces high blood glucose levels by signaling muscle, fat, and liver cells to pull glucose into the cells, and pack it into a unique starch molecule called *glycogen* until it's needed for energy. As explained earlier in this chapter, diabetes results when sufficient insulin isn't available, or when cells don't respond normally to insulin. Your body can compensate for having no glucose available inside of cells for energy production, but only for a short time. The life expectancy of people with type 1 diabetes before treatment was available may be extended by starving them of carbohydrates, but not for long. Carbohydrate — glucose — is necessary.

Fortunately, injectable insulin is available for treating type 1 diabetes, and it works much like natural insulin to move glucose into cells. And, while type 2 diabetes is a loss of the natural response to insulin, it's not a total loss — glucose will still move into cells, albeit slowly. People with diabetes must eat carbohydrate foods to provide energy.

TIP

The amount of carbohydrate, the timing of carbohydrate consumption, and the quality of carbohydrate in the food can either help your body and medication manage blood glucose levels, or complicate the issue. If you eat a lot of carbohydrate at one time, and eat carbohydrate that is digested and absorbed into your blood quickly, blood glucose levels go up very quickly and can overtax your capacity to bring levels down. Even when injecting insulin doses matched to your carbohydrate intake, managing the amount, timing, and quality of carbohydrates pays off. Your personal diabetes meal plan will map this out for you.

So, what about sugar? In some ways, sugar is not much different than any other carbohydrate, and there's a common and dangerous misconception that to manage diabetes one only needs to avoid sugar. You now know that all carbohydrates raise blood glucose levels, and managing carbohydrates, rather than avoiding them, is the best strategy. But sugar does deserve some extra scrutiny. Eating sugar, especially in some industrially produced forms such as high fructose corn syrup, raises glucose levels faster than less refined carbohydrates. For example, cooking pasta al dente (for a lesser period of time) slows down your body's digestion of it and modulates glucose better than well-cooked pasta.

There's mounting evidence that too much sugar is unhealthy for anyone — if sugar causes metabolic disruptions in healthy people, it certainly should be consumed in serious moderation with diabetes. Also, sugar breaks down very quickly during digestion and spikes blood glucose levels — low blood glucose levels can be raised quickly with candy, for instance. Finally, sugar often comes in foods that offer no nutritional value — empty calories and carbohydrates. It's always best to eat carbohydrates that have secondary benefits.

TIP

Some of you may realize that fruit and milk contain simple sugars — fruit even contains free glucose that can be absorbed directly. But Mother Nature has a way, and even though fruit raises blood glucose fairly quickly, the sugar from fruit, which is delivered with fiber and other nutrients, doesn't have the same long-term negative impact on health that refined sugars have.

Keeping your heart healthy

Most people know that diet can contribute to unhealthy cholesterol levels, and those unhealthy cholesterol levels raise the risk for heart disease. A heart-healthy diet can do more than improve cholesterol levels, and a heart-healthy diet is especially important for people with diabetes.

Heart health is so important to diabetes because diabetes itself raises the risk of heart attack or stroke two to four times higher than the risk for people without diabetes. Having high LDL cholesterol, high triglycerides, and high blood pressure along with diabetes multiplies the risk even more. High blood pressure, called hypertension, and diabetes together are double trouble for kidney function, too — the two leading causes of kidney failure working together. Heart disease, however, is by far the greatest threat to a person with diabetes.

Your eating habits can contribute to that risk or can work to reduce the threat. You probably know that saturated fat, and especially trans fat, contributes to heart disease, and a healthy diabetes eating plan emphasizes limiting saturated fat. Excess body weight, common among people with type 2 diabetes, is an independent risk factor for heart disease. But, eating a heart-healthy diet is as much about what you should be including in your meals, as what you shouldn't. Consider the following:

>> Soluble fiber, like the fiber in leafy greens, legumes, whole grains, and beans, sweeps unhealthy LDL cholesterol from your system.

>> The Dietary Approaches to Stop Hypertension (DASH) eating plan developed by the National Institutes of Health, which emphasizes eating whole grains, fruits, and vegetables, and getting high levels of calcium, magnesium, and potassium from food, can lower blood pressure within two weeks.

>> Eating foods consistent with the Mediterranean diet, including fruits and vegetables, whole grains, fish, and olive oil, can reduce insulin resistance, reduce general inflammation (which is now known to be a very important factor in chronic diseases), and reduce the risk of heart attack or stroke.

>> People with diabetes seem to excrete vitamin B1 (thiamine) at a higher than normal level, and the lowered thiamine levels may contribute to the accelerated formation of blockages in arteries among people with diabetes. Whole grains are a source of thiamine.

>> Plant compounds called *polyphenols* found in many ingredients of Mediterranean and vegetarian diets including extra-virgin olive oil, nuts, colored vegetables, green tea, cocoa, and citrus fruits, are antioxidants that improve cholesterol levels, and work to prevent the formation and inflammation of plaques that can block arteries.

The list of how foods benefit heart health and diabetes too, often by improving sensitivity to insulin, goes on and on, and in some cases it's clear the compounds can't come from supplements. There simply is no substitute for a balanced diet rich in whole grains, fruits, vegetables, and healthy fats. You get specific information on how foods can directly benefit your health in several chapters later in the book. Most important, a healthy diabetes eating plan includes foods you are pleased to eat. In fact, if you've fallen into poor eating habits for the convenience, you will be amazed how satisfying real food will be to your tastes.

Making It Easy on Yourself

Managing diabetes well is a commitment that has to be followed by action, but there aren't many commitments of your time and attention that have a bigger payoff. And, if you honestly look at where you invest your time and efforts now, you can surely justify that little more be devoted to your health — Chapter 11 is devoted to strategies that will keep you motivated. The life expectancy of people with diabetes is ten years shorter on average, but it's not diabetes itself that steals those years — it's indifference to self-management responsibilities.

If doing diabetes management well every day can give you those ten years, and it can, then for every two days you attend to diabetes, you get one extra day of living in return if your diagnosis was at age 50. Nothing is guaranteed, of course, but even if your diagnosis was at an earlier age, the return on investment is unbeatable.

What's required of you to get such a deal? Here's the plan for success:

>> See your doctor regularly, ask questions, get your lab work done when requested, and ask to see a registered dietitian and a certified diabetes educator for a personalized meal plan, and for continuing education. If your doctor doesn't take diabetes seriously, find another doctor.

>> Take your medication as prescribed and test your blood glucose often.

>> Make time for 150 minutes of moderate exercise, like walking, each week — only 30 minutes a day, five days a week, and the 30 minutes can be done in 10- or 15-minute segments.

>> Stop smoking, if you do.

>> Get seven or eight hours of sleep each night, and find a way to reduce chronic stress (exercising will help immensely).

>> Nap for at least ten minutes each afternoon if possible.

>> Adopt healthy eating habits.

>> Spend more time doing things you love.

>> Get fresh air and eat communally whenever possible.

This book is dedicated to eating well, and changing old habits for new ones is always tricky. But, there should be no doubt that you can adopt new eating habits. Don't expect to become an expert in one week, and don't let imperfection discourage you. The test for evaluating effective blood glucose control is called A1C, and this test measures your average blood glucose over a couple of months. Averages leave plenty of room for imperfection.

The chapters that follow review diabetes in more detail, explain the importance of nutrition, give you the in-depth story on carbohydrates, walk you through meal planning and shopping, discuss the pitfalls of eating out, and give you one week of meals and some marvelous recipes to start your collection.

Chapter **2**

Understanding Diabetes : A Holistic Approach

n the past 40 years, the number of adults and children with diabetes in the United States has increased by six fold, from fewer than 6 million people in 1980 to more than 37 million estimated in 2022. This represents more than 11 percent of the U.S. population. In addition, 38 percent of the U.S. population have prediabetes, a condition in which glucose metabolism is beginning to be impaired and the risk of developing diabetes is high. The story is much the same in other countries. The World Health Organization estimated in 2022 that 422 million people — almost 10 percent of the planet's population — have established diabetes, with figures rising across the globe.

The most effective way to prevent the spread of this disease and help people live better with it is to treat diabetes with a multisystem and individualistic approach. It isn't just what is going on in the physical body that causes diabetes. Scientifically speaking, *diabetes mellitus* results from the inability to properly process carbohydrate food, specifically the sugar glucose that's set free from carbohydrates during digestion. Glucose is so important that it's delivered to virtually every cell in your body. When the delivery can't be completed for one reason or another, an important balance is lost, and diabetes becomes part of your life.

Looking at diabetes through a holistic lens offers additional ways of understanding the way food is processed in the body. Thoughts, emotions, and beliefs all play a role. Because everyone's DNA is unique, patient-specific treatments are needed to prevent, treat, and even reverse diabetes. The one-size-fits-all medicines are not enough to reduce the growing rate of diabetes cases around the globe.

For the overwhelming majority (with type 2 diabetes discussed later in this chapter), a diagnosis of diabetes is probably related to a less-than-healthy lifestyle over many years, especially how and what you've been eating. But changing how and what you eat can go a long way in minimizing the long-term and life-threatening health effects of diabetes. The good news is that lifestyle changes can reverse a diagnosis of diabetes as well as reduce the risk of complications of diabetes and other chronic conditions. The even better news is that these changes can be sustainable, enjoyable, and rewarding.

Defining Diabetes Mellitus

Diabetes mellitus is defined simply as having higher than normal levels of glucose in your blood too often, a condition called *hyperglycemia*. The term diabetes mellitus is often shortened to simply "diabetes," although this term should not be confused with a different hormonal condition called *diabetes insipidus,* which is not discussed in this book. Blood glucose is sometimes called *blood sugar*, but glucose is a very special sugar when it comes to diabetes, as you discover later in this chapter. For the sake of accuracy, *blood glucose* is the correct terminology, and the term used throughout this book.

TECHNICAL STUFF

The actual words *diabetes mellitus* are Greek and Latin, loosely translated to mean constantly flowing sweet urine. Frequent urination is a common symptom of diabetes as your body works to remove excess blood glucose through your kidneys, and it's reasonable to assume that urine would be sweet. In fact, tasting urine to detect the sweetness of excess blood glucose was a diagnostic test that doctors would perform in the days before the chemistry was well understood. Fortunately, there are now better ways to detect hyperglycemia than urine tasting.

Whereas there are several different ways a person can acquire diabetes — injury or damage by toxins, for example — type 1 and type 2 diabetes are the most common "natural" forms. This book's focus is, therefore, on type 1 and type 2 diabetes and variations of those two conditions.

Explaining the role of glucose

Glucose is a sugar. In chemistry terms, it is a "simple" sugar or monosaccharide. There are many chemical varieties of sugars; for example, you've probably heard of fructose and lactose. But glucose is especially important because it's your body's favorite fuel to provide the energy needed for activity like muscular movement, body heat, and, most important, brain function.

REMEMBER

You may see your brain as mostly used for thinking, but there are many really important activities that depend on signals from your brain that happen with no thinking required. Your brain accounts for 20 percent of your energy use, some of which goes to support rather important activities like automatically breathing.

TECHNICAL STUFF

Sugars are unique chemical compounds. Glucose and fructose, for instance, have exactly the same chemical formula with 6 carbon atoms, 12 hydrogen atoms, and 6 oxygen atoms — $C_6H_{12}O_6$ — but differ remarkably because the chemical bonds between the carbon atoms and other elements are very different. Fructose is much sweeter in taste and doesn't raise blood glucose levels except slightly from a small amount of fructose that is converted to glucose in the liver.

Your body doesn't have a central location where glucose is burned for energy, like a roaring fireplace or the cylinders of a car's engine. Instead, glucose is converted to energy on a microscopic level inside trillions and trillions of the individual cells that make up you.

You can understand how this works by thinking about muscles. When you raise your fist toward your shoulder, your bicep muscle gets shorter; it contracts to bend your elbow and pull the lower arm upward. You can actually measure the difference in bicep muscle length, first with your arm extended straight out and again with your arm bent toward your shoulder. The contraction of your bicep muscle is actually the contraction in unison of millions of individual muscle cells that go together to make a bicep — the cells themselves contract. Movement requires energy, and each individual muscle cell is burning glucose to provide that energy. If you add a 20-pound dumbbell to your muscle movements, it's easy to feel the increasing energy requirement, the heat given off, and eventually the depletion of fuel as the muscle becomes exhausted. The real action to generate this energy takes place inside of individual cells.

Cells come in all shapes and sizes, but most are way too small to see without a microscope. The different kinds of materials and structures that make a cell, including your DNA, are contained within what's called a cell membrane. It's tempting to think of a cell membrane as something like a plastic freezer bag —

you can see what's in there, but it can't escape even if it's liquid. Likewise, you can't put something else in through the plastic without making a hole where liquid can leak out. In reality, cell membranes aren't completely impermeable like the freezer bag and can be influenced to let materials come into or leave the cell through the membrane. And if glucose is converted to energy inside of your cells, it's apparent that glucose found its way into those cells somehow.

Simplifying insulin

Although not always the case, many important cell types including muscle cells won't allow glucose to freely pass through the cell membrane without a mediator. That's where insulin becomes so important.

TECHNICAL STUFF

Insulin is a hormone produced by specialized cells in your pancreas called *beta cells* or *islet cells*. *Hormones* are chemicals released from one location within a body that affect cells in other parts of the body. In the case of insulin and glucose, it's insulin that signals individual cells to allow glucose passage through the cell membrane. This process is often illustrated with insulin as a key unlocking a door that glucose can use to enter the cell, and in many ways this picture is accurate. Both glucose and insulin circulate in your blood to deliver fuel to almost every cell that requires energy to perform its duty.

A more detailed discussion of glucose and insulin comes in the next chapter, and for even more information consult Simon and Amy's book, *Diabetes For Dummies*, 6th Edition (Wiley). The main issue here, to define diabetes, is to understand that if the marvelous and precise ability of insulin to convince cells to open the door and take glucose inside is lost or diminished, glucose remains in the bloodstream. This means cells needing, or at least greatly preferring, glucose for energy don't have any. This also means glucose levels in your blood remain higher than normal, even as your kidneys slowly try to remove the excess. This abnormal state is hyperglycemia, and if this abnormal state becomes your "normal" state, then you have diabetes.

REMEMBER

People who know someone with diabetes may associate low blood glucose, *hypoglycemia*, as a symptom of diabetes. Hypoglycemia deprives the brain of adequate energy, so the signs of low blood glucose are obvious, mimicking alcohol intoxication and leading to unconsciousness. However, hypoglycemia is a result of diabetes treatment, with injected insulin or other medications that stimulate natural production of insulin from islet cells, not diabetes. It's high blood glucose levels, hyperglycemia, that defines diabetes, and this condition can be unnoticeable.

Exploring Type 1 Diabetes

Type 1 diabetes mellitus, formerly known as juvenile diabetes and as insulin-dependent diabetes, is what many people think of as real diabetes. The familiar image is one of an exceptionally thin child taking insulin injections, and that's a fairly accurate image. Type 1 diabetes does tend to occur at a younger age, and insulin injections are a routine part of having type 1 diabetes. Type 1 is relatively rare compared to type 2, accounting for less than 10 percent of diabetes cases worldwide.

Type 1 diabetes also commonly shows itself suddenly, frequently diagnosed only following a life-threatening emergency as the capacity to produce insulin is lost. In retrospect, the signs of type 1 diabetes — constantly flowing sweet urine along with an unquenchable thirst and a never-ending appetite — would have been obvious for weeks. Still, an onset with symptoms building for a week or a month is far more acute than the onset of type 2 diabetes.

Recently, doctors have recognized a variation of type 1 diabetes occurring in adults that doesn't involve the sudden and drastic need for insulin injections.

Losing the capacity to produce insulin

Your immune system protects your body's internal workings from intruders, whether the intruder is a splinter or a disease-causing virus or bacteria. The appearance of an intruder stimulates all-out war. Your immune system can mobilize blood cells immediately with names like killer T-cells and begin manufacturing antibodies specifically designed to target the intruder and finish the job over a period of a few days. Your immune system has probably saved your life many times.

Sometimes, because an intruder contains substances in common with body tissue, this awesome firepower is directed both at an intruder and also at essential parts of the same body the immune system is supposed to protect. When damage is caused by one's own misguided immune system, the condition is called an *auto-immune* disorder. In rheumatoid arthritis, for example, the immune system attacks and damages certain tissue in joints, deforming fingers as a result. In type 1 diabetes, a confused immune system attacks and destroys the insulin producing beta cells of the pancreas. The destruction of pancreatic beta cells means that eventually no insulin is naturally produced, and the body can't move glucose into cells.

That typical sudden and violent onset of type 1 diabetes is not quite as sudden as it seems. The emergency is actually the climax to beta cell destruction that progresses over a period of weeks or months as insulin-producing capacity is steadily depleted. Cells begin to starve for glucose fuel, even as blood glucose levels go higher. Sensing that cells need glucose, hunger hormones stimulate appetite, but additional food only sends blood glucose higher again. Eventually, as blood glucose levels rise to many times normal levels, dehydration from excreting glucose constantly in urine and a buildup of waste products called *ketones* from cells burning fat (an emergency alternative to glucose) cause a condition known as *diabetic ketoacidosis* (DKA). DKA is an urgent medical emergency, and this first DKA event begins what is for all intents and purposes a lifetime of daily insulin injections necessary for survival.

TIP

The major practical difference between type 1 and type 2 diabetes mellitus is the universal requirement for insulin replacement by injection or some other method in type 1 diabetes. Patients with type 2 diabetes usually find their condition can be managed by lifestyle and/or medication, with insulin only being required in the most severely affected patients.

Prior to the mid-1920s when insulin was first isolated, people with type 1 diabetes simply didn't survive. Now, however, medical advances in insulin quality, insulin delivery systems (insulin pumps), and real-time blood glucose monitoring allow people with type 1 diabetes to effectively control blood glucose levels for a lifetime.

Looking for a cure for diabetes is proceeding on many fronts. Some of the more promising directions include the following:

>> A vaccine against the substance that promotes the development of autoantibodies that kill beta cells

>> Use of oral insulin to "quiet" the immune system

>> Use of intranasal insulin to stimulate protective immune cells

>> Development of drugs that block the immunity that kills beta cells

>> Regeneration of beta cells with drugs or stem cells (cells that form many other cells)

TIP

This is a partial list and should give you cause for celebration if you have type 1 diabetes. It should encourage you to control your diabetes as well as you possibly can so that you will be free of complications of diabetes when the cure arrives.

Comparing LADA with type 1

Latent autoimmune diabetes of adults (LADA) has more in common at the start with type 2 diabetes than with type 1 diabetes with one key exception: a berserk immune system. LADA does not come on dramatically like typical type 1 diabetes. In fact, diagnosis and treatment almost always begins as if the patient has developed type 2 diabetes, which doesn't involve autoimmune destruction of beta cells, as explained later in this chapter. DKA doesn't typically occur, insulin therapy is not required, and oral medications with lifestyle changes can often manage blood glucose levels effectively for a time.

LADA is so different from type 1 in these regards that some call LADA "type 1.5 diabetes." However, what puts LADA in the type 1 diabetes category is the presence of beta cell antibodies, and the resulting destruction of these insulin producing cells, albeit ever so slowly. Adults with LADA tend to require insulin therapy for blood glucose control sooner than adults with type 2 diabetes, and antibody studies of patients diagnosed as type 2 suggest that more than 10 percent (in some studies nearly 30 percent) are LADA instead.

REMEMBER

In some circles type 1 diabetes is referred to as "bad diabetes," hinting that type 2 diabetes must be "good diabetes." Type 1 diabetes does require more attention than type 2 because DKA is always possible, as is low blood glucose with insulin injections. But the tools available to control blood glucose levels in type 1 can make that constant attention pay off. Type 2 diabetes can be, and too often is, ignored because the consequences of inattention are often not immediate. But just because you're ignoring diabetes doesn't mean diabetes is ignoring you, and the complications of diabetes discussed later in this chapter aren't concerned with which type diabetes you have.

Puzzling over the causes of type 1

The primary cause of type 1 diabetes is clear — destruction of insulin producing beta cells by the patient's own immune system. The cause of this misguided immune system response is not clear.

There is a genetic component that increases the risk for developing type 1 diabetes, but studies of identical twins, who are literally identical in a genetic sense, demonstrate that genetics doesn't cause type 1 diabetes. Having an identical twin with type 1 diabetes increases the twin's risk of developing type 1 diabetes only to something like 30 percent.

Certain viral infections seem to be a promising suspect in triggering the autoimmune response. Increasing evidence points to a relationship between our genetics, our environment, and a possible viral factor that may lead to Type I diabetes.

Some researchers have proposed that type 1 and type 2 diabetes are essentially the same disease expressed in different ways. Population data hints that inadequate vitamin D is to blame, that persistent organic pollutants like dioxin may play a role, or that excessive hygiene has contributed to an overactive immune system. A long-term study known as TRIGR (which stands for Trial to Reduce IDDM in the Genetically at Risk) is monitoring more than 2,000 babies on three continents to look at a potential connection between some cases of type 1 diabetes and cow's milk or certain infant formulas.

The bottom line is that the cause or causes of the autoimmune response leading to type 1 diabetes is still unknown at this time.

Analyzing Type 2 and Gestational Diabetes

Type 2 diabetes, formerly known as adult-onset diabetes and as noninsulin-dependent diabetes, is by far more common than type 1, accounting for more than 90 percent of diabetes cases. Type 2 diabetes does tend to occur at a more advanced age than type 1, and the onset is slow and steady over a period of years with correspondingly mild, even unnoticeable, symptoms. The American Diabetes Association (ADA) produces statistics every few years revising the estimated number of Americans with diabetes, and the numbers always show about 25 percent of the total cases as "undiagnosed." None of the undiagnosed cases of diabetes can possibly be type 1.

Type 2 diabetes is often called a lifestyle disease, and there is ample evidence demonstrating that type 2 is preventable and potentially reversible with diet and exercise alone. Still, nearly 2 million new cases arise each year in the United States, and the trend is still heading higher.

Prediabetes and the possible progression of type 2

Type 2 diabetes doesn't begin as a problem with insulin production like type 1 diabetes. In fact, the beta cells at the insulin factory are often working overtime. The high blood glucose levels that define type 2 diabetes result from a problem getting glucose into the cells that need it. Remember the insulin-as-a-key-that-unlocks-the-cells image discussed earlier? With type 2 diabetes some of the locks have been changed, and the key (insulin) doesn't work. Type 2 diabetes begins with what's called insulin resistance — normal or above normal levels of insulin finding unresponsive cells leaves excess glucose stranded in the blood.

But this all begins in slow motion. In fact, a recognized condition known as *pre-diabetes* (or impaired glucose tolerance) can be ringing the warning bell for years. Prediabetes is when blood glucose levels are higher than normal, but not high enough to be officially diagnosed as diabetes. A famous study called the Diabetes Prevention Program (DPP) found that people with prediabetes who adopted a healthier diet, lost a modest amount of weight, and exercised regularly reduced their odds of progressing to type 2 diabetes by a whopping 58 percent. The results were even better for participants who were over 60 years of age, and the lifestyle changes were more effective at holding off diabetes than the very effective diabetes medication metformin. Prediabetes is commonly one component of what's called *metabolic syndrome,* a condition that also includes abnormal blood cholesterol levels.

ASK THE DOCTOR

Type 2 diabetes begins and progresses slowly, often without symptoms. If you're overweight, don't exercise, have a family history of diabetes, or belong to certain ethnic groups like African-Americans, Latinos, Asian-Americans, or Native Americans, annual testing for diabetes is a must.

So, why don't more people put a stop to type 2 diabetes before it starts? One reason is because they don't get regular medical checkups that always include a blood glucose level, or the measurement called HbA1C, which indicates blood glucose levels over several weeks; they don't know there's a problem. But even those who know aren't reminded by symptoms. The symptoms of modest hyperglycemia can be unnoticeable, especially because some like frequent urination or fatigue tend to be a natural age-related inconvenience.

In time, however, insulin resistance may increase, and the pancreatic beta cells just get tired of trying to produce enough insulin and wear out. Many people with type 2 diabetes go through a range of medications targeting different pathways for reducing blood glucose levels, and some will eventually end up taking the same kinds of insulin injections as people with type 1. Type 2 diabetes is considered, as this overview suggests, a progressive condition, where progressive actually means getting worse all the time.

TIP

It is essential that you understand this progression (regression) to poorer and poorer health is not inevitable. Just as diet and exercise was amazingly effective at preventing diabetes among participants with prediabetes in the DPP study, so too can diet and exercise along with diabetes medication improve blood glucose control after the diagnosis.

REMEMBER

Exercise and particular foods can improve insulin sensitivity and certain food combinations can influence the speed of absorption of glucose and the rise in blood glucose after a meal. Type 2 diabetes, unlike type 1, can be put into remission.

Weighing the role of body mass

It wouldn't take Sherlock Holmes to figure out that body mass and type 2 diabetes are closely linked. One clue would be that 85 percent of people with type 2 diabetes fall into the overweight or obese range (or higher) on the body mass index (BMI) scale. An above normal weight is something shared by the great majority of people with type 2 diabetes.

Just as the average BMI has steadily risen over the past 20 years or so, where more than two-thirds of the U.S. adult population now falls into or beyond the overweight BMI range, the incidence of type 2 diabetes has risen at almost exactly the same rate. Even more telling — and more concerning — is that rising obesity among children and adolescents has caused type 2 diabetes, once nearly unheard of in this age group, to become relatively common.

In addition, modest weight loss of from 5 to 7 percent of body weight in people with prediabetes can return blood glucose levels to normal. That would be a weight loss of only 10 to 14 pounds for a 200-pound person.

TIP

Scientists are zeroing in on the culprit where excess weight and diabetes are linked, and one hint has been body shape. It seems that weight carried in the midsection of the body, as opposed to legs and posterior for example, increases the risk of type 2 diabetes substantially. Sometimes referred to as an apple shape (where the posterior focused weight is called a pear shape), weight around the midsection represents internal fat deposits, too. This "visceral" fat sends chemical signals that promote insulin resistance, and is much more associated with type 2 diabetes than subcutaneous — under the skin — fat.

Visceral fat explains why people of Asian origin acquire type 2 diabetes at a normal BMI, because body scans have shown they accumulate visceral fat at lower body weight than other ethnic groups. The role of visceral fat also explains why losing a modest amount of weight can have such a striking impact on insulin resistance. Visceral fat, fortunately, is the first to go in a diet and exercise weight-loss effort, and the exercise part is especially effective at eliminating these dangerous internal fat deposits.

Considering ethnicity, genetics, and age

Ethnicity and genetics are associated to some degree, and both have a relationship to type 2 diabetes. There are genetic variations that increase the risk for, or make people susceptible to type 2 diabetes. In fact, the risk that a child will develop type 2 diabetes if a parent has type 2 diabetes is a stronger link than for a parent with type 1 having a child with type 1. But overall, specific genes that are strongly associated with type 2 diabetes have been elusive, even though more than 30 genes have been identified as contributing to an increased risk.

There is nothing elusive about the risk differences associated with ethnicity, however. Whereas again the specific reasons aren't known, essentially every other ethnic group has a higher risk for type 2 diabetes when compared to non-Hispanic whites. Even more troubling, the occurrence and severity of diabetic complications (discussed later in this section) is greater among those groups, too. It's difficult to separate other risk factors such as weight and culture from the data, but researchers who evaluated records on women from the long-term Nurses' Health Study made adjustments for BMI. Following more than 78,000 nurses who didn't have diabetes over a 20-year period saw 3,800 cases of type 2 diabetes develop. In the unadjusted data the risk for type 2 diabetes was 120 percent higher for African-Americans, 76 percent higher for Hispanics, and 43 percent higher for Asians than for whites. However, adjusting for BMI changed the order making risk 126 percent higher for Asians, 86 percent higher for Hispanics, and 34 percent higher for African-Americans. This suggests that BMI is the greatest risk for Asians and a lower risk for African-Americans. The rates of type 2 diabetes are also higher in Native American populations and Pacific Islanders.

It's important to point out that the so-called Western diet, high in processed foods, added sugars, saturated fats, and calories, clearly plays a part in the higher incidence of type 2 diabetes in some ethnic groups. Migrating to the United States and other countries with similarly unhealthy food cultures is actually a risk factor for type 2 diabetes, and as those lifestyle habits spread to other countries, like India, the type 2 diabetes incidence increases there, too. One piece of good news from the Nurses' Health Study, however, hinted that a healthy diet cut the risk of developing type 2 diabetes more for other ethnic groups than for whites. That suggests that a healthy diet can do more to control the course of diabetes in these groups where diabetic complications are so common.

Aging increases the risk for type 2 diabetes in all ethnic groups and both genders. Some of the reasons may be exceptionally complicated biochemical changes having to do with insulin output and glucose transport. But there is a clear relationship with a couple of simple and familiar reasons — diet and exercise.

Senior citizens tend to be overweight, and often that weight is carried in the midsection, suggesting visceral fat with its negative effects on insulin sensitivity. Adults in the 45 to 70 age group have the highest rates of obesity on the BMI scale, more than 30 percent, and weight is a defined risk factor for type 2 diabetes. Not coincidentally, the age groups 65 to 74 and 75+ have the highest rates of type 2 diabetes, more than 20 percent of that population.

Beyond the excess weight, which is likely related to both diet and reduced physical activity, the natural loss of muscle mass that comes with aging may have a role in insulin resistance. Muscles play an important part in getting glucose out of the bloodstream, and fewer muscle cells means fewer places glucose can go.

Maintaining muscle mass with age has many benefits, and preserving insulin sensitivity may be one. Studies measuring insulin sensitivity while building muscle mass with resistance exercise (weight lifting) have shown positive results, and resistance training has become a standard recommendation for aging adults.

REMEMBER

Lifestyle changes (weight loss, improved diet, and exercise) have proven to be even more effective than drugs in preventing the progression of prediabetes to diabetes.

Developing diabetes during pregnancy

Some women without diabetes develop a condition called *gestational diabetes* during pregnancy. Gestational diabetes is almost always a temporary loss of blood glucose balance, and levels return to normal after giving birth. Gestational diabetes isn't the same thing as having diabetes before a pregnancy.

New diagnostic criteria increases the percentage of women considered to have gestational diabetes from less than 5 percent of pregnancies to more than 18 percent, according to the ADA. The new criteria are intended to add emphasis to the issue of blood glucose management during pregnancy, and most women are able to resolve the risks with a focus on lifestyle, especially diet. Of course, women with gestational diabetes should be under the watchful eye of their physician.

WARNING

Having gestational diabetes during a pregnancy increases the likelihood that you will have gestational diabetes in later pregnancies. Having gestational diabetes also increases the risk for developing type 2 diabetes later, especially where other risk factors like excess body weight are in play. Even though gestational diabetes usually goes away after the birth, follow-up screening is recommended to be certain that the abnormal blood glucose levels weren't caused by the coincidental onset of type 1, LADA, or type 2 diabetes during pregnancy.

Summing Up the Potential Complications of Diabetes

Diabetes For Dummies, 6th Edition provides a detailed explanation of the many potential complications of diabetes. The attention and effort you're asked to give to managing blood glucose levels with medication, testing your blood, physical activity, and especially diet, is to reduce your risk for these complications.

TIP

In everyday life you probably use the word *complication* to describe something that disrupts your plans slightly, but can be resolved with a minor adjustment or two. A flat tire, unannounced guests, or a power outage all qualify as a complication in everyday life. Used in a medical context for describing the potential health effects of diabetes, the word has a much more serious meaning. Don't be fooled by the innocent word complication — in diabetes, the stakes are literally life and limb.

In general, the complications of diabetes can be separated into short-term complications and long-term complications. Short-term complications are related to the level of your blood glucose right now. Long-term complications are related to your success managing blood glucose levels and overall cardiovascular health markers, like blood pressure, over many years. This book is aimed at reducing your risk for long-term complications.

There are only two short-term complications — very low blood glucose levels (hypoglycemia), and very high blood glucose levels (hyperglycemia).

» Hypoglycemia is a complication of diabetes treatment, but it can be extremely serious so deserves some emphasis. When insulin levels are too high compared to blood glucose, your brain runs low on fuel. Hypoglycemia can result from too much injected insulin, too little food to match medications that stimulate natural insulin release from the pancreas, or from alcohol consumption. Symptoms may mimic intoxication, and accidents are common on account of disorientation. But hypoglycemia can progress to coma and death without treatment.

» Hyperglycemia results when there is not enough insulin available to reduce blood glucose levels. DKA was explained earlier in this chapter's description of the typical onset of type 1 diabetes, but DKA remains a risk for anyone with type 1 for a lifetime. DKA is a toxic state and can be fatal if untreated. People with type 2 diabetes don't ordinarily experience blood glucose levels high enough to develop DKA, but a similar condition called *hyperosmolar syndrome* can be a life-threatening risk. Usually hyperosmolar syndrome is triggered by dehydration associated with another illness like norovirus, sometimes called stomach flu.

The long-term complications develop where diabetes is poorly controlled over the years, and this is where lifestyle choices like committing to a healthy diet play such a crucial role in preserving health. The damage that excessive blood glucose levels cause over time can have debilitating and deadly consequences, but are preventable in large part.

» Heart attack and stroke are much more common in people with diabetes, two to four times more likely. And, people with diabetes have a higher death rate, and are more likely to have another event if they survive the first. The risk for heart disease is often increased by abnormal cholesterol levels, conditions associated with chronic inflammation and high blood pressure related both to high blood glucose, and to excess weight and a less-than-healthy lifestyle. Treating and managing diabetes with lifestyle must include treating and managing these related risks for heart disease.

>> Kidney disease affects up to 5 percent of people with type 2 diabetes, and up to 30 percent of people with type 1. In fact, diabetes is the leading cause of kidney failure in the United States that eventually may require dialysis treatment or a kidney transplant.

TIP

Anyone who's frustrated following a diabetes–friendly diet to better manage blood glucose should try the renal diet for dialysis patients just for comparison. A renal diet restricts fluid, protein, sodium, phosphorus, and potassium, and may be the most restrictive diet in medical nutrition therapy.

>> Neuropathy describes conditions resulting from damage to nerves, and is a very common complication of diabetes affecting some 60 percent of patients. Neuropathy can result in pain or numbness of extremities (especially the feet), the inability of some muscles to move, digestive problems called *gastroparesis,* urinary difficulties, sexual dysfunction, and a range of other difficulties.

>> Vision is threatened from an increased risk of cataracts, glaucoma, and especially diabetic retinopathy. Retinopathy is another example of how high blood glucose levels can damage small blood vessels.

>> Diabetic foot disease is the leading cause of non-traumatic amputations in the United States, and the progression of foot ulcers is often complicated by the absence of sensation due to neuropathy (and a neglect of routine self-examination of the feet).

Many people with diabetes assume these terrible outcomes are simply part of the normal course of diabetes, but that assumption is dangerously wrong. Controlling blood glucose levels and adopting a healthy overall lifestyle can greatly reduce your risk for these long–term complications, and it's never too late to start.

Linking diabetes and inflammation

Inflammation is the body's natural response to injury or infection. In the short term, the heat, localized swelling, managed cell destruction, and other features of the mobilization of our immune system are very effective in destroying invading organisms and protecting us from harm. The immune cells involved in our protection can even generate powerful bursts of chemicals called *free radicals,* which, through a process called *oxidation,* can attack the cells of microbes. These naturally produced free radicals are highly reactive and disrupt molecules by stealing their electrons, destabilizing them, and setting up a chain reaction, which is an important part of our defense against pathogens. In the short term, *acute* inflammation is followed by healing and repair once the danger is over.

If there is long-term exposure to potentially harmful environmental triggers, chronic infections, or a misdirected or unresolved immune system response, there is a risk that the temporary acute inflammation will not resolve, and chronic low-grade inflammation will continue. Healing and the restoring of a normal state cannot occur. Paradoxically, the processes that are designed to protect our bodies from a temporary threat with limited collateral damage can in these circumstances result in harm to our own cells and organs.

Things that are likely to lead to chronic inflammation are called *pro-inflammatory* factors. Those that reduce the tendency are called *anti-inflammatory.*

We experience many aspects of our lives that may have a pro-inflammatory effect. Smoking, pollution, environmental toxins, and ultraviolet (UV) light are just some of the (sometimes unavoidable) pro-inflammatory factors. Some of these produce their own unstable free radical, electron-hungry chemicals that can result in damaging oxidation reactions in the cells of our bodies. If there is an excess of pro-inflammatory oxidation, this state is called *oxidative stress.*

When we eat, there is a great deal of chemistry to be done to metabolize and convert the "foreign" material that is food into useful compounds. Some foods can have a pro-inflammatory effect and produce electron-hungry free radicals, and others can help to counter excess oxidation and other causes of inflammation through antioxidant effects. These generous donors of electrons to free radicals can balance and stabilize pro-inflammatory elements of our diet and environment. They can quench the fires of inflammation. We discuss antioxidants in greater detail in Chapter 8.

Hyperglycemia, obesity, and diabetes are associated with signs of increased inflammation and are therefore considered to be pro-inflammatory states. The common long-term complications of diabetes are also diseases that are linked with chronic inflammation. It is sometimes difficult to identify which is cause and which is effect. This is important when it comes to choosing a diet and lifestyle that not only reduces the risk of diabetes but also can lower markers of inflammation and so protect from its complications.

Exploring diabetes and immunity: COVID-19 and other infections

Infections can result in disruption to glucose regulation and so it is important for people living with diabetes to be aware of the need for greater vigilance in monitoring their blood glucose levels and adjusting treatment when necessary. In particular, people with type 1 diabetes are at greater risk of short-term complications, including ketoacidosis, during a significant bacterial or viral infection.

It is also true that diabetes can disturb the normal efficient functioning of the immune system. While there is no convincing evidence that people with diabetes are any more likely to catch viruses such as influenza or COVID-19, there is a greater risk of severe disease, hospitalization, and even death. People living with diabetes are also thought to be four times as likely to develop a condition called Long COVID. It is likely that the background inflammation associated with diabetes may be a contributing factor that diminishes the normal protective immune response. You can find out more about inflammation and how activating antioxidants in your diet can help you to protect yourself in Chapter 8.

TIP

Research has shown that people who have a healthy lifestyle, including greater adherence to a Mediterranean diet prior to developing COVID-19, are significantly less likely to have complications from the virus, which makes it even more important to enjoy following the advice we give in this book.

ASK THE
DOCTOR

If you have diabetes, it is especially important to protect yourself from complications such as COVID-19 with recommended vaccinations and to seek any early therapy with anti-viral medications prescribed by your doctor as well as professional support. Keep in mind that over-the-counter medications need to be cleared with your doctor or pharmacist before using them if you have diabetes.

IN THIS CHAPTER

» **Discovering how your body balances blood glucose levels**

» **Seeing how diabetes disrupts blood glucose balance**

» **Measuring blood glucose levels to evaluate your progress**

» **Meeting your medical team and medications**

» **Getting your assignment for diabetes self-management**

Chapter **3**

Managing Diabetes and Blood Glucose

Your body is remarkable in many ways. Chapter 6, for instance, shows how you recycle the complex components of the food you eat to use again as building blocks for your own cells, or as the ingredients of various biochemical recipes. Here's another incredible process you're familiar with, even if you don't realize it — *homeostasis.* Homeostasis means maintaining stable conditions. For example, your body has a complex control system to maintain a relatively constant body temperature of 98.6 degrees Fahrenheit, and you hardly ever have to think about it. But, if your temperature goes much higher or lower than normal you've got potentially serious problems, and you need to help your body regain temperature homeostasis.

You've got another amazing system of checks and balances for maintaining homeostasis with blood glucose levels. Glucose is your favored source of energy — your brain's only source of energy — and it travels around in blood to reach cells everywhere. Blood glucose is a little like the porridge Goldilocks was searching for — everything's best when it's just right. Having diabetes, however, means blood glucose levels aren't just right, and your body needs a little help from you to regain and maintain homeostasis. Fortunately, you have the ability to do just that.

In this chapter, you see why the normal balance of glucose is so important to health, and how diabetes disrupts that crucial balance. More important, you see how you can help recover blood glucose homeostasis, and who can help you along the way.

Regulating Your Body's Blood Glucose Levels

Glucose is a simple sugar that is extremely important to you as a source of energy. It's the key ingredient in a biochemical recipe that produces a powerhouse molecule *adenosine triphosphate*, best known by its initials ATP. ATP is your fuel — the source of the energy you use to move or to think or, for that matter, to generate the heat needed to remain a steady 98.6 degrees Fahrenheit.

TECHNICAL STUFF

The conversion of glucose to energy via ATP takes place inside of the cell membranes of trillions and trillions of individual cells, most all of which are properly equipped to prepare the recipe for ATP in structures called *mitochondria*. And, because blood already visits cells in your farthest outreaches to deliver oxygen and remove wastes, blood also conveniently brings glucose right to the doorstep of cells that need it to make energy. Your body can convert other ingredients to energy if necessary, but glucose is the first choice.

You get glucose from food, and you eat a lot more glucose than you might think, even if you don't have an overactive sweet tooth. Actually, glucose isn't that sweet anyway. Virtually all of the glucose you eat is locked in chains with other sugars or more glucose — *polysaccharides*. If the chains are small, the molecule is still considered a sugar — table sugar (sucrose) is one molecule of glucose and one fructose — a *disaccharide*. If the chains are longer, even to hundreds or thousands of glucose molecules, the molecules are *starch* or *fiber*. Taken together, sugars, starches, and fiber are *carbohydrates*, a word you're surely familiar with if you have diabetes.

Most dietary carbohydrates come from plants. Plants are constructed in large measure of the carbohydrate cellulose, and cellulose can include thousands of linked glucose molecules. As a carbohydrate, cellulose is definitely in the fiber category and not a very digestible fiber at that. If humans could easily digest cellulose, you might have a favorite old-family recipe for cotton ball sauté. Fortunately, plants also make more digestible and more flavorful carbohydrates.

TECHNICAL STUFF

The only dietary carbohydrate you get from animals is lactose, or milk sugar. Lactose in a mother's milk is how infants (and puppies and calves) get carbohydrates for energy, but the ability to digest lactose diminishes in most humans after infancy. As a result, an estimated 65 percent of the human population is lactose intolerant to some degree.

Glucose as a single molecule is liberated from its chain gang polysaccharides by various digestive processes, starting right in your mouth with saliva. By the time your food passes through your stomach, small intestine, and maybe the first portion of your colon, all the easily digestible carbohydrate has been broken apart by specific enzymes, finally freeing the individual glucose molecules. At that point, glucose is ready to be captured.

TIP

Just because fiber is less digestible and may not surrender its glucose easily doesn't mean it isn't a very important part of a healthy diet. In Chapter 6, you discover the many benefits of fiber.

Within your intestinal tract are millions of fingerlike projections called *villi*, which are especially rich in blood supply. Before liberated glucose can escape through the colon as waste material, the molecules are absorbed directly into your bloodstream through small capillaries in a process called *active transport*. Much glucose absorption occurs in the first part of your small intestine, and absorption is very efficient due to the vast surface area of millions of villi. The process is also relatively quick, so eating carbohydrate food results in a surge of glucose entering the bloodstream. Rising blood glucose levels are a serious insult to homeostasis. You won't be surprised to learn that your body has a solution to that problem.

Understanding how insulin works

Specific cells, located in cell clusters in your pancreas known as the Islets of Langerhans, can sense rising blood glucose levels, and these cells — called *beta cells* — are capable of doing something about it. Beta cells produce insulin, and they do their producing in earnest when blood sugar levels are on the rise. High blood glucose levels are an abnormal state, and insulin lowers blood glucose levels simply by helping put the glucose somewhere else — inside of cells.

REMEMBER

You already know that glucose goes toward producing ATP inside of cells, but without insulin as an escort many cells aren't so anxious to invite glucose inside. Insulin is the key that unlocks doors in cell membranes, allowing glucose to pass into your cells and out of your blood.

As blood glucose levels begin to drop, the beta cells sense this favorable change and suppress their release of insulin. In healthy individuals this process is incredibly precise, and blood glucose homeostasis is achieved in a few hours. But, getting glucose into cells and out of the blood is only part of the blood glucose homeostasis story.

Storing glucose for later

If you're following the glucose story carefully, and of course you are, you may have two very insightful questions:

>> If all your excess glucose is escorted into cells to create energy, what happens if you don't need energy at that particular time?

>> If you use all your glucose for energy during the Iron Man Triathlon, why doesn't your blood glucose level drop to zero unless you eat constantly?

Wow — you have asked two excellent questions! It's true that at times you don't need much energy even if you've just eaten and have glucose surging through your system. At other times, as you pointed out, you need a lot of energy with no food in sight. And, it is true that during those times you need a lot — during your triathlon — glucose is drawn into muscle cells from your blood glucose even when your blood glucose levels are normal.

The solution to this problem is storage. Your cells are able to convert excess glucose into a storage molecule called *glycogen*, and to restore this secret stash back to glucose whenever energy as ATP needs to be whipped up. Glycogen stored in your muscle cells provides energy to those muscles when you're working hard and not eating; however, glucose stored in a muscle cell stays in that muscle cell. So, when muscle glycogen is depleted during your triathlon, and your muscle cells are pulling additional glucose from your blood, what keeps your blood glucose stable? In other words, what maintains homeostasis when blood glucose levels should be going down?

One special place where glucose is stashed as glycogen is in liver cells. Glycogen in liver cells isn't obliged to remain in liver cells as it is with muscle cells. Liver cells can release glucose back into your bloodstream.

As blood glucose levels begin to dip, another group of special cells in the pancreas's Islets of Langerhans, this time *alpha cells*, spring into action. Alpha cells secrete a hormone called *glucagon*, which stimulates your liver to release stored glucose back into your bloodstream. Glucagon is so effective that people with type 1 diabetes sometimes carry a dose of this hormone for an emergency injection when their blood glucose levels go dangerously low. The injection can bring levels up much faster than eating even pure glucose. Glucagon's action to raise blood glucose answers the triathlon question.

Insulin and glucagon are secreted more or less constantly to maintain blood glucose homeostasis, even when the circumstances are somewhere in between sedentary and extreme exertion. Like a tightrope walker leaning a little left and then a little right, in normal metabolism these hormones maintain a beautiful blood glucose balance.

TECHNICAL
STUFF

The storage capacity for glucose in muscle cells and the liver is fairly limited. When you consume excess calories, including carbohydrates, insulin will also facilitate glucose storage in fat cells, not as glycogen but as glycerol and triglycerides. Fat molecules store a lot of energy and contribute to energy needs as glycogen is depleted, which explains how exercise really does reduce fat.

Losing the Glucose Balance

Diabetes, however, is a state of blood glucose *imbalance* related to insulin. As explained more thoroughly in Chapter 2, in type 1 diabetes insulin production capacity is completely lost, and in type 2 diabetes cells become resistant to insulin. In both cases, blood glucose levels after eating carbohydrate foods do not come down to normal levels in a normal way.

It's fair to say that what defines a normal level of blood glucose in humans is the level preferred by your brain. Your brain is very important to your existence, does not require insulin to absorb glucose, and usually gets whatever it wants or needs. But your brain is more concerned about operating with low blood glucose levels than about higher levels. High blood glucose causes problems in other ways.

What is a normal level for blood glucose? In common measure, about 1 teaspoon of glucose dissolved in your 1½ gallons of blood is perfect. In laboratory measure, that's 4,000 milligrams (4 grams) of glucose in your 50 deciliters (5 liters) of blood equaling 80 milligrams per deciliter, or 80 mg/dl. Milligrams per deciliter, mg/dl, is the standard measure used in the United States and some other countries. An alternative unit, *millimoles per liter* (mmol/l), is the international standard measure for blood glucose levels and is used commonly in many countries, too. The difference in units is not relevant, but mg/dl can be easily converted to mmol/l by dividing by 18. Therefore, 80 mg/dl and 4.44 mmol/l represent the same concentration when measuring blood glucose.

International diagnostic standards set a normal blood glucose range at between 60 and 99 mg/dl. This standard is for *fasting blood glucose,* which is your level after having no food or drink for 8 hours. A fasting blood glucose level from 100 to 125 mg/dl is known as *impaired glucose tolerance,* commonly called prediabetes. A fasting blood glucose level higher than 126 mg/dl is considered diagnostic for diabetes if that result occurs on more than one fasting blood glucose test.

Another test more representative of a realistic response to food is called an *oral glucose tolerance test* (OGTT). This test measures blood glucose response after ingesting glucose (usually 75 grams) over a two- or three-hour period by testing fasting blood glucose level before the test, and testing at hourly intervals after the oral dose of glucose. A normal result is blood glucose below 200 mg/dl after one hour, and below 140 mg/dl after two hours. If the two-hour result is higher than 140 mg/dl but lower than 200 mg/dl, it represents impaired glucose tolerance or prediabetes. A result higher than 200 mg/dl after two hours is diagnostic for diabetes. A blood glucose level higher than 200 mg/dl on any random test is diagnostic for diabetes.

A variation of the OGTT is recommended for all pregnant women to test for gestational diabetes. The test, given between the 24th and 28th week of pregnancy, uses either a 50-gram or 100-gram oral dose of glucose, and a normal response is a blood glucose level below 140 mg/dl after one hour (50-gram dose) or after three hours (100-gram dose).

These carefully set diagnostic standards measure the extent of blood glucose imbalance. Rarely necessary for diagnosing type 1 diabetes, where blood glucose levels can exceed 500 mg/dl at its sudden onset, people with type 2 diabetes may have a long history of routine lab tests charting the loss of blood glucose balance over many years. When a diabetes diagnosis is made, testing and evaluating blood glucose levels should become a routine part of daily life.

Measuring Blood Glucose

Most people living with diabetes in the 21st century won't fully appreciate being able to test blood glucose levels anytime, anywhere, and with an instrument you can carry in your pocket. But, prior to the early 1980s, blood glucose levels were measured only in medical labs, and estimating blood glucose levels at home involved matching colors of a paper strip dipped into urine. The lab result was, obviously, never a real-time result, and the urine test only signaled approximate levels of hyperglycemia. Glucose doesn't generally appear in urine until blood glucose levels approach 200 mg/dl. In short, people with diabetes 40 years ago, almost exclusively type 1 diabetes, were doing a lot of estimating (guessing) about blood glucose levels, its response to food, and insulin dosing. How things have changed.

Testing blood glucose at home

Guessing about blood glucose levels is completely unnecessary. Now, it's possible to draw a very small amount of blood from your finger or other location (with some meters) and get a relatively accurate measure of blood glucose in ten seconds. Blood glucose meters today also store historical information, which can be downloaded to a computer or transmitted to a physician's office. More and more people with type 1 diabetes are wearing *continuous glucose monitors,* which sense glucose levels through a small wire inserted into the fluid just beneath the skin.

Linking continuous monitoring to an insulin pump that responds and adjusts through an algorithm either in the device or an associated app to give real-time dosing according to need is a recent development that promises to revolutionize the lives of people who have type 1 diabetes. The first system to apply this so-called closed-loop or artificial pancreas technology was licensed in 2016, and systems are being continually refined and developed to give even greater freedom and reassurance of excellent control of blood glucose levels.

REMEMBER

Testing blood glucose levels is extremely important for people with type 1 diabetes because they must make real-time self-treatment decisions about food and insulin dosing based upon the result. People with type 1 who do not have closed-loop technology should test before every meal and approximately two hours after meals with some frequency, a time frame referred to as *postprandial.* They should test before exercising, before bedtime, and anytime they might sense high or low blood glucose levels. They should test anytime someone who knows them suggests they may "be low" — often they lack self-awareness of hypoglycemia clues that are obvious to others. They should also test if consuming alcohol in excess, because alcohol can trigger hypoglycemia, and hypoglycemia can resemble alcohol intoxication.

Testing with type 2 diabetes usually follows a less stringent schedule — maybe only once or twice a day. More testing is recommended if low blood glucose levels are a potential side effect of medication, and Simon and Amy provide guidelines in *Diabetes For Dummies,* 6th Edition (Wiley).

TIP

Many people with type 2 diabetes wouldn't think of testing more often than their doctor prescribes, but one of the great values of home blood glucose testing is looking for patterns. For instance, you can bet there are certain foods that have a dramatic impact on your blood glucose levels, but you can't know which ones without doing some self-experimentation by testing. If you find by some extra testing that Grandma's recipe for rice pudding sends your blood glucose to 320 mg/dl, you could stop eating Grandma's rice pudding. Your doctor may give you a funny look, but think about asking for a few more testing strips each month so you can take advantage of this remarkable technology to better control blood glucose levels.

Getting the averages

Daily blood glucose testing can give you an excellent look at your status at one moment of the day, and that can be essential, especially for people with type 1 who are making treatment decisions. But, in the big picture your success with diabetes is a long distance race — you hope a long, long, long distance race. Minimizing your risks for complications is much less about your blood sugar level at 6:45 a.m. on August 7th than it is about your average blood glucose levels in August, and July before, and June before that.

Fortunately, there's an important blood test that can give you a big picture view of your blood glucose control. Your doctor will order a test for *hemoglobin A1C*, sometimes called HbA1C or simply A1C, at least once a year to evaluate your average blood glucose levels over a two- or three-month period. In technical terms, A1C is a measure of glycated (or interchangeably, glycosolated) hemoglobin — what percentage of your blood hemoglobin has reacted with glucose. A1C is an excellent predictor of your overall blood glucose control, and consequently of your risk for diabetes-related complications.

The A1C test gives a weighted average, meaning your blood glucose control the month of the test has slightly more influence on the result than your control the month before, and so on. This variation is related to the limited life span of hemoglobin. A normal A1C in individuals without diabetes or prediabetes is lower than 6 percent (A1C is expressed as a percentage of hemoglobin that is glycated). Target values for people with diabetes have been established by both the American Diabetes Association (ADA) and the American Association of Clinical Endocrinologists (AACE) at less than 7.0 percent and less than 6.5 percent, respectively. Many other public health bodies in other countries also recommend this lower level, which may be measured in alternative units called mmol/mol. At 48 mmol/mol, this is the diagnostic cut-off level for diabetes, and the ambition to achieve this target reflects the hope that diabetes can be put into remission.

Two important studies have supported the relationship between A1C and diabetes-related complications — the Diabetes Control and Complications Trial (DCCT) in the United States and Canada, and the United Kingdom Prospective Diabetes Study (UKPDS) in the United Kingdom. The DCCT involved more than

1,400 people with type 1 diabetes, and the UKPDS included more than 5,000 people newly diagnosed with type 2 diabetes. Both studies demonstrated clear and convincing reductions in the incidence of diabetes-related complications with better control of blood glucose (lower A1C). The UKPDS of type 2 diabetes projected a 37 percent decrease in eye, kidney, and nerve complications for every 1 percent reduction in A1C, and an 18 percent reduction in the risk for heart attack. The downside in both studies was the risk for low blood glucose episodes. Clearly, consistent blood glucose control, as indicated by the A1C, is an important goal for anyone with diabetes, and a main reason meal planning and nutrition is so critical.

Continuous glucose monitoring is a procedure that is useful for identifying blood glucose patterns from hour to hour over a period of several days, and is becoming a more common test for averages over a short time span as technology improves. This procedure records a blood glucose level every few minutes, although the data is not usually available in real time except to people with type 1 diabetes who wear monitors routinely. Still, downloading data gives a graphic picture of exactly how blood glucose levels rose and fell during the monitoring period, and comparing the graph with the timing of meals, exercise, and medication can be revealing.

Ensuring the Best Diabetes Care

Because an estimated 25 percent of people with diabetes remain undiagnosed, it's pretty clear that a significant number of people with diabetes don't get regular medical care. However, studies of patients under medical care, such as the Diabetes Attitudes, Wishes, and Needs (DAWN) study, have shown a troubling low level of adherence to taking medication; self-monitoring of blood glucose, diet, and exercise; and keeping appointments for medical care. Avoiding the serious complications of diabetes requires a multidimensional approach directed at both prevention and intervention. There are many resources available to help you keep your diabetes from exploding into really serious health problems, and the most important resource is *you*.

Choosing your medical team

You may be inclined to think you can't actually choose a doctor or healthcare team, but like many other responsibilities for diabetes care, it's up to you to know what's necessary and to make some demands if you're not getting the support you need.

Diabetes For Dummies, 6th Edition gives a detailed overview of medical care in one of the chapters, but here's a quick listing of medical resources you can take advantage of:

>> **Primary physician:** Most people with type 2 diabetes work with a primary physician, who prescribes medication and routinely monitors for signs of diabetes-related complications in physical exams and laboratory work. A primary physician may or may not have access to in-house diabetes-related support resources like a registered dietitian, certified diabetes educator, or an organized patient support group. Your primary physician should, however, be willing and keen to recommend or formally refer you elsewhere for these very important support services.

>> **Endocrinologist or diabetologist:** These specialized physicians are most likely working with people with type 1 diabetes, or people with type 2 diabetes who have poorly controlled blood glucose or diabetes-related complications. They are the experts in diabetes treatment and will likely have in-house health professionals to help with diet, exercise, blood glucose monitoring, and emotional support.

>> **Registered dietitian or certified nutrition specialist:** Because food and eating habits are so closely connected with weight, blood glucose, and the risk for heart disease, seeing an expert in *medical nutrition therapy* is very important.

>> **Pharmacist:** Your pharmacist is perhaps your best resource for education about medications, not only those prescribed for diabetes, but also those prescribed for other conditions. Most important, your pharmacist knows how your variety of medications may interact. Diabetes is so prevalent now that many pharmacists are diabetes educators.

>> **Certified diabetes educator:** A wide range of healthcare providers — physicians, registered nurses, registered dietitians, pharmacists, clinical psychologists, podiatrists, and others — have studied and taken a comprehensive certification examination to provide a broad range of education and support to people with diabetes. Spending time with a certified diabetes educator, individually or in a group, for diabetes self-management education (DSME) can be helpful in tying together the many medical and lifestyle responsibilities patients struggle to balance.

>> **Podiatrist:** Getting regular foot exams and early treatment of potential problems by a podiatrist can literally be a limb saver. The loss of sensation and circulation problems makes your feet an easy target for minor infections that can become difficult to control. Anyone with neuropathy (nerve damage) should see a podiatrist regularly.

>> **Dentist:** Diabetes can increase the risk of gum disease, so regular visits to your dentist for examination and cleaning are very important.

>> **Mental health professional:** Diabetes can feel overwhelming, and people with diabetes are significantly more likely to experience depression than the general population. More than 41 percent of the participants in the DAWN study mentioned earlier in this chapter reported "poor wellbeing" even decades beyond their diagnosis. Distress at diagnosis is much higher. Depression and stress deserve attention in their own right, but need particular focus where diabetes is concerned because feeling depressed can diminish with self-care behaviors. Only 10 percent of the DAWN study participants reported ever having sought psychological treatment — don't hesitate to get help with the emotional stresses diabetes can bring.

TIP

Make sure each of your resources sends a report to your primary physician so that your physician knows what's being done for you.

Monitoring your medications

If you're controlling your diabetes with only lifestyle changes, hooray for you! More than likely you've been prescribed one or more medications to help control blood glucose levels, and maybe even medications for blood pressure, cholesterol, or other conditions completely unrelated to diabetes and its potential complications. Rule number 1 is to take your medications as prescribed. Various studies, including DAWN, have shown adherence to medication schedules among people with diabetes range somewhere between 65 percent and 95 percent, often depending upon the complexity (including more than one daily dose) of the schedule. The goal should be 100 percent.

REMEMBER

If medications are causing side effects or you are having problems taking them, it is important to discuss this openly with your medical team so that these issues can be addressed.

Insulin is the most effective controller of blood glucose levels, and the most complicated and burdensome. Insulin is the only option for treating type 1 diabetes, but can be effective in controlling blood glucose levels in type 2 also. Insulin therapy is discussed in the next section.

Most people with type 2 diabetes begin therapy with oral medications — pills. The market for specific diabetes medications is so active, with new additions and, unfortunately, removal for unacceptable side effects, it is useless to offer a list here and call it current. In addition, both brand names and generics are available for many medications, and some newer medications are not pills, but non-insulin injections. Rather than even listing the various classes, which generally include more than one drug and an unpronounceable name like *thiazolidinediones*, here's how diabetes medications work to control blood glucose:

>> Some oral medications coax pancreatic beta cells to produce more insulin. These meds require that beta cells are still working well, and low blood glucose levels — hypoglycemia — can be a dangerous side effect.

>> Other oral medications, including the most common medication prescribed at diagnosis, *metformin,* work to decrease glucose output from liver cells and increase insulin sensitivity in muscle cells. Hypoglycemia is not a side effect of these drugs.

>> One group of drugs helps insulin work better with muscle and fats cells, and decreases glucose output from the liver. Some drugs in this class of pills have been removed from the market due to an increased risk for heart problems.

>> A couple of medications interfere with carbohydrate digestion, reducing the efficiency of glucose absorption, thereby reducing blood glucose spikes after meals.

>> A fairly new category of drugs work in different ways to increase the action of a hormone called *GLP-1*. This natural gut hormone slows stomach emptying, increases insulin secretion, and reduces glucose output by the liver. In people with diabetes, secretion of natural GLP-1 is impaired, and disappears quickly due to the action of an enzyme called DPP-4. One class of type 2 diabetes drugs works to block the action of DPP-4, allowing natural GLP-1 to stay active longer. A second class of injectable drugs is a compound that mimics GLP-1, but lasts longer. Neither class increases the risk for hypoglycemia because the stimulation of insulin secretion is dependent upon blood glucose levels. A drug that acts on a similar hormone called GIP is now used in combination with a positive effect on GLP-1 to boost its effect.

>> A drug called an *amylin analog* is taken by injection by some people who are also taking insulin. This drug slows digestion and decreases glucose output from the liver to help smooth blood glucose spikes after eating.

>> Another relatively new class of diabetes drugs includes *sodium glucose co-transporter 2 inhibitors* (SGLT2 inhibitors). These drugs increase the excretion rate of excess blood glucose through the kidneys by lowering the blood glucose level at which the kidneys naturally begin to remove glucose from your system.

Many of these medications can be given in combination. All of these medications should be taken as prescribed. Whether you take medication or not, you will benefit from a healthy diet and exercise.

Explaining insulin therapy

In January 1922, a young Canadian boy lying near death from type 1 diabetes was injected with insulin from the pancreas of a calf. This moment marked the successful beginning to one of the greatest medical stories of all time, when researchers working at the University of Toronto isolated and purified (to some extent) the secret hormone that lowers blood glucose and saves dying children. Insulin has been saving children (and adults) ever since.

In 1982, purified human insulin became commercially available, and insulin formulations and delivery techniques have improved remarkably over the years. Insulin, which is your body's exact response to rising blood glucose levels, is the most effective treatment for diabetes, but is rarely introduced as an option for type 2 diabetes early on.

Insulin must be taken by injection, some formulations require frequent blood glucose testing to be effective, and insulin therapy comes with a clear risk for hypoglycemia. One common myth holds that insulin causes complications, and more than 70 percent of participants in the DAWN study thought the effectiveness of insulin therapy is low, and that insulin would not help them. This study also found some physicians using insulin therapy as a threat to motivate better adherence to diet and exercise recommendations. Whatever the difficulties and misconceptions, insulin therapy remains essential for people with type 1 diabetes, and an underused option for people with type 2 diabetes.

The most immediate use for insulin is counteracting rising blood glucose levels after eating carbohydrate foods, and the formulations intended for this purpose are called *rapid* or *short-acting*. Rapid formulations begin to act on blood glucose levels quickly, reach peak activity within one to two hours, and are no longer active in four to six hours. Short-acting regular insulin is slower to act, slower to peak, and endures for two to four hours. Rapid- or short-acting insulin is taken at mealtime in a dose matched to the amount of carbohydrate to be consumed. The *insulin to carbohydrate ratio* is specific to the patient and may vary from meal to meal. Two concentrations of insulin are available in the United States — U100 (100 milligrams of insulin per milliliter of injection solution) is more common than U500, which is five times more concentrated for individuals requiring especially large doses.

Intermediate or *long-acting* insulin formulations are intended to provide a steady *basal* rate, or background rate, of insulin throughout the day in the same manner that your beta cells secrete a background level. For people with type 1 diabetes who are already taking injections, intermediate-acting *NPH* can be mixed with doses of regular. NPH is active as a basal level for 10 to 18 hours. Long-acting insulin formulations are usually effective when injected only once each day, and provide a basal level for up to 24 hours. Long-acting insulin, Levimir or Lantus, is the most likely first step for people with type 2 diabetes beginning insulin therapy.

Insulin pumps are becoming more common for people with type 1 diabetes. An insulin pump delivers rapid-acting insulin from a reservoir through a tube inserted beneath the skin. A control device allows the user to initiate a mealtime dose, called a *bolus,* by selecting the desired dose and then pressing a start button. Because the tube remains inserted, an insulin pump can deliver the appropriate basal rate of insulin with rapid-acting formulations. The location of the tube insertion, the infusion set, is changed routinely, generally every three days, but that one operation replaces as many as 15 separate injections. Insulin pumps give the user much greater control, much greater flexibility, and greater comfort and can now be used with closed-loop systems to respond rapidly and accurately to changes in blood glucose.

Seeing a Registered Dietitian or Certified Nutrition Specialist

Adopting and sticking with eating habits that optimize blood glucose control and heart health and blood vessel health is, perhaps, the biggest challenge diabetes presents. First, for most people this represents a significant change. Second, misconceptions abound regarding what a diabetes-friendly diet includes, or more accurately doesn't include — no sugar, no carbohydrates, no this, and none of that. Some give up without ever trying. But, a skillful nutrition professional or diabetes educator not only knows medical nutrition therapy to account for your weight, blood glucose control, and medications, but also knows that enjoying food doesn't have to be surrendered.

FROM THE AUTHORS

We avoid using the phrase *diabetic diet* because it sounds so restrictive. With the minor exception of accounting for and choosing high-quality carbohydrates, there is nothing about an eating plan for diabetes that's different from a healthy diet for virtually anyone. People with diabetes have increased risks of complications, many of which, such as heart disease and stroke, are also common conditions in the general populations.

Achieving and maintaining a healthy body weight

More than 80 percent of people with type 2 diabetes are overweight or obese. There are lots of great reasons for losing weight — better mobility, improved sleep apnea, higher self-esteem, lower blood pressure, and a reduced risk for several cancers to name a few. But, where type 2 diabetes is concerned, losing only a modest amount of weight — 5 to 7 percent of body weight — improves insulin sensitivity and blood glucose control. That means an improved A1C, and a reduced risk for diabetes-related complications.

A registered dietitian customizes an eating plan to help you lose weight, while making certain your food and medication remain appropriately matched. An excellent registered dietitian also works to achieve your weight-loss goals by focusing on foods you can eat, not by declaring groups of foods as off limits.

Reducing risk for a variety of complications

Heart disease is the leading cause of death among the many diabetes-related complications, and heart disease is linked with diet even in the absence of diabetes. Stroke, other circulatory problems, kidney disease, and eye disease are other possible complications of poorly controlled diabetes. These conditions occur because of damage to large and small blood vessels in these organs from prolonged high blood glucose as well as other contributing lifestyle factors that people without diabetes might share. Disease of blood vessels is known as vascular disease. So, you can anticipate that your nutrition professional focuses as much on reducing your risk for heart disease as on controlling blood glucose levels.

A standard set of health indicators for diabetes, known as the ABCs, includes A1C as the A, blood pressure as the B, and cholesterol as the C. The target values are A1C less than 7 percent, blood pressure less than 140/80, and cholesterol LDL (bad cholesterol) less than 100 mg/dl with HDL (good cholesterol) greater than 40 mg/dl or 50 mg/dl for men and women, respectively. Note that two of the three, blood pressure and cholesterol, are independent of diabetes as risks for heart disease and stroke in the general population (although poor blood glucose control worsens the risks). These target figures may vary from person to person depending on overall risk, how difficult they are to achieve, any side effects of treatment, and the age and life expectancy of an individual.

Getting to know quality carbohydrates

Managing carbohydrates — not eliminating carbohydrates — is a key to controlling blood glucose levels, and reducing your risk for diabetes-related complications. And, carbohydrates are everywhere. Not all carbohydrates are created equal, however, and the good news is that many carbohydrate-containing foods enjoyed in a meal are compatible with achieving excellent control of blood glucose levels. Your registered dietitian or nutritionist will help you learn where to find carbohydrates, identify these high-quality carbohydrate foods, and balance your intake of carbohydrate throughout the day in your personalized meal plan.

TIP

You may find a registered dietitian associated with your medical provider, a local hospital, in private practice, or available through your local department of public health. You can search for a registered dietitian in your local area on the website of the Academy of Nutrition and Dietetics (www.eatright.org). Find a registered dietitian who is also a certified diabetes educator by looking for the CDE notation in their title, or by searching the website of the American Association of Diabetes Educators (www.diabeteseducator.org) and look for the RD or RDN designation.

Chapter **4**

Incorporating Easy Lifestyle Hacks

I t is certainly possible to lead a normal, healthy, and active life with diabetes — to even thrive with diabetes. If you've been prescribed medication, then taking it as prescribed is step one. Otherwise, following the advice on healthful eating for diabetes in this book along with the lifestyle hacks we suggest can make a great difference in how well you can perform and avoid negative effects of diabetes. Because everyone is unique, it is up to you to find the best hacks for your wellbeing.

This chapter reviews the incredible benefits of a healthy lifestyle that embraces physical activity, fresh air, community, and pleasurable activities while transforming stress. You also discover the importance of adopting an attitude that makes your long-term health a real priority.

Adopting a Healthful and Enjoyable Diabetes Lifestyle

For many people, *diet* is a word that usually comes to mind when they think about a diabetes-friendly meal plan. Interestingly, the English word *diet* comes from the Greek *diata*, which means way of life. That's because even in ancient times it was widely understood that it wasn't just the food we digested, but also how we ate and with whom, and whether we enjoyed physical activity and engaged in mentally stimulating thoughts as well as relaxation that we could truly thrive as humans.

Nowadays, *lifestyle* is a word without much meaning by itself. But, add something to it — rural lifestyle, casual lifestyle, modest lifestyle, or lifestyles of the rich and famous — and a clear picture pops into your mind. So, what pops into your mind when you hear *healthy lifestyle*? You don't have to live on a diet of sacrifice or practice extreme sports in order to regulate your blood sugar and live well. Research shows that we get the most benefit from activities that we take pleasure in, so it's best to fill your lives with those so that your body, mind, and spirit benefit simultaneously. Adopting a healthy lifestyle isn't about training for the Iron Man Triathlon. It's about making small decisions that fit better choices into your other lifestyle. And, just like pennies make dollars, small decisions can have big results.

TIP

Did you know that a recent study found that those who engaged in one- or two-minute bursts of exercise roughly three times a day, like speed-walking while commuting to work or rapidly climbing stairs, showed a nearly 50 percent reduction in cardiovascular mortality risk and a roughly 40 percent reduction in the risk of dying from cancer as well as all causes of mortality, compared to those who didn't do any exercise? Getting up and moving around throughout the day also has profound effects on blood sugar.

Enjoying physical activity

You can make a long list of reasons why many children and adults get less physical activity now than in days gone by. However, the fact remains that the more we enjoy exercise, the healthier we are.

Walking, swimming, gardening, dancing, going for an evening stroll, playing tennis or golf, cooking, baking, practicing yoga, and weight training are just a few ways to get a great workout. Some other examples of aerobic exercise include biking, shadowboxing, and martial arts, and team sports such as volleyball, softball, and basketball. Resistance training can be effective not only with weights, but also with stretch bands, a gallon or half gallon of milk, rowing, or by doing pushups.

The fact that it's less likely you'll get physical activity during the course of your normal day doesn't make physical activity less important. It simply makes it less likely you'll get the incredible benefits of regular activity unless you're convinced it's worth the effort to find opportunities. Physical activity offers the following benefits to your immediate and your long-term health:

>> Exercise lowers blood glucose and boosts insulin sensitivity. Higher insulin sensitivity can persist for 24 to 72 hours after exercising.

>> Exercise reduces dangerous visceral fat — fat deposited around internal organs, which is associated with insulin resistance and type 2 diabetes — more effectively than diet.

>> Exercise helps prevent high blood pressure and helps lower blood pressure even among people diagnosed with hypertension.

>> Exercise prevents plaque buildup (atherosclerosis) in arteries and vessels, reducing the risk for heart attack or stroke by lowering bad LDL cholesterol and triglyceride levels, and raising good HDL cholesterol.

>> Exercise helps arteries retain flexibility, reducing the potential for plaque buildup.

>> Vigorous exercise helps prevent some cancers, including colon and postmeno-pausal breast cancers.

>> Exercise improves balance, and along with adequate calcium and vitamin D increases bone strength, both reducing the likelihood of a fall and reducing the risk of fracture in a fall.

>> Exercise may reduce the risk of dementia.

>> Exercise improves sleep, reduces the symptoms of stress and depression, enhances sexual enjoyment, improves mobility, and extends lifespan.

That's an impressive list, and you must be anxious to know exactly what you need to do now to get these benefits for yourself. Current recommendations are for 150 minutes per week of moderate activity, like walking, or 75 minutes of vigorous activity. Don't let that number scare you. The 150 minutes per week can easily be broken down into five 30-minute sessions, six 25-minute sessions, or seven 22-minute sessions. (For beginners, 10 to 15 minutes a day can help get you started.) You can even break those times down in half so that you don't have to do all the exercise at one time.

TIP

Choosing enjoyable forms of exercise can help you to stay on track. In addition, many people have a better chance of staying on track when they start increasing physical activity if they have an exercise or accountability partner.

YOU HAVE TO START SOMEWHERE

FROM THE AUTHORS

During the time in her life when she was legally disabled from illness, Amy was in too much pain and was too weak to exercise or even move the way she wanted to. At the same time, she knew that she had to really push herself or she might never gain her mobility back. She heard a story about a man who actually lost weight by closing his eyes and imagining himself running a marathon with great detail. It sounds far-fetched, but Amy saw the evidence, so she figured if she couldn't move, she could start there. So, every day in bed, Amy would imagine herself moving freely. A few weeks later her grandfather came to visit. Then in his late eighties, he encouraged Amy to try walking to at-home exercise videos online. He said they helped him a great deal. She was so impressed with her grandfather's stamina that she promised him she would try. The first week she could only do 1 minute at a time, and then she worked up to 2 minutes, and then 3, and so on. Within a month Amy was walking for 15 minutes — which was a mile — and by the time she transformed her illness she was up to 5 miles with ease. Now Amy reminds herself and others that starting is the most important part.

Lately, resistance exercise — lifting weights is the most obvious example — has been getting more and more attention for offering health benefits that are complimentary to aerobic activity like walking or biking. A review of data from the National Health and Nutrition Examination Survey III concluded that every 10 percent increase in muscle mass corresponded with an 11 percent reduction in insulin resistance. Because insulin resistance is a key cause of type 2 diabetes, the advantages to increasing muscle mass with resistance exercise are obvious.

REMEMBER

Any activity is better than none at all. The American College of Sports Medicine guidelines acknowledge that exercise of less than ten minutes duration may have health and fitness benefits, especially for sedentary individuals. Keep in mind that you can increase your activity levels almost by accident if you change simple daily habits. For instance, make it a point to park a good distance from the door at the mall or grocery store, and take the stairs instead of an elevator or escalator. Recent research is finding that too much time sitting is a special risk beyond not getting exercise, and taking five minutes just to stand or stroll every hour has some benefit.

ASK THE DOCTOR

Be certain to consult with your doctor before changing your activity patterns. Foot health is extra important, so wear comfortable shoes and avoid blisters. But, make it a point to get whatever physical activity you can.

EXTINGUISHING THE SMOKES

Smoking remains a leading cause of preventable death in the United States, although it's notable that contending for the top spot is the group of obesity-related health threats like high blood pressure and diabetes. The combination of smoking and diabetes is a double whammy on your cardiovascular system, when having diabetes has already multiplied your risk.

Smoking damages the lining of arteries and blood vessels, promoting the buildup of waxy plaque (atherosclerosis), and increases the risk for peripheral arterial disease (PAD) and stroke. Smoking reduces levels of good HDL cholesterol, and increases blood pressure and heart rate. Smoking also reduces the flow of oxygen to your heart muscle and reduces your capacity for exercise.

You can simply stop smoking, even though it may not be easy. Give it a try and don't hesitate to get help. Don't let smoking cancel out the gains from all the attention you're ready to give to managing diabetes.

Transforming stress

Everyone experiences stress because some stress is natural and unavoidable. Start with what's called the fight or flight response — pounding heart, dry mouth, perspiration, muscle tension, shaking, lightheadedness, and heightened awareness. These responses are an instinctive physical reaction to a perceived threat, even if the threat is a job interview, a roller-coaster ride, or a public speaking assignment. A rush of adrenaline increases breathing and heart rate, raises blood pressure and blood glucose levels, and can even impair logical decision-making and thinking. Fortunately, the extreme physical response to these states of extreme stress is usually temporary.

Lower levels of stress over the long term can have the same physical effects. The intensity of your response is not as noticeable, but over time chronic stress has a more negative effect on health. It's not possible to eliminate all stress from your life — having diabetes is stressful, as are families, jobs, travel, finances, and hundreds of other circumstances. You can reduce stress, however, by practicing the following simple suggestions:

>> **Identify your main sources of stress.** Write them down, and when you notice them occurring, attempt to change them. If they are chronic issues that cannot be changed, commit to learning to "let go" of their effects on your health or changing your attitude toward them.

>> **Ask to see the hidden blessing.** If you are faced with a difficult situation that you feel you can't change, each morning and night — and when you feel stressed — take deep breaths in and out three times and ask your consciousness to see the hidden blessing in that particular circumstance. If you are willing to listen, the answers you may receive are profound. This does not mean to negate your suffering, but instead helps you look at the situation from a different lens, which may help you better cope with the stressor.

>> **Don't sweat the small stuff.** Little stressors add up. When you find yourself getting anxious, say to yourself, "Is this as important as my health and happiness?" If the answer is no, let it go. If you can't let it go, try breathing exercises, yoga, music, massage, or a quick walk to make dealing with it easier.

>> **Make time for leisure.** It really is good for your health and happiness.

>> **Get enough sleep.** Most adults need seven to eight hours each night, and sleep deprivation has negative effects on your health, too.

>> **Exercise regularly.** It's a healthy way to release pent-up tension, regulate hormones, and promote mental health.

>> **Avoid excess caffeine and don't smoke.** Both excess caffeine and smoking can increase blood pressure and feelings of anxiety.

>> **Eat antioxidant-rich foods.** Such foods can help regulate the body's stress response.

>> **Don't make perfection your goal.** You'll be forever frustrated.

>> **Develop a relaxing ritual that makes you feel safe and comforted.** This is unique to everyone, but you can experiment with cozying up to a cup of herbal tea and a good book, writing in a gratitude journal, or engaging in meditation or prayer. Even a short ritual in the morning and evening can help combat stress.

>> **Seek professional help with severe stress or depression.** Diabetes can feel overwhelming, and you shouldn't have to manage these feelings on your own.

Want another reason to learn how to shed stress? Stress impedes your ability to make wise decisions about diet, and making wise decisions about diet can be an excellent path to losing your stress over having diabetes. It's a circular benefit.

Prioritizing Your Health

Nobody can promise you that diabetes absolutely won't affect your health in some negative way — there are too many variables, including how long your blood glucose levels have been compromised. But, you can be sure that dedicating some time and effort to following through on the responsibilities of diabetes self-management will have a definite positive impact.

Making the commitment

There's nothing about diabetes self-management that's impossible for you to accomplish. In fact, it's not difficult, as really difficult things go. Inconvenient would be a better description. Yet, way too many people with diabetes simply don't commit to the effort. Perhaps the common misconception is that because diabetes is so prevalent, and there's a medicine for regulating blood sugar, nothing else needs to be done. Maybe the absence of attention-getting symptoms in type 2 diabetes has them doubting that diabetes is really all that serious. They may have an opposite view — no matter what they do, there's nothing that will keep the complications away. Others may feel that they genetically inherited diabetes and that it's inevitable.

In all cases, those people haven't made the effort to learn the truth. Learning about diabetes, and the opportunity you have for thriving with this condition, is surely an important commitment. And, making commitments to seize control of your health is what diabetes self-management is all about.

Enjoying the community, fresh air, and pleasurable activities

In many modern societies, the sense of community is not the same as it used to be. Previous generations grew up being able to ask their neighbors for help, rely on people in the area that they live in to support them during times of crisis, and participated in rewarding rituals. Now, things have changed. Eating communally, however, is still one of the main ways we can reap the benefits of being together.

According to a study that appeared in the *Journal of Adolescent Health* and was based on interviews with more than 18,000 adolescents, even teenagers who ate regularly with their parents developed much better nutritional habits. Cornell University research also revealed that coworkers of diverse backgrounds who eat together performed better at work.

REMEMBER

Mental health experts recommend 30 minutes of fresh air a day — and many believe it's more beneficial to the psyche than antipsychotic drugs. Getting more fresh air and spending time outdoors can help to increase your overall health and mental outlook. Research also shows that spending time outdoors leads to more physical exercise.

TIP

Try to spend as much time in nature as possible. Even these small steps can have positive effects:

>> Open the blinds and windows when possible.

>> Try getting your exercise outdoors.

>> Walk to nearby stores, if possible, instead of driving.

>> Sit on a porch, terrace, balcony, or in the yard when possible.

>> Eat outdoors when possible.

>> Seek out new parks or outdoor spaces to visit on your days off.

The activities we enjoy the most are the best for us. All types of hobbies have physical and mental benefits whether it's baking, painting, dancing, gardening, knitting, or hiking. Doing what you love can reduce stress, provide you with a sense of accomplishment, broaden your social circle, lift your spirits, reduce pain, and add quality to your life.

Valuing prevention

The long-term health risks associated with diabetes are a result of years of accumulated damage, which can be occurring day by day with virtually no symptoms. Managing those risks means making commitments and accepting inconveniences day to day and year to year, sometimes with little positive feedback. That is the challenge of valuing prevention — trusting the evidence even when the payoff isn't immediately obvious.

Studies show that diabetes can cut the life span of middle-aged adults by 8 to 12 years if the condition isn't managed effectively. But, at diagnosis those missing years are still 10 to 15 years away. Trusting that what you do today and tomorrow can have a profound benefit to your health many years down the road is best viewed as an investment — an investment in the quality of your future. And, prevention is the best investment you'll ever make.

2

Nutrition with Purpose

IN THIS PART . . .

Ease into the deeper waters of nutrition, discovering the specific needs those with diabetes have and how to meet them with ease.

Find out how the right combinations of macronutrients — carbohydrates, proteins, and fat — will keep your body and mind perfectly fueled.

Activate your digestion by making micronutrients and your gut microbiome work for you.

Unleash the power of bioactive compounds and polyphenols to get the most out of the foods you eat.

Set yourself up for success in all settings — at home, at work, and at restaurants — so that you can maintain your healthful lifestyle everywhere.

IN THIS CHAPTER

» **Understanding the basic principles of nutrition**

» **Aiming for a better A1C**

» **Deflating high blood pressure**

» **Bringing down LDL cholesterol**

» **Adjusting to special situations**

Chapter **5**

Explaining Nutrition Requirements for Diabetes

Where diabetes is concerned, food is medicine. Diabetes, both type 1 and type 2, is all about food. At the most basic level, diabetes is defined by losing the capacity to process the sugars of carbohydrate food in a normal way. But, food is also the key to living healthy with diabetes, helping you control blood glucose levels and reduce your risk for diabetes complications.

This chapter describes how a nutrition plan for diabetes can keep food working for you, and details the importance of aiming to reach certain targets set for specific health markers. These targets are known as the diabetes ABCs — A1C, blood pressure, and cholesterol. There is good evidence that achieving success in these measurements is associated with better outcomes for people living with diabetes.

However, it is an oversimplification (and a missed opportunity) to view food and nutrition just as a way to keep your lab results good to please your health professional! Enjoying and celebrating nutritious food as part of a healthy lifestyle can be so much more than that. It can reduce the risk of many chronic diseases, some of which are particularly associated with diabetes, as well as support improved wellbeing, optimum mental health, and a robust immune system.

For this reason it is important to consider broader aspects of nutrition. For people living with diabetes, it is appropriate to take care to eat the best quality carbohydrates and to monitor their effect on blood glucose, but fundamentally, a diet and lifestyle that is good for a person with diabetes is the same diet that is best for everyone. This chapter gives you the outline for living in good health with diabetes, starting with the five principles of excellent nutrition.

Five Principles of Excellent Nutrition

When considering how we optimize our diet, it is best to take a holistic approach and consider a number of factors that are not limited to a narrow approach but embrace all aspects of our health as well as our environment. An excellent diet should be one that

>> **Provides optimum control of blood glucose.** We explore this more in the next chapters, which consider the role of good-quality carbohydrates in foods.

>> **Helps to achieve and maintain a healthy weight.** This is especially important for those people with diabetes who are overweight.

>> **Has been shown to reduce the risk of other diseases, in particular those that are more common as complications of diabetes.** The components for an excellent diet should include not only good-quality carbohydrates, fats, and proteins, but also be rich in vitamins, micronutrients, and anti-inflammatory and antioxidant "bioactive" compounds that are protective and support optimum mental and physical health. We consider these in Chapters 6, 7, and 8. Processed foods should be kept to a minimum or excluded.

>> **Is sustainable so that its glycemic control, healthy weight, and anti-inflammatory benefits are maintained in the long term.** In other words, it's enjoyable, varied, and tasty, and can be incorporated into daily life.

>> **Is ethical and sustainable for the environment.** Our health depends on the health of our beautiful planet.

Targeting Blood Glucose Control in Type 1 and Type 2 Diabetes

Before you had diabetes two participants worked in tandem to manage your blood glucose levels. First is carbohydrate-containing food, which supplies the glucose that feeds into your bloodstream as it becomes liberated from sugar or starch molecules during digestion. Second is your pancreas, which has *beta cells* that release insulin to lower high levels of blood glucose, and *alpha cells* that release glucagon to raise low levels of blood glucose. This remarkable system kept adequate supplies of glucose stored away in muscle, fat, and liver cells for energy needs, and kept your blood glucose levels balanced in the normal range whether you had eaten recently or not.

After diabetes, this amazing system requires another participant — you. Whether you have type 1 diabetes or type 2 diabetes, your natural system for maintaining blood glucose balance needs help, and unless you're very young or otherwise incapacitated, that help has to come from you. And, taking your medication, including insulin if necessary, is an important but incomplete approach to controlling blood glucose. The main reference book for certified diabetes educators declares that patients need reminding that pharmacologic treatment for type 2 diabetes is only a supplement to lifestyle changes. It is always important to start with nutrition and exercise.

Matching medication and food

It's possible, with an early diagnosis and a strong commitment to lifestyle, to manage type 2 diabetes without medication. However, Type 1 diabetes can't be managed without insulin. So, keeping blood glucose levels in balance almost always involves matching insulin medication to your ingestion of carbohydrate foods. And both the volume and the timing of eating carbohydrate foods are important.

REMEMBER

Everyone's blood glucose levels go higher after eating carbohydrate foods because it takes time to release insulin and for insulin to do its work. The objective of managing diabetes medications and food is to blunt sharp rises in blood glucose levels, and to get levels back down in a way that's close to a normal response.

When your diabetes treatment includes rapid-acting or short-acting (regular) insulin taken before a meal, matching medication with food can and should be done with some precision. That means people with type 1 diabetes, or those with type 2 who are taking these formulations of insulin, must know carbohydrates. Chapter 6 provides more details on carbohydrates.

TECHNICAL STUFF

The relationship between insulin and carbohydrate food is best illustrated by your specific *insulin to carbohydrate ratio* (I:C ratio). That figure is usually expressed as 1 unit of insulin to compensate for a certain number of carbohydrate grams — 1:15, for instance, means 1 unit of insulin for every 15 grams of carbohydrate. A meal that includes 45 grams of carbohydrate requires 3 units of insulin if 1:15 is your insulin to carb ratio. However, your insulin to carb ratio is very much an individual number for you, and your I:C ratio may be different than the I:C ratio for someone else, and may even be different for your breakfast than for your lunch or dinner.

Treating diabetes with rapid or short-acting insulin also requires adjustments. If your blood glucose level is in the normal range at mealtime, your I:C ratio is all you need. But, if your blood glucose is higher than normal, whether at mealtime or not, you need to apply a correction factor. Your correction factor represents how much your blood glucose levels will drop — how many milligrams per deciliter (mg/dl) in the United States — if you take one unit of insulin without food. The number differs from person to person, and may be different according to the time of day.

The individualized numbers are never perfect, but where these insulin formulations are part of your treatment, matching the dose to your food is fairly accurate and extremely flexible.

WARNING

Matching food and insulin always requires knowing your blood glucose level before you take the insulin. Overdosing results in dangerously low blood glucose levels (hypoglycemia), and underdosing leaves blood glucose above normal. Testing blood glucose before every meal and testing again two hours after your meal — called *postprandial* — helps you keep your I:C ratio and correction factors zeroed in.

REMEMBER

In addition, matching food and medication with this kind of precision doesn't apply to other diabetes medications, including intermediate-acting or long-acting insulin formulations. Even diabetes pills that are taken at mealtime aren't dose-adjusted based upon what you're eating at that meal. However, it's important to control carbohydrate consumption in a different way for optimal blood glucose control.

Your diabetes meal plan allocates your daily carbohydrate foods evenly, more or less, to each meal so that your daily dose of glucose from food doesn't all come at the same time. Your meal plan also emphasizes that you get your carbohydrates from foods that are slowly digested, like beans and fruit, rather than from added sugars that can cause blood glucose levels to spike soon after eating. Ultimately, the goal is to help you keep your blood glucose under control, and the benefits of blood glucose control are profound.

Keeping A1C in range

A1C, sometimes called hemoglobin A1C or HbA1C, is the A of the diabetes ABCs. Your doctor orders a lab test of your *hemoglobin A1C* periodically; diabetes professionals pay careful attention to this number. We explain A1C in detail in *Diabetes For Dummies*, 6th Edition (Wiley), but here are two important facts you should know now:

>> A1C measures your average blood glucose levels over the 60- to 90-day period before the test. Even though yesterday's blood glucose level influences the A1C value more than your level six weeks ago — a weighted average — A1C gives the clearest picture of blood glucose control hour to hour, day to day, and week to week. This test is especially important for people with type 2 diabetes who do not frequently test their blood glucose levels at home.

>> A1C values are closely correlated with your risk for many diabetes-related complications, like heart disease and kidney failure. In that regard, the target values set for blood glucose control by the American Diabetes Association (ADA) or the American College of Clinical Endocrinologists (ACCE) are numbers with real meaning. The ADA target is an A1C less than 7 percent, and the ACCE target is less than 6.5 percent.

Table 5-1 shows the correlation between the A1C level and weighted average blood glucose in milligrams per deciliter (mg/dl) and in millimoles per liter (mmol/l). Remember that a normal fasting blood glucose level is 99 mg/dl (5.5 mmol/l) or lower, but levels rise after eating for everyone. The A1C target values represent the level of blood glucose control those organizations view as being both achievable, and effective at minimizing the risk for complications.

Highly respected landmark studies, including the Diabetes Control and Complications Trial (DCCT) in the United States and the United Kingdom Prospective Diabetes Study (UKPDS), demonstrated striking reductions in the risk for complications with improved A1C values. The DCCT showed each 1 percent reduction in A1C represented a 37 percent decrease in the risk for complications of the eye, kidneys, and nerves. A recent study in Sweden tracked 12,000 people with diabetes who all began with A1C values averaging 7.8 percent. Over time, researchers grouped subjects into those with improving A1C (who eventually averaged A1C 7 percent), and those with A1C that remained the same or went higher (averaged A1C 8.4 percent). The group that gained control of blood glucose and improved their A1C showed a 40 percent decrease in the risk for cardiovascular complications and death.

REMEMBER

Controlling blood glucose levels consistently, and achieving the A1C targets is incredibly important to your long-term health. The choices you make every day about the foods you eat have the greatest impact on your A1C and on the quality of your future.

TABLE 5-1

A1C and Average Blood Glucose Level

A1C Value Corresponds To	Blood Glucose	Blood Glucose
5.0%	101 mg/dl	5.6 mmol/l
6.0%	136 mg/dl	7.6 mmol/l
6.5%*	154 mg/dl	8.6 mmol/l
7.0%**	172 mg/dl	9.6 mmol/l
8.0%	207 mg/dl	11.6 mmol/l
10.0%	279 mg/dl	15.6 mmol/l
12.0%	350 mg/dl	19.5 mmol/l

*Recommended target of the American College of Clinical Endocrinologists
**Recommended target of the American Diabetes Association

Losing to Win: Weight Loss

Excess weight is a distinct risk factor for type 2 diabetes, and more than 80 percent of people with type 2 diabetes are, in fact, overweight or obese. The characteristic insulin resistance associated with excess weight can complicate treatment for type 1 diabetes as well, requiring larger and larger doses of insulin, and leaving blood glucose elevated for longer periods waiting for injected insulin to take effect. A nutrition plan for effective diabetes management addresses weight loss if necessary, and modest success in this effort can bring huge rewards for blood glucose control.

Weight status is measured on a scale known as the *body mass index,* or BMI for short. For most adults, BMI is an accurate representation of body fatness, and it is excess fat, for all intents and purposes, that leads to metabolic disorders like diabetes. However, there are some limitations to BMI. It is a less reliable predictor of fitness or risk of lifestyle illnesses for people with high muscle mass, for example, rugby players or U.S. football players. It may also be beneficial to have a higher BMI if you are older because loss of muscle rather than fat may be a reason for a drop in BMI.

BMI takes both height and weight into account, and mathematically is your weight in kilograms divided by your height in meters squared — Kg/M^2. Using English measures, BMI can be calculated by taking weight in pounds divided by height in inches squared, and multiplied by 703 to account for converting to the metric basis. Therefore, for a man or woman who is 5'7" (67 inches) and weighs 200 pounds, the calculation is as follows:

$$200 / (67)(67) = 200 / 4489 = .0446 \times 703 = 31.35$$

On the BMI scale, values between 18.5 and 24.9 are considered normal, or healthy, weights. A value between 25 and 29.9 is considered overweight, and any value higher than 30 places the individual into an obese category. A BMI value greater than 40 is often referred to as *morbidly obese*. A 5′7″ man or woman weighing 256 pounds has a BMI value of 40.1.

Nearly three-quarters of the U.S. adult population falls into the overweight or obese categories, and, alarmingly, one-third of children and adolescents. And, studies consistently show that people underestimate their BMI category, suggesting that the trend toward a heavier population is affecting perception.

Excess weight is mostly the weight of excess fat, which is stored in fat cells called *adipocytes* as energy reserves. Excess calories are stored as fat, whether the calories come from protein, carbohydrate, or dietary fat, and losing weight requires that one begins drawing calories for daily living from that stored fat. It used to be thought that, in general terms, you must burn more calories than you consume by consuming fewer calories, burning more calories, or both. Calorie counting remains an important aspect of weight management; however, other things matter just as much and perhaps even more.

A calorie is a theoretical laboratory measurement of the energy in food, and the body does not simply add up the calories consumed and those used up, putting the difference into body fat. A calorie from one dietary fat does not have the same biological effect as from another. Although carbohydrates have a third of the calories of fats, depending on the food and its context combined together with other foods in a meal, the carbohydrate may make a greater contribution to fat deposition and weight gain. Scientists are recognizing that there are other factors that influence the way we manage the energy from the foods we eat. The effects of foods on our gut microbiome, the presence of compounds that can influence insulin and other hormones, as well as our genetic makeup are just a few of those aspects we explore in future chapters in this book.

The standard formula is that a 3,500 calorie deficit is equal to one pound, so adjusting diet and activity to make a 500 calorie withdrawal from stored calories every day would lead to one pound weight loss every week. In reality, losing weight is more complicated than this simple formula, and metabolic changes can result in plateaus where weight loss tapers off.

REMEMBER

Where diabetes is concerned, the most important step is to get started, because a loss of only 5 to 7 percent of body weight can make a major difference in blood glucose control. The morbidly obese 5′7″, 256-pound subject mentioned previously may hope for a BMI in the normal range by losing 100 pounds, but losing just 18 pounds can improve insulin sensitivity enough to make real improvements in A1C. These improvements are likely related to losing dangerous visceral fat, which accumulates around vital organs, and is the chief suspect for spreading insulin resistance from cell to cell. Visceral fat, however, goes first when a diet and exercise strategy creates a demand for stored calories.

TIP

Having a high-quality diet may be more important than your BMI when it comes to heart disease and overall risk of death. Although it is great to aim for the healthiest diet and also to be in the normal BMI range, in 2020, researchers from Uppsala in Sweden published data in the journal *PLOS Medicine* showing that a person with a normal BMI who was eating an unhealthy diet was more at risk of early death than a person who was overweight but diligently adhering to a healthy Mediterranean-style dietary pattern.

Monitoring Cardiovascular Risks

Having diabetes makes you at least twice as likely as someone who does not have diabetes to have heart disease or a stroke, and you're likely to develop heart disease or have strokes at an earlier age than other people. Some studies suggest that if you've developed type 2 diabetes when middle-aged, your chance of having a heart attack is as high as someone without diabetes who has already had one heart attack.

Women who have not gone through menopause usually have less risk of heart disease than men of the same age, but diabetes cancels the protective effects of being a woman in her child-bearing years. People with diabetes who have already had one heart attack run an even greater risk of having a second one. Heart attacks in people with diabetes are more serious and are more likely to result in death.

Cardiovascular disease is by far the number one cause of death in people with diabetes — 65 percent of people with diabetes will die from heart attack or stroke. This is very serious stuff. The reasons for this elevated risk are many. Persistent high blood glucose levels damage the inside wall of arteries, making plaque buildup more likely. Excess weight and a sedentary lifestyle, common with type 2 diabetes, increase the risks for high blood pressure, high cholesterol levels, and high blood triglycerides. Arteries lose their flexibility, and the characteristics of the lipoproteins that carry cholesterol may even be more prone to building up on artery walls than similar particles in people without diabetes. In addition, having diabetes tends to create a physiological state of oxidative stress. This creates a pro-inflammatory environment. Both of these terms are explained in detail in Chapter 8 of this book, and are considered crucial in the development of heart disease and other chronic illnesses.

TIP

Both regular aerobic exercise and weight training exercise can reverse the increased cardiac risk associated with diabetes. The effect of both together is greater than the sum of the effect of each individually.

REMEMBER

Eating habits play a huge role in improving your increased risk for cardiovascular disease, and meal planning for diabetes management should always have heart health as one goal. Getting regular physical activity, not smoking, and reducing stress are also essential elements of an effective diabetes management lifestyle, not only for better blood glucose control, but also to further reduce cardiovascular risks.

Normalizing high blood pressure

Blood pressure is the B of the diabetes ABCs. Your circulatory system is something like the waterlines that run through your town or city, pushing water through large and small pipes with enough pressure for you to have an invigorating shower. Your arteries, veins, and tiny capillaries deliver materials, like glucose and oxygen, to cells all over your body under the pressure provided when your powerful heart muscle contracts. Water pressure is measured in pounds per square inch, but your blood pressure is measured in millimeters of mercury with a *sphyg-momanometer,* and you may have seen devices that actually have a tube of mercury.

Blood pressure always includes two numbers — your *systolic* pressure over your *diastolic* pressure. The *systolic* pressure is the pressure against the wall of your arteries when your heart pumps. The *diastolic* pressure is the pressure in your arteries between heart beats. A normal blood pressure is less than 120/80, and the target blood pressure for people with diabetes is 130/80 or lower.

WARNING

Chronic high blood pressure, when blood pressure measures 140/90 or higher most of the time, is called *hypertension,* and hypertension is a major risk factor for heart attack, stroke, heart failure, aneurysms, peripheral artery disease, and kidney failure. These are many of the same problems that can be caused by diabetes, too, so high blood pressure added to diabetes is a real double whammy.

It's likely that your doctor will prescribe medication to help control your high blood pressure if you have diabetes. However, just as lifestyle choices play a major role in managing diabetes, those same choices can have a major impact in improving your blood pressure. Exercise, not smoking, and what you choose to eat make a real difference. The effectiveness of eating habits to reduce high blood pressure has been most effectively demonstrated in clinical trials conducted by the National Institutes of Health beginning in 1992. From those studies came an eating plan known as DASH — dietary approaches to stop hypertension — and following the DASH eating plan clearly has a direct impact in improving blood pressure.

As well as highlighting whole-grain carbohydrates, vegetables, and fruit, the DASH diet emphasizes a reduction in salt and sodium intake and a higher potassium intake from fruits and vegetables. The potassium-to-sodium ratio is important, and for many people this can have a significant positive effect on reducing blood pressure. Chapter 14 looks at the DASH diet in more detail.

TIP

Of course, your use of the salt shaker adds sodium to your diet, so replacing salt with other spices is one key to reducing blood pressure with diet. But, the real secret to limiting sodium is to read nutrition facts labels, because most dietary sodium is likely to come as added salt from prepackaged or canned foods. Look for no-salt-added packaged foods.

The Mediterranean diet has also been extensively studied and has been found to reduce blood pressure. Many of the principles are shared with the DASH diet with plentiful whole grains, vegetables, and fruits, but there may also be specific benefits of the regular consumption of extra-virgin olive oil. The combination of naturally occurring and healthy vegetable nitrates (distinct from potentially unhealthy nitrites combined with meat proteins in artificial preservatives) with the fat of olive oil results in nitro-fatty acids that can reduce blood pressure.

Lowering LDL cholesterol

Cholesterol is the C in the diabetes ABCs, but this subject can be a little complicated. Cholesterol is essential for a number of cellular functions, playing important roles in building and maintaining cell membranes, synthesizing bile for fat digestion, manufacturing vitamin D, and building certain hormones.

Cholesterol is ferried around in your bloodstream by special carriers called *lipoproteins*, and these lipoproteins come in assorted varieties. Low-density lipoproteins, abbreviated LDL (and commonly called bad cholesterol), circulate in the blood to deliver necessary cholesterol to cells around your body. There's nothing bad about that; however, there's a limit to how much cholesterol your cells require, and when that limit is reached, your cells close down the receiving department. When cells won't take delivery of more cholesterol, LDL cholesterol continues circulating in the bloodstream where an inflammatory immune response can make it more likely that LDL particles accumulate inside of artery walls, forming waxy plaques. This process is called *atherosclerosis*, and it's the principal cause of heart and cardiovascular disease. The inflammatory processes are key to plaque and clot formation and we consider the importance of incorporating ingredients in your diet that have extraordinary protective anti-inflammatory effects. So whatever your LDL cholesterol levels, the degree to which your diet is suppressing inflammation is perhaps more important.

High-density lipoproteins, abbreviated HDL (and commonly called good cholesterol), seem to collect excess cholesterol from your blood, thereby reducing the
risk for atherosclerosis. Target cholesterol values aimed at reducing your risk for
heart disease, therefore, look at both LDL and HDL. Your medical team looks to
lower your LDL while raising HDL levels with medication, exercise, and diet. With
diabetes, these cholesterol targets are as follows:

>> LDL levels less than 100 mg/dl (often less than 70 mg/dl if other risk factors
are elevated)

>> HDL levels greater than 40 mg/dl for men, and greater than 50 mg/dl
for women

>> Triglycerides, another blood fat, should be less than 150 mg/dl

Similar to blood glucose control and high blood pressure, lifestyle choices, like
regular physical activity and not smoking, go a long way in keeping your LDL
lower and your HDL higher. Diet plays a key role as well, and you should be seeing
a consistent pattern by now about how these same lifestyle choices preserve your
health on several fronts.

Objective number one for controlling cholesterol is to reduce saturated fat in your
diet and eliminate trans fat. It is important to note, however, that the saturated fat
in naturally fermented yogurts and cheese have not been shown to be associated
with an increased risk of heart disease. It is probably the combination of genetic
susceptibility, particular dietary saturated fats, artificial preservatives especially
with processed meats, and methods of preparation in unhealthy oils that contribute to unhealthy LDL-to-HDL ratios.

REMEMBER

Healthy eating isn't completely about what you shouldn't eat; it is equally about
what you should eat. For cholesterol management, eat soluble fiber, like the fiber
in oats, beans, and barley, and eat lots of fruits and vegetables, especially the leafy
greens. Unless there's a reason your doctor says you shouldn't, have alcohol in
moderation to help raise HDL. And fish, which is high in omega-3 fatty acids, can
raise HDL and make an enviable dinner.

Insulin resistance (including type 2 diabetes), high blood pressure, and high levels
of LDL cholesterol are key elements of a broadly defined medical condition known
as the *metabolic syndrome*. Although people with metabolic syndrome may not
have diabetes, these and other abnormalities associated with metabolic
syndrome — such as an increased tendency to form clots and evidence of increased
inflammation — are all associated with increased heart attacks. Improvement in
lifestyle with a better diet and more exercise is the first step in reversing metabolic syndrome, just as it is for diabetes.

Looking at other risks

Complications of diabetes are not limited to heart disease and stroke. The damage caused by prolonged high blood glucose levels can be experienced in large or small blood vessels in numerous organs including the kidneys, eyes, and brain. Obesity, which often accompanies type 2 diabetes, is associated with an increased risk of many types of cancers. This is why it is so important to enjoy a diet that not only allows optimum regulation of blood glucose, but also has evidence to support protective effects against blood vessel damage, heart and kidney disease, and stroke. Even better if such a diet reduces the risk of cancers and dementia, improves mental wellbeing, nurtures a healthy gut microbiome, and promotes the achievement and maintenance of desirable weight, aligning with the five characteristics of an excellent diet.

Being Aware of Special Circumstances

People with diabetes are people first, so they span the entire spectrum of what people are, from babies to the elderly, from Olympic athletes to the sedentary, and virtually everything else you can imagine. Some circumstances may deserve special consideration when it comes to diet, however.

Children

Type 1 diabetes can strike children at almost any age, and type 1 diabetes always requires insulin injections matched with carbohydrate intake to balance blood glucose levels. Although the foundation of maintaining long-term health in spite of diabetes is *self-management,* young children are unable to take on that responsibility. Therefore, with type 1 diabetes in children, parents or other caretakers must play the primary role in balancing food and insulin, and experts suggest that some parental oversight is important into the teen years as well.

WARNING

The biggest concern with children taking insulin, and especially young children, is severe hypoglycemia, or low blood glucose. There is evidence that hypoglycemic events can do permanent damage to young, developing brains, and avoiding such occurrences may require frequent blood glucose monitoring and eating on demand — and getting toddlers to do anything on demand can be challenging. Unpredictable activity levels can make blood glucose control even more challenging.

Ultimately, kids and adolescents are growing, and it takes adequate food with adequate nutrients to support this rapid growth. Because tight blood glucose control is so difficult, A1C targets for children and adolescents are set higher than for adults. For children under six, where hypoglycemia can be so dangerous, an A1C less than 8.5 percent is considered satisfactory. The A1C target is gradually brought in line with the recommendation for adults as teens become adults.

Type 2 diabetes in children has become much more common in recent years as childhood obesity rates have risen sharply, and these children may also have high blood pressure and high cholesterol levels. Because children have unique dietary requirements to support growth, it's extra important that a diet and exercise program for diabetes self-management involve a medical team with a registered dietitian. A study conducted by the National Institute of Diabetes and Digestive and Kidney Diseases compared the effectiveness of common type 2 diabetes pills for controlling blood glucose levels in children 10 to 17 years of age. The results showed that these medications were much less effective in children, suggesting that insulin therapy early in the course of type 2 diabetes in children may be the most effective long-term option for preserving health.

Elderly

The incidence of type 2 diabetes is highest in the senior population, as high as 20 percent of the population over 65, and managing diabetes in seniors presents its own set of challenges. In addition, management is important because people aged 65 have the potential for 20 or more additional years of quality living. Diabetes complications can certainly develop in that span of time, and seniors with diabetes may well bring other risk factors, like high blood pressure and elevated cholesterol, into the mix.

Effective diabetes management for healthy seniors is not terribly different than for younger adults, keeping a focus on controlling blood glucose, blood pressure, and cholesterol with medication, exercise, and diet. Adequate calcium and vitamin D are necessary for bone health, and seniors also need to manage weight. Typically, a loss of muscle mass and added body fat comes with aging, and added fat can increase insulin resistance.

Treating diabetes in elderly adults who are frail or mentally impaired is the greatest challenge, complicated by multiple health conditions and drugs, an undependable memory, a lack of mobility for beneficial exercise, changes in normal metabolism, and inconsistent help by caregivers. Treatment decisions often aim primarily at avoiding the potential for low blood glucose, and dietary concerns may require a greater focus on malnutrition than on blood glucose control.

Individualizing treatment is especially important for seniors. The ADA sets a goal of a hemoglobin A1C in order to prevent long-term complications. Because these may take 20 years to develop, intensive measures to get A1C to target levels may be unnecessary. It is much more important to focus on quality of remaining years of life and to avoid the risks of hypoglycemia from overambitious targets.

Athletes

Exercise is a crucial element of effective diabetes self-management, and something most people with diabetes don't do enough. The case with athletes, however, is the opposite — more than normal levels of exercise. And, the dietary challenge is in balancing the calorie and carbohydrate requirements for energy with safe blood glucose levels, both during athletic activity, and in between training or competition. Maintaining safe blood glucose levels means avoiding both extremely low and extremely high blood glucose levels, both of which are risks.

A low blood glucose level, called *hypoglycemia,* can occur when exercise depletes glucose stored in muscle and liver cells, and insulin is still available. A high blood glucose level, called *hyperglycemia,* can happen when there is inadequate insulin available to move glucose into cells. Both conditions can be dangerous. Excessively low blood glucose deprives the brain of the glucose it needs to manage everything that goes on in your body. High blood glucose levels require muscle cells to burn fat, and the buildup of waste products called ketones can turn blood dangerously acidic in athletes with type 1 diabetes. Intense exercise can affect blood glucose levels not only during activity, but for hours afterwards.

The key to balancing blood glucose and carbohydrates in athletes is monitoring blood glucose levels frequently — before, after, and, if possible, during intense activities. Blood glucose monitoring during normal activities as well helps establish routine energy needs necessary to support the more extreme activity level.

Celiac and gluten sensitivity

Like type 1 diabetes, *celiac disease* is an immune system glitch, where a person's own immune system attacks the lining of the small intestine in response to a protein found in grains called *gluten.* Damage to the intestinal lining can interfere with the normal absorption of vitamins and minerals, and even carbohydrates needed for energy. Having type 1 diabetes increases the likelihood of having celiac disease, or a less severe gluten sensitivity, with estimates putting the risk at five to ten times higher than the general population.

The challenge for people with diabetes and celiac is diet — specifically, grains. The only effective treatment for celiac disease is strictly following a gluten-free diet, and even though the market for gluten-free products is rapidly expanding, balancing two different eating plans can be burdensome. The best choices for whole grains when managing diabetes and celiac disease, or an unspecified gluten sensitivity, are brown rice, quinoa, amaranth, or gluten-free oats. Support from a registered dietitian can be helpful in establishing an eating plan for effectively managing both conditions.

Gastroparesis

Gastroparesis means stomach paralysis, but in practical terms it's a potential complication of diabetes resulting from damage to the nerve that controls stomach emptying — gastroparesis is an *autonomic neuropathy* that causes your stomach to empty slowly. The general problem where gastroparesis is concerned is the disruption of normal eating patterns and the potential for inadequate calories, insufficient macronutrients, vitamin and mineral deficiencies, and even dehydration from lack of fluids. Food high in fiber, like grains, fruits, and vegetables, can be especially difficult to eat (digest) and so are meats and high-fat foods.

Managing gastroparesis can include eating smaller, but more frequent, meals, getting some essential nutrients from liquids, and eating pureed food. It's essential to balance these dietary changes with diabetes medication, and the nutrition requirements for blood glucose control. Again, guidance from a registered dietitian is critical.

Kidney failure

Poorly controlled diabetes is the leading cause of kidney failure, followed closely by high blood pressure, also too common among people with type 2 diabetes. Your kidneys filter waste products from your blood, including excess glucose, and high blood glucose levels over time cause kidney damage that reduces their filtration capacity. This damage is referred to as the complication *nephropathy*. Controlling blood glucose levels can help prevent nephropathy from advancing to kidney failure, but when the filtration rate (called GFR for *glomerular filtration rate)* of your kidneys is degraded to a point considered to be kidney failure, a special diet is necessary to delay progression.

In the earlier stages of kidney disease it's likely that your diet limits protein amounts and provides only high-quality protein. This diet also assures adequate fat and carbohydrates provide for your energy needs so that protein is not metabolized for energy.

When kidney disease progresses to end stage, where dialysis or a kidney transplant is necessary, your diet restricts fluids, phosphorous, sodium, potassium, and protein. This diet requires a registered dietitian with input from a specialized kidney doctor called a *nephrologist*. The take-home message about kidney failure is that controlling blood glucose, blood pressure, and LDL cholesterol from the early stages of your diabetes can go a long way in saving you from confronting this very difficult complication.

IN THIS CHAPTER

» **Understanding why macronutrients matter**

» **Recycling food to build what you need**

» **Getting to know quality carbohydrates**

» **Recognizing fats that are good for you**

» **Choosing healthy and sustainable proteins**

Chapter **6**

Meeting the Macronutrients: Carbohydrates, Fat, and Protein

Many people don't realize the crucial role consuming balanced amounts of macronutrients plays in the diet of someone with diabetes. The term *macro* means big, and macronutrients are certainly of big importance. But the term macro is used to describe carbohydrates, fat, and protein primarily because you need them in big amounts. The macronutrients are what build you, protect you, and fuel your many activities. And the macronutrients store energy you know as *calories*.

In this chapter, you discover why carbohydrates, fat, and protein are so important, and how your body has a specialized demolition crew ready to deconstruct each of the three macronutrients into its absorbable components so you can build what you need from the pieces.

The quality and quantity of macronutrients is important to diabetes, and to overall health. And, because you get the majority of your macronutrients from food, the meal-planning information in this chapter gives you a little what and why, as well as the where, which, and how much about each of these three essential nutrients.

Food Is More than Macronutrients

It is all too common to hear people say that, for example, they don't eat pasta because it is a carbohydrate, or cheese because it's a fat. In recent decades we were all encouraged to have a "low-fat" diet to reduce the risk of heart disease, and now, with a rise in obesity and type 2 diabetes, many health professionals are recommending a "low-carb" diet. There are variations on these themes, with "keto" diets advocating replacing carbohydrates with proteins, and others suggesting that it is best to increase fat consumption. We call these arguments "the macronutrient wars" because protagonists of such diets can get so fired up. We look more closely at some of these diets in Chapter 14, but we recommend avoiding macronutrient food fights!

When talking about macronutrients, it's important not to oversimplify what we eat and define food simply in terms of carbohydrates, fats, and proteins. Consider the following factors:

>> **Foods may not be exclusively made up of a single macronutrient.** Is a bean a protein or a carbohydrate? The truth is the bean is a great source of both. Let's not fall out over it.

>> **There are different types of carbohydrates, fats, and proteins that may be healthy or less healthy.** Foods can be described in nutritional terms as containing "high-quality" carbohydrates, fats, or protein types.

>> **We eat food, not macronutrients.** There is more to food than the largest macronutrient proportion it contains. Take the humble potato. When it comes to macronutrients it is mainly made up of carbohydrate; however, it is rich in important micronutrients such as vitamin C, potassium, and magnesium (see Chapter 7), and bioactive compounds with antioxidant and anti-inflammatory effects (see Chapter 8).

- **The way a whole food is physically and chemically organized (the food matrix) is important.** The structure of a food and the complex interactions between its component nutrients affects how it is absorbed and metabolized and ultimately how healthy it is.

- **We are not the only ones who eat our food.** Before our metabolism kicks in to convert the macronutrients we absorb into useful components, our food undergoes significant processing by our trillions of gut microbes, which need to be healthily and happily balanced. Fermented foods such as yogurts and quality cheeses may be high in fat, but the beneficial effects they have on our microbiome are excellent for health (see Chapter 7).

- **If we are not eating this, we must be eating that.** If we eat less of one macronutrient, unless we are cutting down on our overall intake, chances are we are replacing it with a different macronutrient. Arguably, one of the possible causes of the increase in rates of obesity, type 2 diabetes, and other chronic diseases may stem from the advice that eating fat caused heart disease. Later in the chapter, we discuss how this is an oversimplification — it depends on the type of fat, and some fats are harmful and others protective. The marketing of low-fat foods that had a higher proportion of refined carbohydrates and the increased use of refined vegetable oils may have had a detrimental effect on health. With some low-carbohydrate diets advocating increased consumption of fat and protein, perhaps in the form of processed meats, there are clear risks that the resulting diet may increase the risk of heart disease and cancers.

- **There is no "right" macronutrient proportion.** Traditional diets from across the world have been shown to be healthy. They share some important characteristics such as being low in processed foods and refined carbohydrates, as well as comprising of healthy (high-quality) macronutrients, but they can vary in terms of the overall proportions of carbohydrates, fats, and proteins.

Building a Complete Meal Is Important

In our professional experience, we continue to meet with people who aren't familiar with what constitutes a "complete meal." In highly industrialized societies, people are familiar with the examples that television commercials and billboards give them, and believe that specific marketing tactics are what constitute a meal. A burger, fries, and soft drink, while containing some degree of fat, carbohydrates, and protein, are not what we are considering to a be a complete meal for the purposes of this book.

TIP

A healthy meal can be created using a combination of foods from the three macronutrient groups to provide a balance. The key is always to get the best types and amounts of those foods that help someone with diabetes stay properly nourished while keeping their blood sugar levels regulated.

Your need for varying amounts of carbohydrates, fats, and protein may vary depending on your physical activity, but this can easily be built into meal planning and food choices. Believe it or not, consuming the tasty meals featured in this book (and others that follow these same principles) can help you to achieve your health goals.

TECHNICAL STUFF

The degree to which a carbohydrate results in a rise in blood glucose is called its *glycemic index,* but a more realistic measure of the effects of eating a food considers how quickly it causes a rise in blood glucose against the amount in a serving. This is described as the *glycemic load.* An example frequently used is watermelon, which has a much lower "real-world" glycemic load than its higher glycemic index would suggest due to its high water content.

The interactions between the macronutrients also have interesting effects. If a fat is added to a carbohydrate, for example, extra-virgin olive oil drizzled over pasta, the rise in blood glucose can be slowed due to delayed gastric emptying, beneficially influencing the speed and extent of the curve of blood glucose rise with a meal. Fats are also satiating, so in combination with other carbohydrates and proteins in a meal they help us to feel fuller more quickly. For this reason, each of Chef Amy's recipes in Chapter 18 is not just a dish, but a balanced meal that you can savor with the confidence that you are enjoying delicious food while getting your nutritional needs met.

Energizing with Quality Carbohydrates

Contrary to popular belief, carbohydrates, or *carbs,* when they come from good sources, are good for you. We live in a media-driven world, which for a variety of reasons likes to isolate specific different foods at different times and villainize them. But true, positive nutrition has stood the test of time for millennia. Before labeling carbs as off-limits, or labeling specific foods as carbohydrates and others as not, it is important to know what carbs truly are. Carbohydrates aren't just in junk food; they're also present in vegetables, fruits, and whole grains that our bodies need.

TECHNICAL
STUFF

Carbohydrates, specifically molecules of the carbohydrate glucose, are your body's favored fuel, and even though your cells can, and do, extract energy from protein and fat, glucose is choice numero uno. Glucose enters your bloodstream after you eat carbohydrates through absorption sites in your small intestine, and the rising glucose level in your blood signals special *beta cells* in the pancreas to release the hormone, insulin. Insulin stimulates cells, especially muscle, fat, and liver cells, to allow glucose molecules to pass through cell membranes where it can be stored inside of these cells for fuel when needed.

Cells store glucose in a molecule called *glycogen,* and glycogen is ready at a moment's notice to jump into a metabolic cycle that spits out the power pack molecule *adenosine triphosphate* (ATP), the real fuel for everything requiring energy. Glycogen is your most accessible source of energy, and carbohydrates in your diet keep the supplies ready when needed.

The role of carbohydrates in your body is not limited to energy, by the way, although diabetes tends to focus attention on that role. Glycolipids (glucose plus lipids) are a component of cell membranes, glycoproteins help protect your sensitive tissues with mucus, and the five-carbon sugar ribose is a component of DNA. The sugar lactose is produced in the milk of nursing mothers, and helps humans and animals get the energy needed for growth, temperature regulation, and strenuous activity like crying.

Milk sugar is the only significant carbohydrate component of your diet that is from an animal source, however, and most adults lose the ability to digest lactose. Plants are your carbohydrate factories, and you can thank plant carbohydrates for the wood that built your house, and for the fuel you need every day to run your body. And many plant foods that contain carbohydrates also happen to come along with essential vitamins, minerals, antioxidants, and other compounds that work to keep you healthy.

Carbohydrate stores four calories of potential energy per gram, and excess carbohydrate in your diet is stored as fat. Excess consumption of carbohydrate, especially fructose, can also act to raise levels of low-density lipoproteins, the so-called bad LDL cholesterol, and blood triglycerides.

REMEMBER

Beyond being an important macronutrient for energy and nutrients, dietary carbohydrates are overwhelmingly the macronutrient most related to blood glucose levels. And, whether your love for carbohydrates and the calories they provide was important in contributing to your risk for diabetes or not, carbohydrates are certainly important now. Both type 1 and type 2 diabetes are characterized by blood glucose levels that don't come back into normal balance after eating carbohydrate foods.

CONSIDERING PREDIABETES

It is now recognized that there may be circumstances when a person is not diagnosed with type 2 diabetes but their body's ability to handle carbohydrates with an efficient rise in insulin and blood glucose stabilization is impaired. This is called *prediabetes,* and someone with this condition may pass the threshold for a diagnosis of type 2 diabetes unless lifestyle changes can reverse the situation and improve glucose handling. Just as we all can have a measurement of our blood cholesterol levels whether low or high, we all have an HbA1C measurement, and some of us may be closer than others to the levels consistent with a diagnosis of prediabetes or type 2 diabetes.

In type 1 diabetes your body loses the capacity to produce insulin, whereas in type 2 diabetes the cells needed for glucose storage become resistant to the influence of insulin. In both cases, your normal processes for converting food to energy are disrupted. A certain level of blood glucose is necessary to supply cells that don't store glucose, like brain cells, with fuel whenever it's needed. But over time, persistently higher-than-normal levels of blood glucose damage tissues and significantly raise the risk for heart attack, stroke, nerve damage, vision loss, kidney failure, and other negative health impacts, innocently called complications. Controlling blood glucose with diabetes is a balancing act, and you're the acrobat.

Your task after a diabetes diagnosis is to manage your intake of carbohydrates in a way that keeps those variations in blood glucose levels close to normal. Your meal plan recommends you get as much as 50 percent of your daily calories from carbohydrate foods, but not all carbs are created equal. Carbohydrates include simple sugars like glucose, and also sugar molecules joined in chains that form starches and fiber. Depending on how quickly the carbohydrates you eat are broken down during digestion and on the mix of carbs with other macronutrients when you eat, blood glucose can rise very rapidly or very slowly. Managing your diabetes means managing carbohydrates.

REMEMBER

Effective diabetes meal planning and nutrition involves identifying healthy carbohydrates and working them into your diet in a way that best controls your blood glucose. The following sections help you identify carbohydrates and get the right carbohydrates on your plate.

Looking at sugar and diabetes

Virtually everyone knows that sugar has something to do with diabetes — sugar diabetes, the sugar, or a touch of the sugar are all colloquial phrases that mean diabetes in some communities. *Blood sugar* is a common phrase substituted for the more precise *blood glucose*. Sugar affects diabetes, but sugar's role in diabetes may not match what you think of when you hear the word *sugar*.

To you, sugar most likely means common table sugar. To biologists and chemists, the word *sugar* describes a particular kind of organic molecule belonging to a category of similar molecules called carbohydrates. Carbohydrates — the word actually means carbon with water — often follow the formula $C-H_2O$, and the numbers of carbons and hydrogens and oxygens can go into many thousands when joined together. Sugars are the simplest carbohydrates, and in the world of food, the simplest of the simple sugar molecules are called *monosaccharides*. Glucose and fructose are two monosaccharides that may be familiar to you.

Disaccharides, which are two monosaccharides joined together, include *sucrose,* common table sugar, the milk sugar *lactose,* and *maltose,* a sugar familiar to beer drinkers. Table sugar is one molecule of glucose, and one molecule of fructose. *Oligosaccharides,* containing up to ten monosaccharides in a chain, are common in legumes like beans.

Carbohydrate digestion works to break chains of sugar molecules into their monosaccharide building blocks. In your diet, simple sugars and disaccharides can be absorbed rapidly, and the glucose component can have an immediate effect on blood glucose levels. When sugars are not naturally packaged in their original state like an apple or a beet, such as the added sugar sucrose, their sole nutritional benefit is in the calories. But, in an affluent society, added sugars usually add up to excess calories, and with diabetes in the equation, the rapid rise in blood glucose levels makes control more difficult. Even among individuals without diabetes, this spiking of blood glucose and insulin levels seems to have long-term consequences. And diets high in excess, added sugar clearly contribute to obesity and increase the risk for diabetes and heart disease.

In *Diabetes For Dummies,* 6th Edition (Wiley), we explore how people are "hard wired" to seek out energy-dense foods because of the need to be protected from times of scarcity that no longer exist in most developed countries today. The sweetness of simple sugars, which can provide easily available fuel, is a taste that is instinctively attractive. There are even suggestions that our affinity for sugary foods might be considered to have addictive characteristics. However, it is possible to learn to enjoy foods with flavors other than those that just appeal to a "sweet tooth." As the relationship between high consumption of simple sugars and obesity and type 2 diabetes has become clearer, manufacturers of some products like sodas have introduced artificial sweeteners. Unfortunately, these come with their own problems, including the possibility of negative effects on our all-important gut microbiome. We discuss our food environment in more detail in Chapter 10.

TIP

The bottom line on sugar is that it's best eaten in its natural form, for example from fruit, instead of as a refined, added sweetener. Longer-chained saccharides, like the oligosaccharides in legumes, are another excellent dietary source of sugars.

Not all carbs are created equal: Complex carbohydrates

As the number of chained together molecules of simple sugars gets longer, the carbohydrate foods are sometimes called *complex*. Starches are where plants store their excess glucose, and the chemical bonds connecting the simple sugars in starch are easily broken by your digestive system.

Whereas starches can be refined and isolated from their source for dietary purposes like sugar, their use is usually limited to thickening agents like corn starch. You are much more likely to get your dietary starch from the whole food, because starch itself is relatively tasteless. Starches are prevalent in potatoes, corn, peas, beans, lentils, hard-shell squashes, quinoa, rice, wheat, barley, oats, and the flours and refined products from grains. Because starches are packaged with protein, fat, and fiber, and because the chain length of simple sugars is more complex, starches often have a less dramatic impact in blood glucose levels.

TIP

It's important to mention nonstarchy vegetables in this discussion about complex carbohydrates. Nonstarchy vegetables contain much less carbohydrate than the starchy ones, and in that regard are essential parts of diabetes management by contributing volume without fat, and by having a reduced impact on blood glucose. Greens of all varieties, peppers, cucumber, summer squashes, green beans, carrots, broccoli, cauliflower, artichoke, turnips, fennel, and asparagus are a few of the nonstarchy vegetables that can color your plate and deliver vitamins and healthy phytonutrients to your body.

Evaluating glycemic index and glycemic load

Earlier in this chapter, we mention how it is possible to describe the effect of a carbohydrate on blood glucose. Here we describe in a little more detail the measurements of glycemic index and glycemic load.

The glycemic index (GI) of carbohydrate-containing foods was originally developed in 1981 at the University of Toronto. Recognizing that different foods affect blood glucose differently, researchers fed carbohydrate foods to fasting volunteers and monitored their fasting blood glucose response over the following two hours.

The blood glucose response to eating pure glucose serves as a benchmark, affecting levels more quickly and more profoundly, and a little math produces a GI number that compares other foods to glucose. The GI number of glucose is set at 100. GI values between 70 and 100 are labeled as high, values between 56 and 70 are labeled as medium, and values of 55 and below are considered low.

Figure 6-1 illustrates the blood glucose response of a high GI food, and a low GI food. Note with the higher GI food blood glucose levels not only go higher, but also begin to rise more quickly.

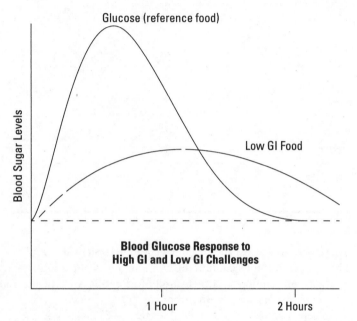

FIGURE 6-1:
Blood glucose levels in response to both high GI and low GI food.

Table 6-1 shows the GI value of common foods, but before you look at that comparison, consider why these numbers vary so much. The impact of a food on blood glucose depends upon the speed of digestive processes, how efficiently free glucose is absorbed into the bloodstream, and how quickly insulin begins to help move glucose out of the bloodstream and into cells. High fiber content, longer-chain carbohydrates, how starch molecules are entrapped within the food, whether a food contains both carbohydrate and fat, and unknown factors can slow stomach emptying, slow the liberation of glucose from carbohydrate chains, or interfere with glucose absorption in the small intestine to impact the blood glucose response. Your insulin status is a key issue when evaluating what the glycemic index means to you.

TABLE 6-1 Glycemic Index (GI) Value of Common Foods

Food	GI Value
Glucose	100
Instant white rice	87
Baked potato	85
Watermelon	72
White bread	72
Pineapple	66
White spaghetti	64
Ice cream	61
Banana	54
Skim milk	32
Lentils	29
Grapefruit	25
Edamame (green soybeans)	18
Lettuce and cabbage	10

There are two issues to consider about the practical use of the glycemic index. First, different foods contain different amounts of carbohydrate. The blood sugar response of volunteers is measured after eating a particular food in an amount that contains 50 grams of carbohydrate. For glucose this is 50 grams (about 4 tablespoons), because it's all glucose. For cabbage, getting 50 grams of carbohydrate means eating 10 cups of shredded cabbage, or about 800 grams (the GI of cabbage was probably estimated). There is simply not nearly as much glucose in cabbage as there is in glucose.

A second calculation takes this variation in the amount of carbohydrate in the same weight or volume of different foods into account. Glycemic load (GL) is designed to estimate how much a certain amount of a certain food raises blood glucose compared to eating 1 gram of glucose.

Glycemic index numbers, like those in Table 6-1, reflect both the blood glucose response and the insulin response of volunteers who don't have diabetes. If you have diabetes, these numbers don't necessarily reflect your insulin response.

To be clear, knowing the glycemic index of foods gives you a great tool. Eating foods with a low glycemic index value that gradually release glucose into the bloodstream may allow your abnormal response to insulin to still keep pace with rising blood glucose levels when you have type 2 diabetes. If you take insulin by injection or through an insulin pump, knowing the GI of foods can be useful in timing your injections or bolus. Just be extremely cautious about taking glycemic index and glycemic load as absolute numbers.

ASK THE
DOCTOR

Because different foods affect the absorption of carbohydrates differently, the glycemic index also varies according to the accompanying food. It's not an exact science, but lower glycemic foods are generally better for your blood glucose control than higher glycemic foods.

Counting Carbs

Another way to assess the impact of your food on blood glucose levels is to count the carbohydrate content of the food you eat.

Counting to 15 grams

Carbohydrate counting (*carb counting* for short) doesn't have you count each gram of carbohydrate one by one. Instead, carbohydrates are packaged into 15-gram *carb choices*; one carb choice for a particular food always includes approximately 15 grams of carbohydrate.

The counting part is easy. If your meal plan calls for four carb choices at your evening meals, you simply include a total of four carbohydrate foods, each in a serving size that equals approximately 15 grams of carbohydrate. Here's how you can break this down:

>> You can eat four different carb choices.

>> You can have two servings of the same food that are each 15 grams of carbohydrate (along with two more carb choices of different foods).

>> You can have four carb choice servings of the same food (although variety is best).

Your meal plan will make a recommendation for a specific number of carb choices at every meal, and will probably wedge a carb choice snack or two in somewhere. Just imagine that every morning you find that a fairy has left 12 or 13 tokens on your dresser, each one good for a 15-gram carbohydrate serving during the day — 4 grams for breakfast, 4 grams for lunch, 4 grams for dinner, and 4 grams for a snack.

Comparing carb choices

Now for the harder part — not hard, just harder. The measure of carbohydrate-containing foods — dairy or plant — that includes your 15 grams of carbohydrate is not the same from food to food. Table 6-2 shows the weight, volume, or size of one carb choice for some different foods.

TABLE 6-2 **Measuring a 15-Gram Carb Choice**

Food	One Carb Choice
Maple syrup	1 tablespoon
Oatmeal	¼ cup, dry
Beans	⅓ cup, cooked
Rice or pasta	⅓ cup, cooked
Unsweetened cereal	½ cup
Milk	1 cup*
Yogurt	1 cup
Baked potato	3 ounces
French fries	10 fries
Bread	1 slice
Bagel	½ small bagel
Popcorn	3 cups popped
Apple	1 medium sized
Banana	½ medium banana
Raspberries	1 cup
Honeydew melon	1 cup
Nonstarchy vegetables**	1½ cups cooked
Nonstarchy vegetables**	3 cups raw

1 cup milk is actually 12 grams carbohydrate, but is considered 1 carb choice.

**Nonstarchy vegetables include asparagus, artichoke, beets, green beans, broccoli, cabbage, carrots, cauliflower, cucumber, greens, jicama, mushrooms, okra, pea pods, peppers, radishes, rutabaga, spinach, tomato, turnips, yellow and zucchini squash, and many more.*

Knowing which portion size of a food you'll eat to get each 15-gram carb choice is really necessary if you're serious about blood glucose control. You may feel unnatural thinking so much about food. Yes, it would be nice if one carb choice for all carbohydrate foods was the same serving size, but there's a big difference between a tablespoon of sugar and 3 cups of shredded cabbage. If the serving size on nutrition labels always equaled 15 grams of carbohydrate it would help, but every can of beans gives nutrition information for ½ cup, and that's 22 grams of carbohydrate. And what about those recipes or restaurant meals where one serving of the dish has 60 grams of carbohydrate?

REMEMBER

There's no need to panic. First, this isn't rocket science, as the saying goes. Anyone who's managed type 1 diabetes for a while, where you can carefully match grams of carbs and a precise dose of insulin, already knows that the variations in both food and your metabolism put perfection way out of reach. What's most important is knowing what you need to know. Remember, the all-important A1C is about averages.

There's one final calculation that's like a discount coupon for you with some carbohydrate foods. *Dietary fiber* and *sugar alcohols* are carbohydrates that are not efficiently digested — you can find the grams of these listed on nutrition labels under total carbohydrate. Anytime the dietary fiber or sugar alcohol amount is 5 grams or more, you can deduct one half of the amount from total carbohydrate. Often the deduction isn't much — kidney beans have 22 grams total carbohydrate and 7 grams fiber in the nutrition label's ½-cup serving size, so you can deduct 3½ grams from the 22 grams for an adjusted total carbohydrates of 18½ grams per ½ cup. Likewise, a ½-cup serving of a particular *no sugar added* ice cream has 17 grams total carbohydrate and 8 grams sugar alcohol. Because the sugar alcohol is 5 grams or more, deduct one half, 4 grams, from total carbohydrate to get net carbohydrate in the ½-cup serving of 13 grams.

TIP

Memorizing the one carb choice portion for foods you eat all the time is easy enough, but nobody can know everything. A good starting place is to practice visualizing the correct measurements of foods for one carb choice while you are at home. To help you with carb food choices you may not eat as often make yourself a cheat sheet, buy a pocket-sized carb counting reference, or download a carb counting app to your smart phone. If you're determined to be successful, easy solutions are available for you.

Insulin bolus dosing

Everyone with type 1 diabetes takes insulin with meals to compensate for the carbohydrate total of the meal. You may take an injection, or you may initiate a bolus from your insulin pump. Some people with type 2 may take insulin injections related to food also, although it's much more common for people with type 2 to take long-acting insulin, which is unrelated to meals. If you take short- or fast-acting insulin before meals, there are a few things that need consideration.

>> You need to know your current blood glucose level.

>> You need to estimate how many grams of carbohydrate you intend to eat.

>> You need to know your insulin-to-carb ratio — one unit of insulin accounts for how many grams of carbohydrate?

>> You need to know how to correct for your current blood glucose — less insulin if your blood glucose level is on the low side, and more insulin if blood glucose is elevated.

That is a bunch of need-to-knows. If you're using an insulin pump, your insulin-to-carb ratio and correction factor should be programmed into the control.

A book on meal planning for diabetes is not a good place to give you your insulin-to-carb ratio or your correction factor. These numbers are unique to you. Your doctor will start you with dosages based upon your size and age, and together you can fine-tune based on trial and error. Eventually, your dosages for eating or correcting blood glucose may be different depending on the time of day. The key where meal planning is concerned is you won't know where you're going if you don't know where you're starting — test your blood glucose before meals.

Putting Carbs on Your Plate

Whether you consider in great detail the glycemic index of a food or make it a life goal to precisely "carb count," there are some obvious ways to achieve a healthy carbohydrate intake: eating modest portion sizes, making good meal ingredient combination choices, and abiding by the following carbohydrate guidelines, which are seen in healthy heritage diets like the Mediterranean diet:

>> **Choose whole grains.** Whole grains contain everything that makes up the grain, which is the *bran,* the *germ,* and the *endosperm.* Refined grains generally only contain the endosperm. Choosing whole grains simply means choosing whole-grain breads, crackers, and pastas, or whole grains such as oatmeal, barley, quinoa, and brown rice instead of the alternatives — a different package in your regular grocery.

>> **Choose whole fruit.** Whole fruit contains healthy dietary fiber and no added sugar. You don't have to choose fresh fruit, by the way. Canned or frozen fruit is excellent as long as there are no added sugars (packed in syrup). The no

added sugar warning goes for fruit drinks, too, but you may be surprised to know that eating the fruit itself is a better choice than 100 percent fruit juice.

>> **Eat lots of vegetables.** Vegetables are especially important to diabetes because of their low carbohydrate content and rich nutrient content. Again, frozen or canned vegetables are excellent if you avoid added sugar, fat, or sodium. Always choose the *no salt added* option for canned vegetables. Pick a wide variety of textures and colors, and avoid adding sugar, fat, or sodium at home with salt, butter, and margarine, or add-ons like salad dressings.

>> **Limit sweets.** Added sugar not only pours concentrated carbohydrates into your diet, but also delivers no nutrients to make it a fair trade. Many processed foods contain ingredients such as high fructose corn syrup. If you want a little sweetening, add raw (unprocessed) honey, which has the added benefit of containing natural compounds that may protect from infections and have anti-inflammatory properties. Some of Chef Amy's recipes include natural honey for precisely these reasons.

Filling Fiber and How to Use It

Fiber is the most complex of carbohydrates, often forming the structural elements of plants. Fiber is relatively indigestible by humans, but is still an extremely important part of your diet. Insoluble fiber provides bulk, which helps to move food residues through your digestive system. But some fiber — soluble fiber — also has beneficial physiological effects. The most accepted benefit of soluble fiber is in lowering bad LDL cholesterol levels — oat bran is well recognized for this benefit, and beans are a tasty source of soluble fiber, too.

Specific benefits to health from the fiber component of your diet are challenging to isolate because foods that offer fiber are also rich in biologically active phytochemicals and antioxidants. But having adequate fiber in your diet may lower blood pressure, reduce the risk for some colorectal and breast cancers, improve your immune system, and improve blood glucose control.

Americans typically consume only about 15 grams of fiber per day, but the recommended daily consumption is 25 grams for women between 19 and 50 years of age, and 38 grams per day for men in that age range. The recommended amount decreases for both men and women over 50, but the more the merrier. While a huge volume of fiber may lead to digestive irritation, if you can tolerate more fiber, get more fiber.

TIP

Fiber only comes with plant-based foods, but you can increase your fiber consumption by making different choices. For instance, white bread from refined flour only contains one third the fiber of whole wheat bread — brown rice contains almost six times more fiber as white rice. Oatmeal, beans, and peas are excellent sources of fiber, too. Remember that grains, beans, and peas are also starchy, and need to be accounted for in your diet to control blood glucose.

Embracing Healthful Fats

Dietary fat is kind of complicated. To start with, the proper terminology is *lipids* — lipids include both oils and solid fats. But lipid is a technical term not used too often in dietary jargon, so just remember that the term *fat* includes oils, too (remember lipid, however, for a discussion about fat imbalance later).

You may be under the impression that fat should be eliminated completely from your diet, but if you can do that, and it wouldn't be easy, you would soon find that you're having skin problems, weakened bones, vision issues, and maybe even trouble thinking. Fats are an essential part of your diet, and with diabetes it's likely your meal plan recommends that you get 25 to 35 percent of your calories from fat. Too much of the wrong kind of fat, however, has clearly negative health implications.

Most of the fat you get from foods comes in the form of *triglycerides,* which is glycerol chemically bound to three individual fatty acids. Fats are hydrophobic, meaning they don't mix with water, and you probably know that already, having looked at salad dressings where the oil has separated. This property makes fat digestion a little tricky, but the enzyme bile works to break fat globs into smaller bits so *lipase* can detach the fatty acids. Fat digestion and absorption takes place primarily in the small intestine, and the free fatty acids are absorbed into the bloodstream of the lymph system, depending upon the molecule size.

TECHNICAL STUFF

You may already know *glycerol,* the molecule that binds the fatty acids as triglycerides in your diet, from your soap, shaving cream, or other personal care products. It often goes by the alias *glycerin* in its more glamorous roles.

Fats, or fatty acids, are chained, organic molecules with the typical carbon and hydrogen elements, and depending upon how many hydrogen atoms are included, a fat is either saturated (with hydrogen) or unsaturated. Saturated fats are solid at room temperature, whereas unsaturated fats are liquid, and unsaturated fats are generally healthier in your diet.

Going beyond insulation

Most people have a good idea where some of the fats from food go when they've been absorbed into the body. *Adipocytes* (fat cells) store fat in layers beneath your skin for cushioning and insulating your entire body, and you've likely noticed that some people have more fat in storage than others. Men and women also tend to accumulate stored fat in different areas, giving adults distinctly different shapes.

But fat is doing a lot more than just lounging around looking cuddly. Adipose cells actually release some hormones, including leptin, a hormone that signals the brain when you've had enough to eat. Key vitamins, including vitamins A, D, E, and K, are fat soluble and transported to cells by fat molecules. Your brain is about 60 percent fat, and fat in the material that insulates nerves, called myelin, helps protect the electrical signals from interference. Fats constitute a part of every cell's membrane, and fat can segregate toxins.

Fat also stores energy, and the role of fat for producing energy is relevant to diabetes. You have already heard in previous chapters how glucose, a carbohydrate, is your body's favored fuel for energy production. But you store a relatively limited amount of glucose in muscle, fat, and liver cells. When glucose isn't available, your cells can convert fat into energy. Fat molecules store 9 calories per gram of fat, more than twice as much energy, twice as many calories per gram, as either carbohydrate or protein.

WARNING

The byproduct of burning fat, however, is compounds called *ketones,* and if the concentration of ketone wastes becomes too great, blood can turn dangerously acidic. Ketoacidosis from excess ketones can be fatal, and is a risk for people with type 1 diabetes where glucose isn't available to cells because insulin concentrations are insufficient. Ketoacidosis is common at diagnosis, when natural insulin production suddenly stops, and therapeutic insulin has not been initiated, but can occur anytime blood glucose levels get very high due to an imbalance of blood glucose and insulin.

Highlighting unsaturated fat

Most all fat-containing foods are a mixture of saturated and unsaturated fats, but if less than one third of the fats are saturated, the fat or oil can be considered unsaturated. Monounsaturated fats and polyunsaturated fats are healthier fats in your diet than saturated fats, and it's recommended that two thirds of your daily fat consumption be from unsaturated fats. Unsaturated fats include the well-known omega-3 fatty acid, which means a double carbon bond is on the third carbon in the fatty acid chain.

The health benefits related to unsaturated fat are both in the reduction of the risk for cardiovascular disease, and for diabetes management. Unsaturated fats improve the ratios between bad LDL cholesterol and good HDL cholesterol (see the discussion of cholesterol in the next section), and polyunsaturated fat is associated with improved insulin sensitivity. The health benefits of unsaturated fats first gained attention from the Seven Countries Study, which is described in Chapter 14.

TIP

Different types of dietary fats appear to carry a different risk of adding to visceral fat — that is the tummy fat especially present in obesity and type 2 diabetes, known to be associated with an increased risk of heart disease and breast cancer. It turns out that eating monounsaturated fats found in olive oil, avocados, and nuts, for example, reduces the amount of visceral fat.

Table 6-3 provides a list of dietary sources for unsaturated fat, and notes whether the food is predominately a source of monounsaturated or polyunsaturated fatty acids.

TABLE 6-3   ## Dietary Sources of Monounsaturated and Polyunsaturated Fats

Monounsaturated Fatty Acids	Polyunsaturated Fatty Acids
Almonds, peanuts	Corn oil
Avocado	Flax*
Canola oil	Salmon*
Olive oil	Soybean oil
Sesame seeds	Walnuts*

*Walnuts, cold water fish like salmon, and flax are sources of omega-3 fatty acids.

TECHNICAL STUFF

Some research hypothesizes that an imbalance between unsaturated omega-6 fatty acids and omega-3 fatty acids can actually increase general inflammation and chronic disease risk. Although both are polyunsaturated fatty acids, the so-called Western diet tends toward more than a ten-fold higher intake of omega-6 fats over the omega-3 fats. The difference is attributed to some extent to the high consumption of omega-6 fats from corn oil and soybean oil in processed and convenience foods.

Debating saturated fat and cholesterol

Saturated fats are carbon chains with no double bonds between the carbon atoms; therefore, the molecule is saturated with hydrogen bonds. *Trans fats* result when unsaturated fats are *hydrogenated*, making the fat saturated. Saturated fats are generally solid at room temperature, and hydrogenation of food products like stick margarine was specifically for this purpose.

WARNING

Trans fats or *hydrogenated fats* were commonly used in processed foods for decades until their relationship with heart disease was finally established beyond doubt. Many countries now ban their use, though they are still present in many foods around the world. According to the World Health Organization (WHO) in 2023, these fats, which have no benefit other than for the processed food industry, are still responsible for up to half a million premature deaths from heart disease around the world. The WHO called for their global elimination in 2018, yet 5 billion people remain at unnecessary risk because countries have failed to comply with this recommendation.

Current guidance is to limit saturated fats to less than 7 percent of daily calories, and to strictly limit trans fat to less than 1 percent of daily calories or eradicate entirely. The reservations about saturated fat relate historically to the relationship of elevated blood cholesterol level to cardiovascular disease, especially to the buildup of waxy plaque in arteries (atherosclerosis). More recently, the focus on your total cholesterol level has evolved.

Cholesterol is a type of fat called a *sterol*, and it has several crucial and necessary roles in your biology including roles in the production of vitamin D, testosterone, and estrogen. Cholesterol is manufactured in your cells, but can also be taken in our diet with some animal and plant fats, along with saturated fat, from foods of animal origin. Where the total cholesterol level was formerly viewed as the measure most significant to heart disease risks, the focus now is redirected at the difference between the particles that ferry cholesterol around in the blood — lipoproteins. In that regard, references to bad LDL cholesterol and good HDL cholesterol actually refers to the *low-density lipoprotein* or *high-density lipoprotein* particles transporting cholesterol, not to cholesterol itself. And, from the perspective of heart disease risk, it is the levels of LDL, and the ratio of LDL to HDL that seem most significant. Saturated fats, and especially the manufactured trans fats, raise LDL levels and lower HDL levels, and LDLs tend to form arterial plaques whereas HDLs actually remove plaque forming materials.

There is also an important link between the *oxidation* and inflammation of LDL cholesterol, which is part of the process of heart disease, and the extent to which this occurs is influenced by other aspects of our lifestyle and diet including what we eat that can reduce these effects. We consider this in more detail in Chapter 8.

TIP

Dietary cholesterol, such as the forms found in eggs, shrimp, and dairy, are not thought to affect your blood cholesterol levels as much as many types of saturated fat, so just because you might read that these foods are high in cholesterol, there is no need to cut them out from your diet completely.

The research on these issues is always ongoing, and inconsistencies always show up in complicated studies of human diet and health, often related to the difficulty in excluding other potential health factors unrelated to diet. There is solid agreement on the dangers of trans fat, which clearly raises LDL and lowers HDL. There is general agreement that reducing saturated fat is beneficial, but especially beneficial if the calories are replaced by adding monounsaturated fat, like olive oil, instead of adding additional carbohydrates.

With diabetes, polyunsaturated fats have a favorable impact on insulin sensitivity, and trans fats are especially unfavorable. Interestingly, regular consumption of red meat is associated with an increased risk for type 2 diabetes, and the risk is even greater for processed red meat.

Finally, hyperlipidemia (there's the lipid word) is the medical term describing abnormally high levels of lipids (fats) in blood — hyperlipidemia is an element of metabolic syndrome. Managing your level of blood lipids is important for managing the risk for diabetes complications. Current target values are LDL lower than 100 milligrams/deciliter (mg/dl), HDL higher than 40 mg/dl for men and 50 mg/dl for women, and triglycerides lower than 150 mg/dl. Triglycerides are a blood fat not as specifically related to fat in the diet.

TIP

Knowing that food is more than its macronutrient content, it is important to choose fats that deliver the most for health. Full-fat fermented dairy foods may contain saturated fat but have been shown to reduce the risk of developing diabetes. Nuts are a source of healthy unsaturated fats and also combine micronutrients, fiber, and compounds called stanols that reduce the absorption of dietary cholesterol. When it comes to the main source of fats in the Mediterranean diet, extra-virgin olive oil delivers not only healthy predominantly monounsaturated fats, but also contains abundant amounts of the antioxidant vitamin E and polyphenol bioactive compounds from the olive fruit.

Identifying the Best Quality Proteins

In our modern societies, we are pretty aware of the importance of protein in our diet. If you're someone with diabetes, it's important to avoid the wrong types of protein and to make sure that you are getting the proper amounts of proteins. Proteins are extraordinarily complex, and the blueprint for assembling all of the proteins you require is coded into your DNA.

Proteins are the jacks of all trades in human biology. Proteins are especially efficient in binding tightly to other molecules, often assisted by pocket-shaped depressions in the protein molecule created by its special folding pattern. The following describes some of the more important functions and roles of protein in your body:

>> Protein is necessary for growth, critical for children, teens, and pregnant women, but important to everyone in this regard for tissue repair.

>> Protein provides structure, both on a cellular level to help maintain cellular shape and on a whole body scale where protein makes up hair, nails, tendons, and ligaments.

>> Special *motor* proteins are responsible for the contraction of muscle cells. Muscles are the largest accumulation of proteins in your body, and remember that it's specialized muscles that pump your blood and move air into and out of your lungs — important stuff, to say the least.

>> Proteins called *enzymes* speed up chemical reactions, and include the digestive enzyme pepsin, which works specifically to break down protein. The function of enzymes to facilitate and accelerate chemical reactions is crucial to life, and as many as 4,000 enzyme involved biochemical reactions have been identified.

>> Proteins serve as transporters and messengers. Antibody proteins, part of your immune system, capture and hold foreign bodies, including bacteria and viruses, and hemoglobin transports oxygen to cells around the body. Important protein hormones, like insulin, send signals to cells — insulin signals cells to allow glucose molecules to pass through the cell membrane, and it's a pretty important function with diabetes.

That's an impressive list of responsibilities, and gives a glimpse into why protein in your diet is so important. It's necessary to have all the right raw materials available to keep all of your working proteins in production.

Recycling amino acids from food

Amino acid molecules are what characterize proteins. *Amino acids* primarily consist of carbon, hydrogen, and oxygen like most organic compounds, but always include nitrogen in what's called an amino group. Many of the proteins in your body turn over rapidly, degrading into their amino acid constituents. An average adult may turn over 250 grams of protein every day, mostly from muscle. Some of the amino acids are reincorporated into new protein, and some is burned as energy (protein stores 4 calories of energy per gram). The nitrogen becomes a waste product from protein burned for energy, and is excreted in urine as urea. This constant turnover is why protein is such an important part of your diet — new amino acids are always necessary to build new protein. Your dietary protein recommendations are calculated to resupply amino acids for rebuilding protein that has been burned for energy, or otherwise lost.

Hundreds of specific amino acids have been identified, but only 20 are specifically coded into human DNA for inclusion in protein assembly. Other amino acids do play important roles in metabolism, however. Your body can actually produce some of the 20 protein coded amino acids from other amino acids, or from protein degradation products. But you cannot produce 9 of the 20, and these are, therefore, called *essential amino acids*. These amino acids must be acquired from food. The essential amino acids are histidine, isoleucine, leucine, lysine, methionine, phenylalanine, threonine, tryptophan, and valine.

REMEMBER

Managing diabetes with diet includes getting an adequate intake of high-quality protein in your diet to maintain important muscle mass, and to keep important metabolic functions humming along. The highest quality protein has amino acids that are readily available and easily absorbed during digestion. Some foods, called *complete protein* foods, contain all of the essential amino acids in sufficient amounts. Foods that don't contain all nine essential amino acids are called *incomplete,* and the missing essential amino acids are called the *limiting* amino acid. Lysine, threonine, and tryptophan are the most common limiting amino acids.

Identifying the best animal sources of protein

Nutrition researchers can give protein sources a score, based upon the abundance of essential amino acids, relative abundance of nonessential amino acids, the digestibility of the protein food, and the presence of allergens or compounds that inhibit amino acid accessibility. In the scoring contest, animal sources of protein often score highly.

Protein deficiency in a healthy person with a varied (and that includes a vegetarian or vegan) diet is very rare, as an adequate supply of amino acids can come from different sources. Many people choose meat as a substantive supply of protein in their diet. Others may have a vegetarian or vegan diet that excludes animal products for personal ethical, religious, or other reasons.

ASK THE DOCTOR

There have been concerns that vegetarian or vegan diets might be deficient on the essential amino acids that we must get from our food. However, in an article published in 2019 in the journal *Nutrients,* authors Mariotti and Gardner cited robust evidence confirming that eating protein-rich foods, such as traditional legumes, nuts, and seeds, is sufficient to achieve full protein adequacy in adults consuming vegetarian or vegan diets.

WARNING

Despite the "completeness" of animal proteins, there are reasons to be cautious about the overall amount we consume. In 2015, the WHO declared processed meat to be *carcinogenic,* which means having the potential to cause cancer, in the same category as smoking, with red meat also likely to be linked with some cancers. This does not mean that eating a sausage today results in developing bowel cancer tomorrow, but the associated risk certainly does need to be taken seriously.

The reasons for the link is not fully understood. Some researchers suggest that the combination of preservatives such as sodium nitrite (additive E250 on food labels), used to protect processed meat from carrying harmful bacteria, when combined with the amines in proteins forms carcinogenic compounds called nitrosamines. Some traditional hams do not use sodium nitrite and there are now some companies that are finding alternative ways to ensure a safe shelf life of their products and are marketing nitrite–free bacon and sausages.

LEANING TOWARD LEAN: A DIABETES PRIORITY

Here's the thing about animal sources of protein — they almost always come with a dose of unhealthy saturated fat. And, because diabetes significantly increases your risk for heart disease, eating in a heart-healthy way by limiting saturated fats is an important assignment for maintaining your overall health.

You can reduce the fat content of the meat you eat by making simple choices. For example, remove the skin from poultry, select leaner cuts of beef and pork (and trim excess fat), buy 90 percent lean ground beef or ground turkey, and eat especially fatty meats like bacon and pastrami only occasionally. Balancing the rich source of protein in meat with saturated fat is one reason to look for some of your protein from plant sources, and your grocery may offer a variety of ever-improving meat substitutes from soy, flavored and textured for uses reserved for meat.

However, with increasing vegetarian and vegan substitutes on the market, there is a tendency for manufacturers to add artificial preservatives and flavor enhancers, the effects of which on health may be detrimental. Some of these products can be classified as processed or ultra-processed foods. We advise caution if you see a long list of additives. It is better to opt for whole foods such as beans, legumes, soy, and those mentioned earlier in this section than to eat artificial items just because they have protein added to them.

There are also some concerns about chemicals called heterocyclic amines (HCAs) that are formed from animal proteins during cooking, especially at high temperatures and when cooked "well done" or char-grilled. Some studies have shown that the cooking medium and ingredient interactions may be important as well. For example, a marinade of extra-virgin olive oil, wine, herbs, and spices has been shown to significantly reduce the formation of HCAs in meats during cooking.

Using plants for protein

As a rule, plant proteins are not complete proteins, containing all of the essential amino acids in suitable amounts. Plant protein also tends to be less accessible in digestion, ultimately scoring lower on scales rating biological value or amino acid content. It's perfectly possible and indeed usual to get all the necessary amino acids in a vegetarian (or vegan) diet, but it generally requires consuming complementary foods over the course of the day, where one food provides an adequate source of the amino acid that is deficient in the other. A vegetarian or vegan diet should therefore be varied and incorporate a variety of different plant foods. There is one notable exception to that generalization, however — soy.

The soybean, often served green as edamame or prepared as tofu, is a high-quality and complete protein. Four ounces of edamame or tofu give you 14 grams of high-quality protein, twice the protein of a large egg or an 8-ounce glass of milk. Incorporating soy into a vegetarian or vegan diet can assure that all essential amino acids are consumed in sufficient amount. If you live in the United States, we recommend seeking out organic soy.

Many other plant sources of protein are available as well. Beans and other legumes, nuts, and grains all can contribute to daily protein requirements. The grain quinoa offers 6 grams of protein in a ¼-cup (dry) serving, along with the essential amino acids to make it a complete protein, for instance, and a healthy diet should always include plant sources of protein. Vegetarians who do not consume eggs or milk and vegans do need to get protein from a variety of complementary sources to assure they get a complete range of essential amino acids, or learn to love soy.

Chapter **7**

Making Micronutrients Work for You

You've likely heard the phrase *big things come in small packages.* That would be a perfect description for micronutrients. *Micro* comes from the Greek word *mikrós,* which means small, as in microscopic. In nutrition, the word micronutrients refers to vitamins and other compounds that are essential to your health, but only in very, very small amounts. Where your dietary needs for the macronutrients carbohydrates, fat, and protein are calculated in grams per day, the daily requirements for micronutrients is in milligrams (mg) or even micrograms (mcg or μg) per day. There are 1,000 milligrams or 1,000,000 micrograms in one gram.

This vast difference may have you thinking that micronutrients are insignificant, but don't be fooled. A failure to get adequate vitamin B12, even in this unimaginably small amount, can lead to severe disorders of the nervous system, including dementia. Big things really do come in small packages.

In this chapter, you see how important these powerful compounds are to your health and to diabetes management. More important, you see how you can be certain you're getting enough, or not getting too much, of the micronutrients that keep the machinery of your marvelous body humming along.

Introducing Versatile Vitamins

Vitamin is a word you probably already know. In biology, a vitamin is an organic compound required in small amounts as a vital nutrient that can't be produced by you in sufficient quantities. Vitamins, therefore, are compounds you must get from food, or from another external source.

Currently, compounds recognized as vitamins are grouped as vitamins A, B, C, D, E, and K — there are 13 different vitamins within these major groups. Here are some interesting facts about vitamins:

>> The vitamin letter can represent several different compounds, some that are simply the raw material you need to make the actual vitamin compound. Vitamin A, for example, can be retinol, retinal, or any of four different *carotenoids,* including beta carotene.

>> The six vitamin groups haven't always been the same. There were once vitamins F, G, H, J, L, M, N, O, P, S, and U. Some compounds were reclassified into the B complex (there are currently eight different B vitamins recognized), and scientific advances showed that others can be manufactured by your body.

>> The discovery of different vitamins has often come from studying the symptoms of a particular vitamin deficiency. In the mid-1750s, a Scottish doctor proposed that the disease *scurvy,* a terrible and deadly illness that plagued long ocean voyages, can be prevented by eating lemons and limes. Although vitamin C wasn't actually identified until 1920, the association of this certain illness with deficiencies of certain foods saved the lives of many British sailors, who had been nicknamed *limey.*

Humans need vitamins from conception for healthy growth and development, and throughout life for the maintenance of cells, and, most important, for sustaining a healthy *metabolism* — properly using the energy provided by the macronutrients carbohydrates, fats, and protein. Because diabetes is a metabolic disorder, you might imagine that getting adequate vitamins would be an important part of diabetes management — and you would be absolutely correct.

Give me a "B" (vitamin or two)

Eight different vitamins are grouped into what's called the vitamin B complex — B1, B2, B3, B5, B6, B7, B9, and B12. Some you may know better by their actual names — thiamine (B1), riboflavin (B2), and niacin (B3). Others, like pyridoxine (B6) and cobalamin (B12), you're more likely to know by the number. The B vitamins are important in diabetes management for two reasons.

First, all B vitamins participate in the chemical reactions taking place in your cells to harvest the energy from carbohydrates, fats, and protein, the energy that fuels everything from muscle movement to body heat to transporting glucose from your small intestine into your bloodstream during digestion.

The second reason B vitamins are important to diabetes management relates to where you find them and how to make the healthiest choices. Most likely you recognize thiamine, riboflavin, and niacin because a long-standing Food and Drug Administration bread enrichment program requires the addition of these B vitamins to refined (white) flours and bread products. Why? Because refining whole grains by removing the bran and germ also removes the natural B vitamins you could have gotten by choosing whole grains in the first place. Choosing carbohydrate foods like grains is an important part of managing diabetes in your daily eating, and getting naturally occurring B vitamins along with your carbohydrate choices is one reason choosing whole grains is so important.

Table 7-1 lists the eight B vitamins, their function, and the best dietary sources for getting these essential nutrients.

REMEMBER

It should be noted that the daily recommendations for these vitamins vary between men and women, and generally are significantly greater during pregnancy. Folate is especially important during pregnancy for preventing neurological birth defects.

It's also important to point out that vitamin B12 is almost exclusively derived from meat and dairy products rather than plants, with some exceptions such as a fermented soy-based food called tempeh and nori — a seaweed sometimes used in sushi. Some species of mushrooms, which are fungi and so neither plant nor animal, also have reasonable levels of B12. That makes this crucial compound a challenge for vegans to acquire, even in the tiny amount necessary. Strict vegans have to consume foods fortified with vitamin B12 such as cereals, or take supplements to meet their daily recommended allowance.

TECHNICAL
STUFF

Recent research has focused on thiamine, vitamin B1, as being especially important to diabetes health — thiamine is a key component of normal carbohydrate metabolism. A 2007 study published in the *International Journal of Clinical Practice* found that a sample of people with both type 1 and type 2 diabetes showed blood levels of thiamine 75 percent lower than normal because they were excreting thiamine in urine at a higher than normal rate. A 2011 study published in the journal *Diabetologia* suggested that the metabolism of carbohydrates when thiamine levels are low produces byproducts that may contribute to serious complications of diabetes, including arterial plaque buildup and neuropathy.

TABLE 7-1　　　**A Review of the B Vitamins**

Vitamin and Daily Amount	Compound	Function	Food Source
B1 (1 -1.5 mg/day)	Thiamine	Central role in extracting energy from carbohydrates, production, and cell metabolism DNA	Whole-grain and enriched grain products, pork, liver
B2 (1.1-1.3 mg/day)	Riboflavin	Helps produce energy in cells, supports cell growth, helps regulate metabolism	Beef liver, milk, yogurt, spinach
B3 (14-16 mg/day)	Niacin	Energy production and cell growth, facilitates glucose and fat metabolism, helps enzyme function	Turkey breast, peanut butter, beans, yogurt
B5 (5 mg/day)	Pantothenic	Helps produce energy in cells, involved in synthesizing amino acids, fatty acids, neurotransmitters, and antibodies	Yogurt, salmon, sweet potato, corn, egg, whole grains
B6 (1.3-1.7 mg/day)	Pyridoxine	Helps synthesize amino acids, helps immune system, helps produce hemoglobin, antibodies and insulin	Potato, banana, garbanzo beans, fish
B7 (30 µg/day)	Biotin	Helps produce energy in cells, regulates hormone synthesis, key role in metabolizing carbohydrate, fats, and protein	Egg, cottage cheese, peanuts, whole grain
B9 (400 µg/day)	Folate	Makes new cells, helps form hemoglobin, reduces risk for heart disease, crucial to fetal development	Spinach, beans, avocado
B12 (2.4 µg/day)	Cobalamin	Makes red blood cells, helps form protective sheath for nerves, crucial role in cell division	Salmon, beef, yogurt, shrimp, no plant sources

The jury is still out as to whether thiamine supplementation is directly beneficial to diabetes health, and, if so, at what level. A review of studies published in the *British Medical Journal* in 2022 demonstrated no improvement of glycemic outcomes with supplementation but suggested that further research was needed. However, it seems clear that working plenty of thiamine-rich foods into your diet is a wise strategy. Whole or enriched grain products, lean meats (especially pork), fish, nuts, seeds, and beans are great dietary sources of thiamine.

A sunny day with vitamin D

Vitamin D is unique in that you can, and in how you can, make your own. Remarkably, exposure to sunlight turns a form of cholesterol stored in your skin into a precursor of the active form of vitamin D. However, the advertised dangers of overexposure (or any exposure) to direct sunlight keeps many people from getting sufficient exposure for adequate vitamin D production year round. Plus, other factors, like where you live, the color of your skin, and how much body fat you store (body fat captures and holds vitamin D) make consistently adequate production of vitamin D by exposure to sunlight nearly impossible for many people.

Although most people can get enough natural light by walking outside every day even on a cloudy day, many of us commute to work in vehicles and sit indoors for much of the day. The same factors that tend to reduce our outdoor exercise also limit our enjoyment of outdoor light.

REMEMBER

Getting adequate vitamin D is crucial to bone health because vitamin D is essential for adequate absorption of calcium and may have many more benefits to your health. For the purpose of this book, the following two aspects of vitamin D are most important:

>> Beyond its crucial role working in tandem with calcium and phosphorous for bone health, evidence that vitamin D has much broader positive impacts on your health is growing. Vitamin D appears to help regulate your immune system and reduce inflammation responses; may work to prevent several cancers; seems to reduce the buildup of dangerous plaques in arteries and help reduce blood pressure; may work to prevent the metabolic syndrome, which is often associated with type 2 diabetes; and may even reduce the risk for both type 1 and type 2 diabetes.

The relationship between low levels of vitamin D and metabolic syndrome (or type 2 diabetes) are confounded by the fact that fat cells tend to capture vitamin D, keeping blood levels depressed. Lower vitamin D levels may simply be a result of obesity, which may be the real culprit behind these related conditions, and there's not much evidence that vitamin D helps control blood sugar levels after diabetes is diagnosed. Inadequate levels of vitamin D, however, does suppress insulin production, and the potential positive effect of adequate levels of vitamin D on heart health and general inflammation would suggest that maintaining adequate levels of vitamin D may help reduce the risk for diabetes complications. Excess weight, however, works against your efforts to increase levels of vitamin D.

>> It's very difficult to get adequate vitamin D from food. Because vitamin D is a *fat-soluble* vitamin, fatty fish like salmon and mackerel tend to be the best natural sources, and animal sources contain the most active form of vitamin D, called D3. Non-animal sources of vitamin D are a different, less active, form known as D2, but mushrooms exposed to ultraviolet light can provide significant amounts of D2. Plant-based foods supply virtually no significant vitamin D (mushrooms are a fungus). Many foods, like milk and orange juice, are fortified with vitamin D, but you may have to drink six cups of milk each

day to reach the daily recommended intake for people 1 to 70 years of age of 600 international units, or IUs (an IU for vitamin D equals .025 µg, so the daily recommendation is for 15 µg). The daily recommendation rises to 800 IUs at age 70, but people with diabetes may need even more. If in doubt, it is advisable to ask your doctor for a blood test.

The daily recommended intake for vitamin D is targeted to achieve a minimum blood level of 20 nanograms per milliliter (ng/ml) of 25-hydroxyvitamin D (the active compound that should be measured in the lab). Ultimately, the cautions and challenges with getting adequate sun exposure, coupled with the relative difficulty of consuming an adequate dose of vitamin D from food, makes vitamin D supplementation necessary for many people to maintain an appropriate blood level. Although overdosing on vitamin D is possible, unless you spend a lot of time outside in the sun without sunscreen and take high doses of supplements too, it is highly unlikely. Most instances of vitamin D toxicity are related to accidental consumption of huge doses. For adults, the upper limit for recommended daily intake of vitamin D is 4,000 IUs.

TIP

The fat-soluble vitamin D in foods like mushrooms and oily fish is more easily absorbed when cooked with extra-virgin olive oil.

Finding Marvelous Minerals

You've probably heard the words *vitamins* and *minerals* spoken together since childhood, but *mineral* is actually a term from geology. The truth is that the nutrients discussed in this section — calcium, chromium, magnesium, potassium, sodium, and zinc — are basic chemical elements like oxygen, gold, or uranium. Each of these is listed on the periodic table of elements, and technically they're all metals. In fact, pure elemental sodium is not only a metal, it's explosively reactive when mixed with water. Calcium is a soft, gray metal that's slightly harder than lead, and magnesium is a metal that burns so brightly it's used in fireworks and flares.

So, why don't you spontaneously erupt into bright white flames as soon as you step into the shower? Because when basic elements combine with other basic elements, they can become stable and even lose the typical metal appearance. Sodium, an explosively reactive metal, combines readily with chlorine, a poisonous gas, to form table salt — sodium chloride. Chemistry is amazing, and biochemistry even more amazing. These important metals play crucial roles in your metabolism, and you find them in the foods you eat.

Calcium: More than strong bones

Most everyone knows that calcium is a necessary nutrient for bone health, and getting adequate calcium in your diet is important for maintaining bone health as you age — even more so for women than for men. Calcium and phosphorous work together to form bone, and vitamin D plays a crucial role in managing calcium in your body. The process of bone building never ends, because calcium and phosphorous are removed from bone and re-deposited regularly.

Your body works to maintain consistent levels of calcium in your blood. Approximately 99 percent of the calcium in your body is stored in bones and teeth, but if dietary calcium is too low, processes remove calcium from bones so it's always available for other important functions. What could be so important to sacrifice bone strength? How about the following:

>> Calcium plays a key role in normal brain and nerve function, specifically in the release of chemicals that allow nerve signals to travel.

>> Calcium keeps you moving and keeps your heart beating by helping muscle cells contract.

>> Calcium is essential for proper blood clotting.

>> Calcium helps to control blood pressure.

>> Calcium works to make cells receptive to taking glucose inside of the cell membrane.

It should be obvious that getting enough calcium is important. The current recommended daily intake, or recommended dietary allowance (RDA), ranges from 700 milligrams per day (mg/d) for children aged 1 to 3, 1,000 mg for children 4 to 8, 1,000 mg/d for everyone aged 19 to 50, 1,200 mg daily for women aged 51 and above and men older than 70, and 1,300 mg per day for rapidly growing kids ages 9 to 18.

How do you get your recommended calcium from food? Dairy products like milk, yogurt, and cheese are the richest sources of dietary calcium — one cup of milk or yogurt contains as much as 300 milligrams — check the nutrition facts label for the exact number. Some tofu is processed with calcium, and many foods or drinks are fortified with calcium as well. Canned sardines or salmon can provide significant calcium, but only if you eat the bones along with the fish. Frankly, for strict vegetarians or people with significant lactose intolerance, getting 1,000 or more milligrams of calcium per day can be challenging. Once again, the importance of getting adequate calcium in your diet may require taking a calcium supplement.

It's possible to get adequate calcium from non-dairy, non-fortified foods with careful planning. A lunch of two bean and vegetable burritos in corn tortillas, diced avocado and salsa, a leafy green salad with raw broccoli, and a poached pear would add 380 milligrams of calcium to your daily quest.

TIP

Calcium supplements come in many varieties, including, by the way, calcium/vitamin D combinations. Calcium supplements should be taken with meals for better absorption, but there's a catch on dosing. Your body cannot properly absorb more than 500 milligrams of calcium at one time, and that includes calcium from both food and your supplement. If your intake of calcium-containing foods is almost always very low, you still need to take more than one supplement to get your daily requirement and stay under 500 milligrams per dose. Taking a 1,000 milligram dose is wasting the money you spent on the supplement. If your meals often include calcium, purchase smaller doses of calcium supplement, maybe 250 milligram formulations, so you stay under the 500 mg per dose limit when you include the calcium in your meal. Finally, look for supplements that provide calcium in the form of calcium citrate, which is the most readily absorbed calcium compound.

Chromium: From the Emerald City

Chromium is an interesting element. Elemental chromium is used industrially in making stainless steel and for chrome plating, and variations of the chromium element (called isotopes) give rubies their red color and emeralds their characteristic greenness. In your biology, however, chromium plays a role in helping insulin regulate glucose levels, and one compound containing chromium has been designated as *glucose tolerance factor*.

There's agreement that chromium is essential in trace amounts, but research regarding beneficial effects on blood glucose from increasing chromium intake above usual dietary levels through supplementation have been inconsistent.

At this point there is not enough evidence to recommend chromium levels greater than the current adequate intake recommendation, which ranges between 20 and 35 µg per day for adults, depending upon age and gender. An adequate intake level is established when there is not sufficient research for an official recommended dietary allowance. Proponents of chromium supplementation, usually with *chromium picolinate*, generally speak in ranges between 200 and 1,000 micrograms per day, and there is general agreement that these ranges are safe.

In general, the amount of chromium in food is small, but only a small amount is necessary for healthy people. Foods that provide chromium include whole eggs (chromium is in the yolk), whole grains, beef, liver, cheese, black pepper, wine, broccoli, and brewer's yeast.

Magnesium: A crucial player

If you've ever had, or longed for, *mag wheels* on your car, or powdered your hands before mounting the uneven parallel bars, you're already a magnesium lover. But aside from hundreds of industrial and pharmaceutical uses (for example, milk of magnesia), magnesium is essential to health and life.

Magnesium, for instance, works hand in hand with more than 300 enzymes to facilitate biochemical reactions, including those that create *adenosine triphosphate,* the energy molecule made from carbohydrates and the other macronutrients, and in assembling DNA, the molecule that carries the instructions for building and operating you. Adequate levels of magnesium play a role in controlling blood pressure, too, and increasing dietary intake is a key element of the Dietary Approaches to Stop Hypertension (DASH) eating plan, described in detail in Chapter 14.

Low levels of magnesium have been associated with type 2 diabetes and metabolic syndrome, as well as being a side effect of medications commonly prescribed for indigestion or alongside other drugs to protect the stomach from ulcers and bleeding. Magnesium deficiency is more common than was previously recognized, and low levels may contribute to the formation of calcium plaques in arteries, which is a risk for heart attack. Having diabetes can result in an increased excretion of magnesium as well, so getting enough magnesium should be a clear priority.

The recommended dietary allowance for magnesium is 320 milligrams per day (mg/d) for women, and 420 mg/d for men, and surveys tend to show that American adults don't get enough magnesium in their diets. White fish, dark greens, broccoli, beans of all varieties, almonds, pumpkin seeds, artichokes, rice and barley, and wheat bran or whole wheat flour are all rich in magnesium. Eating a balanced diet of whole foods provides the appropriate level of magnesium for most people. The upper limit for magnesium from supplements has been set at 350 mg/d, but unless diabetes is poorly controlled, supplementation is probably not necessary. Your doctor should decide whether you need a magnesium supplement, which type you need and the amount, and that may depend upon medication, other conditions such as Crohn's disease, alcohol abuse, infections, or the status of calcium and potassium levels in your blood.

TECHNICAL STUFF

There are different forms of magnesium supplements and if you are advised to take supplements, your individual needs must be taken into account. For example, magnesium citrate (magnesium combined with citric acid), commonly found in its natural form in fruits, is easily absorbed. It can help constipation as well as cause diarrhea in excessive doses. Magnesium chloride, lactate, malate, taurate, glycate, L-threonate, and other salts of magnesium with varying absorbability may help with magnesium levels if you are found to be deficient, and some of these specific examples have had limited research to show that they might be useful for conditions such as fibromyalgia and improve cognition and even sleep. More research is needed to understand the potential use of magnesium supplementation beyond simply supporting general health by reversing established deficiency.

Potassium: Too much, or too little

Potassium is an essential element of fertilizer for plants, particularly with heavy crop production. Its chemical symbol K is the third number listed for fertilizers containing nitrogen, phosphorous, and potassium — 15-30-10 fertilizer has 10 percent potassium in the bag (the remaining 45 percent is inert ingredients), and it's often listed as potash on the label. Plants tend to accumulate potassium in their cells, and that might lead you to speculate that plants are a good source of dietary potassium. You would be correct.

Potassium plays key roles in your body by regulating fluid and nutrient balance inside and outside of cells, by facilitating nerve signals, by helping muscles contract, and by counteracting sodium to help maintain normal blood pressure. Potassium is an *electrolyte*, participating in the electrical communication between nerves throughout your body. Studies have shown that low potassium levels negatively impact blood glucose control as well.

If you have access to blood test results taken by your doctor, chances are you may see that your potassium level is probably within the normal range. Our bodies (and in particular our kidneys) are remarkably skilled at balancing out our electrolytes. If they are not in the normal range then there can be serious consequences. So, most people would not be classified as being deficient in potassium based on blood levels. But that does not mean that increasing potassium intake from vegetables and fruit is not beneficial.

Almost 75 percent of adults with diabetes also have high blood pressure, and increasing potassium intake is another objective of the DASH eating plan. Most Americans don't consume enough potassium in their diets — the recommended dietary allowance for adolescents and adults is 4,700 milligrams per day — but this key nutrient is not one that should be ignored. So, regarding the title of this section — too much, or too little — it's almost a certainty that you're getting too little potassium in your diet.

WARNING

There's one circumstance, however, where only a little potassium is too much — a renal diet prescribed for kidney failure. It's ironic that choosing not to eat the kinds of foods that are beneficial to diabetes and high blood pressure now may result in having them virtually eliminated from your diet for dialysis. Don't forget, diabetes and high blood pressure are the number one and number two causes of kidney failure.

So, maybe you should think about increasing potassium in your diet right now by increasing your intake of potassium-rich foods. White beans, lentils, edamame (green soybeans), potatoes and sweet potatoes, salmon, canned tomatoes, dates and raisins, spinach and greens, Brussels sprouts, hard-shell squashes, yogurt, bananas, and cantaloupe are all foods that can add more potassium to your diet today. Note that many of these are carbohydrate foods, illustrating why it's important to plan your carbohydrates carefully, and focus on whole foods in your daily eating.

REMEMBER

Your preconceived notions about food may not always be accurate. Bananas have a legendary reputation as a potassium powerhouse, but a plain, boring, white potato has almost twice the potassium ounce for ounce.

Sodium: A little goes a long way

It's appropriate that this discussion of micronutrients puts sodium and potassium together because they work together in your body in many ways. And both are dietary concerns — potassium because you almost certainly get too little, and sodium because you almost certainly get too much unless you are receiving specific advice to the contrary from your medical professional.

This variation actually tells the story of the so-called Western diet, because although you may be getting sufficient potassium from vegetables and fruits, instead you're likely getting significantly excess sodium from — well, nearly everything else. In fact, of the more than 4,000 milligrams of sodium the average American consumes each day, only 10 percent or less comes from the sodium chloride in your salt shaker; maybe another 15 percent is naturally occurring in the foods you eat. That leaves 75 percent that's added by someone else, like a food processor or a restaurant. In an interesting turn, therefore, this discussion about sodium doesn't focus on how you can find more, but rather on how you can reduce your daily intake.

So, what good is sodium anyway, how much do you need, and how much is recommended for people with diabetes? Remember, 75 percent of people with diabetes also have high blood pressure, so much of the story of sodium focuses on that other significant risk for heart attack, stroke, and kidney failure.

Sodium, like potassium, is an electrolyte, facilitating the transmission of electrical messages throughout your nervous system, participating in the balance of fluids in your body, and helping in the transport of other compounds through cell membranes. So, sodium is essential, and a deficiency of sodium can be very serious. A sodium deficiency, called *hyponatremia*, usually occurs as a result of fluid retention, where the amount of sodium is not affected, but the concentration of sodium is reduced by excess bodily fluids. It's possible to lose too much sodium through perspiration, but this is something that would most likely be seen in marathon runners or other extreme endurance athletes. It's the concentration of sodium that's important, and maintaining your normal concentration of sodium requires only about 200 to 300 milligrams of sodium per day from diet — most Americans get 20 times more sodium than necessary.

TIP

It's important to remember that not all sodium is created equal. Much of the table salt we find in dining rooms and kitchens today is chemically processed. This means that it has been stripped of its natural nutrients and contains chemical anticaking agents that are not only not good for us, but also they make the sodium more difficult for our bodies to break down. Unrefined sea salt, however, contains trace minerals such as magnesium and potassium that have been shown to counter the negative effects associated with sodium, so choose it whenever possible.

WARNING

Excess sodium in your diet, especially when potassium is deficient, is closely associated with high blood pressure, called hypertension. Excess sodium contributes to high blood pressure by requiring more blood volume to keep sodium concentration in a normal range. Moving more fluid through the same-sized arteries requires more pressure, and when other lifestyle factors promote narrower arteries by the accumulation of arterial plaques (atherosclerosis) and less flexibility of the arteries, blood pressure can skyrocket. Consistently high levels of sodium, high blood pressure, and diabetes eventually cause kidney damage.

For years the daily recommendation for sodium intake was set at 2,300 milligrams per day (mg/d) for anyone under 51 except in the case of existing high blood pressure. Recognizing the dual risk of diabetes and high blood pressure, a 1,500 mg/d limit was set by the United States Department of Agriculture's Center for Nutrition Policy and Promotion in its 2010 Dietary Guidelines for Americans for anyone with diabetes. (Note that 1,500 mg of salt is equivalent to just three quarters of a teaspoon.) And while salt (sodium chloride) is your most likely source of dietary sodium, preservatives and additives like sodium nitrate can add to the load.

Reducing sodium in your diet can be challenging, but because your most likely sources come from foods in the grocery or at a restaurant you have the information you need, in most cases, from a nutrition facts label, or from the restaurant's website. You just need to be sure to use the information that's available, and don't just look at foods you perceive as salty — sodium is virtually everywhere, and it all adds up. Fortunately, food manufacturers have focused on producing low sodium formulations of many foods in response to public health concerns.

You can find discussions about sodium throughout this book, and a detailed discussion about the DASH eating plan in Chapter 14. The effectiveness of this clinically tested diet at reducing blood pressure almost immediately is one of the best examples of how food can be medicine.

Insulin and zinc: Two peas in a pancreas

Zinc is the grayish metal that coats roofing nails, the key ingredient in the white paste you may see on lifeguards' noses, and may even help to dampen the symptoms and duration of the common cold. And zinc is an essential micronutrient.

Zinc is crucial to your immune system, enhances your senses of smell and taste, is involved in the metabolism of the macronutrients, promotes tissue growth and cell reproduction, is an antioxidant working to protect cells from damage, and is involved with hundreds of enzymes. And zinc plays a very important role in your body's production, storage, and use of insulin, the hormone that lowers high blood glucose levels.

TECHNICAL STUFF

Zinc in pancreatic beta cells binds to several insulin molecules, six to be exact, forming what's called an insulin *hexamer* for storage. In fact, long-acting insulin formulations for injection — NPH or Lantus, to name two — contain zinc so that the insulin is bound in hexamers that convert to the active insulin *monomer* (a single insulin molecule) slowly.

There is not sufficient evidence to suggest getting more than the recommended dietary allowance of zinc brings additional benefits to blood glucose management, and excess zinc can cause imbalances with copper and other micronutrients. It seems prudent, however, to include foods or a multivitamin that puts adequate zinc into your diet. The current RDA is 8 mg/d for adult women and 11 mg/d for adult men — the RDA varies for children, adolescents, and pregnant or nursing women.

TIP

Foods that contain zinc include oysters (the richest source), crab, beef, beans, yogurt, cheese, oatmeal, and almonds. The absorption of zinc from many plant sources is inhibited by phylates, which are also present in the grain, so the bioavailability may be less than zinc from animal sources.

Sorting Out Supplements

Dietary supplements are a complex issue, but registered dietitians have a simple, two-word starting point — food first. That doesn't mean that supplements of one kind or another aren't suitable, or even necessary for you. It means that taking supplements as a substitute for a healthy, balanced diet is no way to achieve good health, and it's certainly no way to prioritize diabetes management.

In the previous sections of this chapter you saw time and again how research hints at profound benefits for a particular nutrient, but the effect of that particular nutrient can't easily be separated from everything else that comes in its natural packaging. It may be that another active compound, or something as simple as fiber, gives nutrients like phytochemicals the key to their effectiveness. In some cases, beneficial effects were seen only from the natural, whole food, and specifically not from the nutrient supplement. In other words, it is important to consider nutrients in the food matrix.

The bigger issue is that your focus on micronutrients can't divert your attention away from your primary objectives with diabetes management — blood glucose control and heart health. Discounting how a healthy diet and overall lifestyle can help resolve diabetes-related concerns is failing to see the forest for the trees. Many of these micronutrient compounds work to prevent health problems, not to cure them. Plus, poorly controlled blood glucose levels inhibit the activity of some micronutrients, and accelerate your excretion of others. With vitamin D, you even learned how excess weight stored as body fat can capture the active compound so it's not even available to exert its powerful influence on your health.

REMEMBER

Getting your micronutrients from food first when you have diabetes is one specific and practical example that meal planning pays off. The essential nutrients and powerful phytochemicals that come from dairy products, whole grains, beans, vegetables, and fruit also come along with carbohydrates. Working these foods into your daily eating means making sure your daily carb choices include a wide and varied selection of these healthy options. Appreciating the importance of natural micronutrients in healthy carbohydrate foods can help you make wiser choices too, like when you're tempted to dedicate 25 percent of your daily carb choices to a sugar-sweetened soft drink.

So, who needs supplements? There is relatively general agreement in the medical community that supplementation of one kind or another may be appropriate for the following circumstances:

>> People who are on medications that are known to deplete vitamin or mineral levels in the body may find benefit in taking a supplement.

>> People dealing with chronic health issues, stress, weakened immune systems, or who are malnourished may find benefit; however, the scientific evidence is not well established for their general use and care should be taken to avoid side effects or interference with medications.

>> People who may become pregnant should get folic acid daily from a supplement, in addition to eating foods that contain folate, to prevent certain birth defects.

>> Pregnant individuals should take a prenatal vitamin that includes high-strength folic acid, and they may also need additional iron (seek the advice of

your doctor and pharmacist). For those who experience heavy bleeding during their menstrual cycle, an iron supplement may be advised.

>> People nursing an infant may require supplemental vitamins, and their infants need a vitamin D supplement as well.

>> Children and adolescents who can't, or don't, drink milk need a vitamin D supplement during seasons they can't get sufficient sun exposure, or if direct sun exposure isn't advised.

>> People with lactose intolerance, food allergies, or who are on a very strict diet limited to 1,600 calories per day, or less, may need appropriate supplements.

>> People who can't properly absorb vitamins, as a result of bariatric surgery or a digestive disorder like Crohn's, celiac, or other inflammatory bowel disease, may need supplements, sometimes by injection.

>> Vegans may require supplemental vitamin B12, calcium, and vitamin D.

>> People over age 50 need additional vitamin B12 from fortified foods, or from supplements and may need Vitamin D supplements.

>> People with an identified vitamin deficiency or with a condition (such as macular degeneration) that is treated with vitamins may likely need a supplement.

REMEMBER

Always seek advice from a regulated and trusted practitioner if you are considering the use of supplements. You may notice that most all of these circumstances would, or should, involve a physician's care for the underlying condition. So, in these cases you're likely to get specific instructions on which vitamins or nutrients, and how much, you should take.

If you are taking supplements, or planning to take supplements, without specific instructions from your medical provider, at least discuss your daily intake with your doctor and your pharmacist. It's important that your medical providers assess your particular health issues, and evaluate potential interactions with any other prescription or over-the-counter drugs you're taking.

WARNING

Drug interactions with vitamin supplements can take many forms. Niacin in combination with statins to lower cholesterol can cause serious muscle problems. Calcium supplementation can prevent the proper absorption of certain antibiotics if taken together. And some prescription drugs for acne or psoriasis are chemically similar to vitamin A and pose a risk for vitamin A toxicity if used while taking a supplement.

The likelihood of vitamin toxicity is fairly small unless you're taking doses of the fat-soluble vitamins A, E, D, or K, that are significantly beyond the amount your body needs. These compounds are stored in fat, and can accumulate in your body because you excrete excess amounts slowly. The water soluble vitamins, all of the B vitamins and vitamin C, are more easily excreted when you consume amounts in excess of your needs. Of course, that means excessive doses in a supplement are literally flushing your money away.

If this section on supplements sounds like it's all caution and no cheerleading it's because the scientific evidence for mega doses of vitamins and other nutrients rarely supports the popular claims. But dietary supplements are not held to the same kinds of rigid regulatory standards as pharmaceuticals, and manufacturers' claims can push the limits of verifiable results. Plus, consumers are irresistibly attracted to the possibility of a simple solution to good health, and are ever more willing to invest billions of dollars every year on products with completely unsubstantiated promises. The National Institutes of Health, Office of Dietary Supplements, maintains a webpage that provides a world of information on supplements at https://ods.od.nih.gov.

TIP

That said, there are two specific supplements that many people should consider — vitamin D and calcium. And you can probably get both in one. The purpose and function of both is discussed earlier in this chapter.

The Gut Microbiome and Its Role in Diabetes

How many of us wake up each morning and wonder what we are going to feed our 100 trillion gut bacteria today? And how many people with diabetes consider the state of their gut microbes as being crucial to diabetes, its onset, and its management? Although that may sound a strange way to think about the bacteria that inhabit large parts of our intestines, scientists are increasingly understanding the crucial role they play in our health and how the food we eat affects the composition and diversity of what is called our *gut microbiome*. We often think about microbes including bacteria as the causes of infections and disease, but in this case, they are often referred to as "friendly" bacteria.

TECHNICAL STUFF

The first research into the microorganisms that are found in our intestinal tract began in the late 1800s. In recent years there has been an explosion in evidence to show that this symbiotic relationship we develop in our infancy and maintain through our lives affects virtually every part of our health including our immune system and our risk of chronic diseases, obesity, metabolic syndrome, and diabetes. The way in which the gut microbiome acts even influences our mental health, cognition, and risk of dementia. These microbes act as protectors, metabolizers, and signalers, interacting with numerous organs and systems, regulating and supporting multiple aspects of health.

Several factors determine the nature of our gut bacteria population including genetic and environmental. Research is beginning to help us to understand the effects of different species of microbes, including the patterns and composition associated with better markers of health and also where there is a loss of a healthy microbiome, called *dysbiosis*. Dysbiosis can exist where there is an overgrowth of populations of potentially harmful microbes, where there are fewer species that are known to be beneficial, or when there is a loss of overall diversity. When this is the case, there is an increased risk of oxidative stress (we consider this more in Chapter 8), inflammation, and a number of chronic diseases. There are some species present in our guts that influence, positively or negatively, aspects of diabetes such as glucose absorption, metabolism, and insulin sensitivity.

Dysbiosis can be linked with many factors that are also associated with cardio-metabolic risk including obesity, low levels of exercise, chronic stress, some medications, poor sleep rhythms, and hormone dysfunction. Establishing our healthy gut microbiome is important in early infancy as we are born from a sterile environment into one where our future health depends on healthy bacteria. A normal delivery and early breast-feeding help with this exposure.

Of the factors that may affect the microbiome such as our genes, age, exposure to antibiotics, exercise, stress and sleep, our diet is possibly the most important area we can influence. Diets like the Mediterranean diet have been shown to promote a healthy gut microbiome, and it is thought that this is related to the wide variety of foods in the diet that nurture and "feed" our gut microflora — so called *prebiotics* and *probiotics,* which are foods that contain live beneficial bacteria to supplement and maintain a diverse and healthy microbiome.

We each have an individual gut microbiome that depends on genetic and environmental factors. The idea of "personalizing" our nutrition to understand the link between our genes, microbiome, and foods and how we might optimize our diet is of increasing interest, but meanwhile there are some general principles that can help us to achieve our most healthy state.

FROM THE AUTHORS

Both prebiotics and probiotics play an important role in general health and more specifically in weight and diabetes management. Studies have shown that prebiotics can lower fasting and postprandial (after a meal) glucose levels, improve insulin sensitivity, improve lipid profiles, lower inflammatory markers, and stimulate production of the naturally occurring hormone GLP1, which influences appetite and glucose metabolism. Some medications for weight and type 2 diabetes management have been designed to mimic this effect. You can read more about this in *Diabetes For Dummies,* 6th Edition (Wiley).

Understanding the role of prebiotics

Prebiotics are plant-based fibers that pass through the stomach undigested and broken down or fermented by gut microbes, increasing the growth and activity of beneficial strains of intestinal bacteria. They can be considered as good "food" for good microbes. Examples of prebiotics include onions, garlic, artichokes, bananas, whole grains, green leafy vegetables, soybeans, almonds, oats, and apples. The fiber in these foods gives it the prebiotic effects; however, compounds called *polyphenols* in many vegetables and fruits also interact with the gut bacteria. (See Chapter 8 for more on polyphenols.)

Good sources of prebiotics include the following foods:

Artichoke	Eggplant	Radishes
Asparagus	Flaxseed	Root vegetables
Avocado	Fruit	Plantains
Bananas (under ripe)	Garlic	Potatoes
Barley	Green tea	Rye
Beet root	Honey	Sea vegetables
Bran	Jerusalem artichokes	Soybeans
Burdock root	Jicama	Spices and herbs
Chia seeds	Kefir	Sugar maple
Chicory	Leeks	Sweet potatoes
Chinese chives	Legumes	Tomatoes
Cocoa	Lentils	Vegetables
Cottage cheese	Onions	Yams
Dandelion greens	Peas	Yogurt

Learning how probiotics can help

Probiotics are live bacteria or yeasts that exist in fermented foods either occurring naturally or having been added in their production. You may have heard of examples like *Lactobacillus* and *Bifidobacterium*. The most common foods that contain probiotics include yogurt, some cheeses, kefir, sourdough bread, miso, tempeh, kombucha, sauerkraut, and some other pickles. The exact contribution these cultures make to our health is not firmly established. There is some evidence that probiotics can help conditions such as irritable bowel syndrome and restoring the natural balance of gut bacteria following an illness or treatment, but there are many claims made about their effects that have been difficult to prove beyond doubt.

Some studies have been published suggesting a possible slower rate of decline for people with early Alzheimer's dementia who increased the probiotics in their diet and others appear to demonstrate improved mental health and a decrease in perceived stress. It is clear that many heritage diets associated with good health outcomes are rich in fermented probiotic foods that often contain other nutrients of benefit as well.

Good sources of probiotics include the following foods:

Beer	Miso	Root and ginger beers
Buttermilk	Natto	Sauerkraut
Essene bread	Olives	Sourdough
Fermented anything	Pulque	Tempeh
Fermented sausages	Raw pickles	Wine
Fermented vegetables	Raw vinegars	Yogurt/kefir
Kombucha	Raw whey	

Chapter **8**

Eating a Rainbow: Bioactive Compounds and Polyphenols

B ioactive compounds are perhaps the most important things you eat that you have probably never heard of. As more is discovered about the best diets that can add years to life and maximize the quality of life during those years, it is easy to appreciate that it's not just the macronutrients and micronutrients that count. The interactions between ingredients when they are combined, the role of an individual's gut microbiome, genes, and the way they eat all play an important part in the way diet impacts health.

Some of the most exciting discoveries relate to the powerful effects of chemicals found in very small amounts in plants called *bioactive compounds.* There are 26,000 known bioactive compounds in food. Scientists are just beginning to reveal how even small amounts of these compounds may play a protective role in reducing the risk of developing diabetes, heart disease, cancers, dementia, and chronic inflammation. We know the basics about the nutrients we should eat — high-quality, low glycemic, and high-fiber carbohydrates with proteins predominantly from plants, fish, or poultry accompanied by healthy fats. Our foods should be natural, sustainably sourced, rich in micronutrients and vitamins, and unprocessed with no added sugars or artificial additives. We should enjoy alcohol in moderation, mainly wine with a meal, use supplements only when we have a reason to, and we should value what we eat. But this is certainly not the end of the story. It is just the beginning.

The potential for bioactive plant compounds having a significant role in protecting us from a wide range of common chronic diseases is exciting researchers around the world. This chapter explores what is known, as well as what isn't yet known about these compounds, including where they come from and why they exist, how they might reduce inflammation, and even what they look and taste like.

Defining Bioactive Compounds

Bioactive compounds is a term used to describe groups of plant chemicals that are found in small amounts in our diet. They are biologically active, meaning they have effects that can impact health. They are not classified as types of micronutrients because a *nutrient* is defined as a food component that is necessary to sustain life or growth. It is increasingly recognized that bioactive compounds, although not necessary for sustaining life, may well be very influential in sustaining health.

TECHNICAL STUFF

The terms used to describe bioactive compounds can be confusing and misleading. Some people use the word *phytonutrient* for these chemicals. *Phyto* means plant. But strictly speaking they are not nutrients, so many chemists feel this is not correct terminology. *Polyphenols* are bioactive compounds, most of which contain more than one hexagonal ring of carbon, hydrogen, and oxygen. Terms used for this group can include *polyphenol, phenols, phenolic acid,* or *biophenols*. In this book, we refer to this group as polyphenols. Beta-carotene is a bioactive in a group called the *carotenoids*, but it is also converted to vitamin A, which is separately classified as a vitamin.

Most bioactive compounds fall into one of three main chemical groups (with notable exceptions such as capsaicin from chili peppers that has been used as pain killer):

>> **Carotenoids:** These are plant pigments that are yellow, orange, or red. More than 1,000 carotenoids have been identified. Examples of carotenoids include the orange beta-carotene found in carrots as well as many other vegetables, and lycopene, which is the red pigment in tomatoes.

>> **Glucosinolates:** These are pungent compounds based on glucose and amino acids that contain nitrogen and sulfur atoms. They are commonly found in the vegetables like broccoli, kale, and Brussels sprouts. They are related to the sulfur-containing compounds called *allium* in garlic and give mustard seeds and horseradish their unique flavor.

>> **Polyphenols:** These are the most common bioactive compounds in our diet. Over 8,000 individual polyphenols have been identified to date. They can be divided into *flavonoids* and *non-flavonoids,* and further subdivided to include polyphenols called *phenolic acids, lignans, secoiridoids, phenolic alcohols,* and *stilbenes.*

TIP

Although, as the name implies, the glucosinolates are derived from a glucose molecule, the quantity of glucose in these compounds is tiny and does not affect blood glucose levels.

Understanding Bioactives and Their Role in Health

To understand how bioactive compounds might act to protect us, it is helpful to consider why plants go to the trouble to make them in the first place. Bioactive compounds are *secondary metabolites,* which means they are produced not for survival but for the additional benefit of protection, and perhaps even giving the plant a competitive benefit in its potentially challenging environment.

The story of bioactive compounds and the way they work is an evolving one. There is plenty that isn't known. How they are handled by our gut microbiome, whether it is the compounds themselves or those formed after they are broken down, whether our genes affect this process, exactly where and how they act, and precisely what quantities can be helpful to health, are all areas of ongoing research. What is clear is that a diet rich in polyphenols is linked to reduced markers of inflammation and *oxidative stress* (circumstances where there is an excess of reactive, potentially damaging molecules), so there is certainly evidence to support their important protective role, but there is no evidence to suggest that we should be taking high-dose supplements or binging on one or more polyphenol, carotenoid, or glucosinolate.

TECHNICAL STUFF

Plants produce polyphenols and other bioactive compounds to protect themselves and their fruit from the potentially damaging chemical reactions set off by exposure to ultraviolet (UV) light, heat, and oxygen. They can also have the added benefit of antimicrobial effects to prevent the plant being attacked by harmful bacteria, viruses, or fungi. These compounds are often needed most in the exposed outer layers, and can have advantages if they are sometimes bitter in taste to deter animals from eating the plant. In addition, plants, existing in a dynamic and ever-changing environment, can produce more polyphenols for added security if the circumstances are more challenging, perhaps when there is a drought or at higher altitude with more UV exposure, and they can even change the combination of polyphenols to alter the taste and color as a signal to animals their fruit is ready to be eaten and seeds dispersed.

A few years ago, any serious scientist would have laughed at the suggestion that plants help each other by communicating either through releasing invisible chemicals in the wind or in root systems that "talk to each other." However, current evidence supports the notion that plants under stress release polyphenols or other chemicals to let their neighbors know of a risk so that they can raise levels of other protective polyphenols in anticipation. Plants are very smart and they have to sometimes work together to survive. In case you are thinking that this is all very interesting and increasing your respect for plants, but not very relevant, later in this chapter you will see that we too can benefit from the protective effects of bioactive compounds and recognize the clever ways that nature presents their potential to us in the foods we eat.

SMART AND POWERFUL PLANTS

Plants are smart and they can kill! A story that illustrates the protective and adaptive powers of bioactive compounds for plants is one that involves a murder mystery from South Africa, finally solved by sleuths from the University of Pretoria. One very hot summer, rangers in parts of the Transvaal National Park reported the deaths of 3,000 elegant antelopes called kudus over a period of just a few months. Apparently healthy animals were dying, especially in regions where they were in high numbers. What became clear is that high concentrations of kudus were eating more and more acacia tree leaves, threatening the very existence of the trees in their finely balanced environment. In a dramatic response, the trees reacted to the stress by increasing the concentration of types of polyphenols called tannins (familiar to us in tea and wine) in their leaves to such an extent that they caused acute and fatal effects on the kudus' intestines. The acacia trees also adopted a strategy of sending chemical signals to other trees even outside the confines of the park, which resulted in acacia trees increasing their tannin levels in anticipation of the danger over overgrazing coming their way. Polyphenols and other bioactive compounds can have very beneficial effects, but it must always be remembered that first and foremost they are produced for the protection of plants.

Bioactive compounds may work to protect us from various diseases in several different ways. They may work as food for our gut microbiome. There is certainly evidence that polyphenols increase levels of particular microbes that are associated with maintaining a healthy weight. An article published in the journal *Molecules* in 2018 described the role of polyphenols from plants present in honey relevant to its use on wounds to reduce infections. Research has shown the capacity of polyphenols to influence the way our genes are expressed, with interest in the possibility they may have the power to "turn off" genes that increase the risk of developing certain cancers. Polyphenols may also have the capacity to increase insulin sensitivity, which may explain the 57 percent reduction in relative risk of developing type 2 diabetes between people consuming high- or low-polyphenol diets described in a study published in 2017 in the *British Journal of Nutrition*.

Many studies have shown associations between consumption of foods that are rich in bioactive compounds and reduced risk of many chronic diseases. Other research focuses on extracting specific compounds and, for example, targeting them at cancer cells in a laboratory. And while it is not unusual for one study to contradict a previous one, or for the media to pick up on a headline that may exaggerate the findings, there is a consistent accumulation of research that shows that diets rich in a variety of bioactive compounds can offer protection against diabetes and many of its complications including heart disease, strokes, dementia, and some forms of cancer.

The specific ways in which polyphenols in particular help diabetes and glucose regulation include lowering insulin resistance, encouraging a healthy gut microbiome, and through stimulating a hormone called GLP-1, which improves insulin function and a feeling of fullness. Drug companies produce injectable medications such as Ozempic that mimic the effects of natural GLP-1 and that are used in the treatment of type 2 diabetes and obesity.

TIP

Diets like the Mediterranean diet that are rich in plant polyphenols are known to reduce the risk of obesity and diabetes. This may be one of the ways in which such diets have their beneficial effects. Unlike medications, they are free of side effects and can be maintained for a lifetime.

Analyzing Oxidation and Antioxidants

How can you keep a sliced apple from turning brown? You can add an antioxidant like the vitamin C in lemon juice. *Antioxidants* are compounds that can help reduce cell damage caused by the byproducts of reactions in your cells that use oxygen. These byproducts are called *free radicals,* and they are looking to steal electrons, often from the fats that are present in cell membranes, in reactions that are called *oxidation.* An excess of free radicals can result from environmental factors such as smoking, pollution, UV light, radiation, and chronic inflammation. It can also be caused by the chemistry of our own metabolism, where the conversion of the compounds from the "foreign materials" in food to beneficial nutrients for our bodies involves considerable processing and can increase oxidative stress.

Where there is an excess of free radicals, their disruptive electron stealing potential can set up a chain of harmful reactions that can in turn cause cell damage and inflammation. This is described as a state of *oxidative stress.* We have evolved to counter this with our own innate protective systems of *reduction* or *redox*, which can neutralize oxidation reactions.

Our cells are in a constant flux of repair and replacement in a chemical environment where we are converting compounds from our food to create energy. We are protecting ourselves from pollutants, attack from harmful microbes, UV light, and radiation. The chemistry that gives us life can also overwhelm us. Protecting ourselves from oxidative stress through our own redox systems and with the help of the foods that we eat is vital to sustaining health. Exercise is very good for us. We rebalance the intensive energy producing reactions though with an antioxidant response and the net effect is that vigorous activity is usually followed by a reduction in oxidative stress. Why we sleep remains largely a mystery, but we do know that it provides an opportunity for rebalancing oxidative stress.

Inflammation: The Good, the Bad, and the Ugly

Doctors are increasingly recognizing that many chronic diseases such as heart disease, stroke, dementia, arthritis, inflammatory bowel disease, and diabetes are associated with ongoing low- or high-grade inflammation. Sometimes this inflammation is obvious (for example with symptoms of swelling and pain of joints in arthritis), but on other occasions it is less overt, though it can sometimes be detected in the blood with chemical *biomarkers* of inflammation such as C reactive protein (CRP), tumor necrosis factor alpha (TNF- alpha), and interleukin 6 (IL-6). Diabetes is a disease with increased inflammation.

Acute inflammation is part of our body's response to an infection or incursion by potentially harmful material from the outside world. Our response is to mobilize our immune system and to chemically attack the invading pathogen or foreign particles. This is often accompanied by redness and swelling of surrounding tissues. Damage to our external surfaces presents a risk of bleeding, so there is an increased "stickiness" of our blood cells to form clots and avoid hemorrhage.

Once the threat is neutralized, inflammation recedes and cells that may have been damaged in the process undergo healing and repair. Our immune system stands down, often committing to memory the structure of a bacteria or virus so that it can be dispatched quickly if it returns.

Chronic, longer-term, low-grade inflammation occurs when we are unsuccessful in fully eradicating an infection, when our immune system is not working correctly (perhaps misdirecting reactions to normal cells in an autoimmune reaction), or when our body is in an abnormal chemical state of oxidative stress. High levels of free radicals that are not neutralized by our internal rebalancing redox systems or the bioactive compounds we get from our diet can be an important factor in chronic inflammation. Certain patterns of gut microbes in our microbiome are also associated with chronic inflammation.

Chronic inflammation and disease

Chronic inflammation has been linked to many diseases, including obesity, diabetes, and many of the complications of diabetes. Heart disease and stroke were previously considered to simply be the result of cholesterol clogging and blocking blood vessels, but it is now understood that the inflammation of cholesterol plaques on artery walls is key. LDL cholesterol under oxidative stress results in damage to arterial walls and inflammation, which can result in blood clots responsible for strokes and heart attacks.

Chronic inflammation can also damage DNA in cells, which might be vulnerable to cancerous changes. This is possibly the reason why people with chronic inflammatory bowel conditions resulting from autoimmune chronic inflammation are at greater risk of developing bowel cancer.

TIP

The good news is that not only do we have systems to protect us from oxidative stress and the drivers of chronic inflammation, but there are also foods that have antioxidant and anti-inflammatory effects. It is important when choosing a diet to include the foods that have these beneficial effects and to limit those that have the opposite effect and have been shown to be *pro-inflammatory*.

WARNING

Pro-inflammatory foods tend to promote chronic inflammation. Such foods include those that cause a spike in blood glucose levels such as refined carbohydrates, ultra-processed and processed foods, red meat, an excess of vegetable oils, cookies, cakes, and sweetened beverages.

Foods rich in bioactive compounds such as polyphenols have been shown to reduce oxidative stress, many have been shown to inhibit the chemical pathways of inflammation, and others even have chemical structures similar to anti-inflammatory medications such as aspirin (a small daily dose of which has been prescribed by doctors for decades to patients to prevent strokes and heart disease). Examples of this include the action of rosemarinic acid found in rosemary and oleocanthal, which is a polyphenol present in extra-virgin olive oil and which has the same mild throat-irritating sensation and similar anti-inflammatory effects as ibuprofen. Polyphenols may also play a role in reducing the increased risk of blood clots associated with inflammation, moderating the immune system, and even acting at a genetic level to inhibit chronic inflammation.

The Dietary Inflammatory Index

Measuring the tendency of a diet to contribute to chronic inflammation is not an exact science. The Dietary Inflammatory Index, or DII, is one measure that has been used by researchers to try to quantify a diet in terms of its effects on inflammation. Highly processed diets with added sugars and saturated fats common in the United States and Europe tend to rank highly on a DII scale, whereas heritage plant-based diets have a healthier, lower score.

A study published in 2020 in the *Journal of the American College of Cardiology* reported from the large Nurses' Health Study a 38 percent reduction in relative risk of developing heart disease in those who consumed the most anti-inflammatory diet in comparison with the least anti-inflammatory. In addition, a review article published in the *International Journal of Clinical Practice* in 2022 showed a reduction in the incidence of type 2 diabetes in people who were choosing a diet ranked low on the DII scale, though this was difficult to quantify due to inconsistencies of the DII scores.

Researchers are trying to accurately standardize the DII. A diet ranked low on the DII in principle limits pro-inflammatory foods and promotes increased consumption of anti-inflammatory ingredients such as green leafy vegetables, dark yellow vegetables, chocolate, red wine, and extra-virgin olive oil. Many foods included in commonly used DII rankings are high in bioactive compounds such as carotenoids and polyphenols. Some might be recognized as "superfoods," although we should be cautious using this term because there is no accepted definition and the term is often used for marketing processes.

TIP

Diets like the Mediterranean diet are naturally aligned with the principles of low DII diets, show reduced biomarkers of inflammation, and are associated with reduced risks of chronic diseases as the benefits of an anti-inflammatory diet are experienced.

What has surprised many researchers is the power and speed at which these effects can be seen. One experiment involved denying participants access to anti-inflammatory foods for a short period of time, measuring their baseline biomarkers of inflammation and then providing them with one meal of "sofrito" — a polyphenol compound–rich combination of extra-virgin olive oil, onions, tomatoes, and garlic (sometimes with celery and bell peppers) that is often used on the scoring for adherence to the Mediterranean diet. There was a significant and rapid decrease in biomarkers of inflammation within hours of the meal. This suggests that what we eat today can have an influence on our levels of inflammation and that the regular consumption of bioactive compounds at every meal may be protective against the problems caused by chronic inflammation.

WARNING

Some medical conditions of chronic inflammation, especially those of an autoimmune origin, need medications that sometimes act to reduce the inflammation and to control symptoms. Other diseases discussed in this chapter such as heart disease, stroke, cancers, and of course diabetes usually require medical therapies. While it's important to understand and enjoy a healthy anti-inflammatory diet and understand the link between foods, oxidative stress, and inflammation, this should always be in conjunction with the advice and prescribed medication from medical professionals.

Getting to Know Carotenoids, Glucosinolates, and Polyphenols

The simple way to classify the most common bioactive compounds is to divide them into family groups of carotenoids, glucosinolates, and polyphenols. They each have different characteristics and are present in different foods.

Colorful carotenoids

Carotenoids are plant pigments, and hundreds have been identified. In plants, carotenoids absorb sunlight for photosynthesis, the process by which plants build carbohydrates from sunlight, water, and carbon dioxide. The pigments also protect chlorophyll in the plant cells from sunlight damage. Carotenoids are divided into two groups — one group that includes oxygen called *xanthophylls*, and a group that does not include any oxygen called *carotenes*.

The class of xanthophylls includes *zeaxanthin* and *lutein*, and the pigmentation is generally yellow. Xanthophylls give egg yolks their yellow color, but the compounds aren't produced by the chicken — they come from plant materials in chicken feed. In humans, these carotenoids accumulate in the eye, where they absorb damaging UV light and protect the retina from damage. One large study that included lutein in a mix of other nutrients showed that this carotenoid along with vitamins C and E, zinc, and copper, slowed the progression of macular degeneration, a leading cause of blindness in seniors. The richest food sources for the xanthophylls are dark leafy greens like kale, spinach, Swiss chard, and turnip and collard greens. Zucchini, broccoli, Brussels sprouts, pistachios, and kiwifruit also contain these carotenoids compounds.

The carotene pigments tend toward orange and red, and include *beta-carotene* and *lycopene*.

Beta-carotene

Beta-carotene is rapidly converted to vitamin A in the small intestine, and functions in your eyes to improve night vision and color vision. Vitamin A also is essential for your immune system, works in transcribing instructions from DNA, maintains normal skin, and has antioxidant properties. Beta-carotene seems to protect premenopausal women from breast cancers, slow the progression of (but does not prevent) osteoarthritis, and prevents exercise-induced asthma attacks.

TIP

Good sources of beta-carotene tend to be orange or dark green fruits and vegetables — carrots, apricots, winter squashes, cantaloupe, sweet potatoes, pumpkin, dark greens like kale and spinach, and herbs like basil and parsley. For some foods, lightly steaming them can improve beta-carotene absorption, but in most cases prolonged cooking or the canning process reduces the concentration of available beta-carotene. Fat-soluble carotenes are also better absorbed if the foods are eaten at meals that include some dietary fat.

WARNING

Beta-carotene supplementation should be done only under the supervision of your doctor. Fat-soluble vitamins like vitamin A can accumulate to toxic levels over time. And in a study to look at the potential benefits of beta-carotene supplementation for smokers, supplementation actually increased the risk of lung cancer, where intake from natural food sources did not.

Lycopene

Lycopene is a carotenoid associated with bright red colors, and tomatoes serve as the standard bearer for the group. Lycopene is an effective antioxidant, and has been studied extensively for a potential benefit in reducing the incidence of cancers, particularly prostate cancer. Much of the evidence for lycopene's possible effect in reducing or improving cancers comes from population studies of cancer incidence among people who eat lots of tomatoes, or have high lycopene blood levels.

Unfortunately, much of the evidence is inconsistent, and many of the more positive results suggest that tomatoes are more effective than lycopene alone. That may mean that lycopene has no beneficial role, or that its effectiveness is also related to other compounds, like vitamin C, also found in tomatoes. But the absence of compelling evidence from controlled clinical trials doesn't mean lycopene isn't beneficial to health. A recent study suggested that a variation in a gene called XRCC1 may influence whether lycopene can influence prostate cancer risks. Other research hints that lycopene may reduce the risk of nonalcoholic fatty liver disease. Research on lycopene is ongoing, including a role in glucose control and reducing oxidative stress in diabetes.

TIP

Foods rich in lycopene include tomatoes, pink grapefruit, watermelon, pink guava, and papaya. Unlike carotenoids, cooking increases the availability of lycopene, especially with the addition of a monounsaturated fat like olive oil. The concentration of lycopene in canned tomatoes, tomato sauce, or ketchup might be ten times that in a raw tomato.

Glucosinolates and garlic

Another class of bioactive compounds is the glucosinolates. These pungent sulfur-based compounds are present in the brassica family of foods such as broccoli, cauliflower, mustard, rapeseed, and horseradish. Allium is a related sulfur compound present in onions and garlic, along with other bioactive compounds including polyphenols.

Vampires (and loved ones) beware — garlic is on the menu. But is garlic actually beneficial to diabetes?

Garlic, as you may guess, is in the onion family and is another food with an interesting history spanning thousands of years. Garlic is also another food that has been touted for its inherent medicinal properties, and the active ingredient is thought to be *allicin,* a sulfur-containing compound with antioxidant properties.

Garlic has been shown in studies to exert a modest effect in lowering blood pressure, and it seems to reduce atherosclerosis. Both effects may be by increasing the flexibility of arteries. Some cancers may be reduced by eating garlic but not garlic supplements, and regular consumption of garlic over a period of several months is positively associated with reduced tick bites.

However, in spite of the fact that the Internet is awash with websites testifying to the benefits of garlic to diabetes, no reputable studies have been able to demonstrate any beneficial effect to blood glucose control. Garlic is, however, a wonderful flavor enhancer and condiment that may help you reduce sodium, and even fat, in your diet.

TIP

It won't do much good to try and freshen your breath after eating garlic. The chemical that gives your breath that special odor, allyl methyl sulfide, actually moves through your bloodstream to your lungs. So, the problem is not in your mouth, but actually in the air you exhale.

Powerful polyphenols

Polyphenols are present especially in colorful vegetables and fruits. Polyphenols have antioxidant and anti-inflammatory properties and can also improve insulin sensitivity and promote a healthy weight.

A study of twins published in the journal *Nutrients* in 2020 showed that a high-polyphenol diet was associated with a 20 percent reduction in risk of obesity. Polyphenols have also been linked with possible antimicrobial, anticancer, anti-thrombotic (reducing blood clotting), and anti-aging actions as well as protective effects on our brains and mental health. They also reduce insulin resistance, improve glucose control, help us to feel full, and benefit our gut microbiomes.

Polyphenols are molecules that have a hexagonal combination of carbon and hydrogen atoms with an additional pairing of oxygen and hydrogen atoms. This structure enables them to generously donate electrons, neutralizing free radicals and limiting their capacity to damage other stable molecules. Polyphenols probably work in a number of ways that aren't yet fully understood, and their biological activity may not be solely down to their antioxidant capacity.

Flavorful flavonoids

Flavonoids are polyphenols, once labeled vitamin P. They are often responsible for providing the color to flowers and help filter UV light from the sun. In general, flavonoids are antioxidants and often seem to work with vitamin antioxidants, such as vitamins C and E, to enhance the function of both compounds. There are more than 4,000 flavonoids, broadly divided, without unanimous agreement, into *flavonols, flavones, flavanones, isoflavones, catechins, anthocyanidins,* and *chalcones.*

Flavonoids have been reported to reduce the incidence of coronary heart disease; have antibacterial, anti-viral, antitumor, anti-inflammatory, and antiallergenic effects; and help improve the flexibility of arteries. As with the other bioactives, research on flavonoids is complex and complicated by the range of other nutrients in flavonoid-containing foods. Some specific flavonoids of note include the following:

>> *Anthocyanins* are active compounds found in blueberries, blackberries, cranberries, cherries, and the pigment in the fruit of blood oranges and the peel of eggplant. These compounds have been shown to exhibit anti-aging properties, reduce inflammation, and have promise in preventing and treating certain cancers. Black raspberries, a rich source of anthocyanins, have been shown to increase the death rate of cancer cells, inhibit the formation of blood supplies to tumors, and minimize DNA damage. Cancer research involving anthocyanins is an active field.

- >> *Hesperidin* is a flavonoid found abundantly in citrus fruits, such as oranges and lemons. Because hesperidin may improve blood vessel health, it's used to treat internal hemorrhoids and small leg ulcers caused by poor circulation. Hesperidin is also touted as a treatment for varicose veins, but the jury is still out on whether it's effective for that purpose.

- >> *Catechins* might remind you of an informal get-together with friends — tea, a little wine, and some chocolate. But this class of flavonoids has some impressive potential health benefits. Unfermented green tea is the winner for total catechin content, and green tea has amassed some pretty strong evidence of benefits for heart disease, some cancers, and even Alzheimer's dementia. People who regularly drink green tea have less heart disease, fewer strokes, lower total and LDL cholesterol, and recover from heart attacks faster. Some evidence suggests that tea may help fight ovarian and breast cancers as well. Catechins are anti-inflammatory, and a review of the effectiveness of weight-loss supplements found that green tea had a statistically significant benefit to weight loss.

- >> *Epicatechin*, a specific catechin found naturally in dark chocolate, reduced the brain damage caused by strokes in mice, and an observational study of heavy cocoa drinkers in Panama found striking reductions in that group's risk for heart failure, stroke, diabetes, and cancer. A recent study published in the *Journal of Neurovirology* found that epicatechins protected brain cells from damage by the human immunodeficiency virus (HIV) in AIDS patients. Also, a small study of profoundly ill patients administered epicatechin-enriched cocoa noted improved muscle cell function, and indicators that muscle cells were producing new mitochondria (the structures where macronutrients are converted to energy).

TECHNICAL STUFF

Quercetin, a flavonoid in vegetables, fruit skins, and onions, exhibited the highest antioxidant properties in preventing the oxidation of low-density lipoprotein (LDL cholesterol) in the laboratory. The oxidation of LDL in your body is a reaction known to promote arterial plaque buildup. However, coming in a close second place were two flavonoids contained in hops, a key flavoring ingredient of beer — xanthohumol and isoxanthohumol.

TIP

Genistein, a flavonoid in soy called an isoflavone, is a powerful antioxidant as well, and has been shown to inhibit arterial plaque formation.

Non-flavonoid polyphenols

Many of the foods described in the previous sections contain other polyphenols as well including *stilbenes, lignans, secoiridoids, phenolic alcohols,* and *phenolic acids.*

Stilbenes are polyphenols present in berries and grapes. One stilbene called resveratrol is present in cocoa, peanuts, blueberries, strawberries, cranberries, and grapes, and has been studied in relation to the potential benefits of red wine, although always in the context of the possible harms of excess alcohol consumption.

You may have seen, or at least know of, the famous movie *The French Connection*, but have you heard of the French paradox? The French paradox describes observations that captured public attention in the 1990s showing that despite their higher consumption of saturated fat, the French seem to have a lower incidence of heart disease than people in the United States. When a 1991 story on the television news show *60 Minutes* left an impression that red wine was the key to the French paradox, red wine consumption in the United States increased by more than 40 percent. Eventually, the public's attention turned to *resveratrol*, a natural plant phenol found in the skin of red grapes.

Resveratrol slowly became recognized as an anti-aging substance, based to some extent on reports that doses of this compound extended the life expectancy of yeast cells, nematode worms, and eventually a short-lived fish — in some cases the doses were equivalent to 30,000 milligrams per day for a human, so it may be that the breakdown products of resveratrol are more important for any effects in humans than the compound itself. Resveratrol has been cited as beneficial for heart disease, diabetes, cancer, and Alzheimer's dementia, and is said to be antiviral, able to increase testosterone levels, an anti-aging miracle for skin, and a treatment for acquired tolerance to opiates in people with chronic pain.

Noting the relatively low levels of resveratrol in wine, researchers are looking at a different group of polyphenols in grape skins and seeds — oligomeric procyanidins, which have been shown to improve the functioning of blood vessels. Levels in wines depend on the grape variety, maceration time (how long the grape skin is in contact with the juice), and the conditions of cultivation. There is a fascinating observation that some regions known for the longevity of their residents such as Sardinia and South West France also consume particularly high procyanidin wines. It is not possible to say that it is all down to the red wine, but it makes for interesting research.

WARNING

If you're visualizing a resveratrol supplement as just another way to have a relaxing glass of wine, your mental image might be a fantasy. The resveratrol in some supplements is derived from the unpurified extract from Japanese knotweed, and may include emodin, a compound that can have a laxative effect. Relaxation is not usually associated with a laxative effect.

Lignans have also been shown to possess anti-inflammatory, antioxidant, and antitumor activity and are possibly protective against cardiovascular disease. They are found in various seeds, grains, legumes, vegetables, and fruits. Sesame seeds and their paste, which is called *tahini* and used in traditional Middle Eastern and Mediterranean recipes such as hummus, are a great source of lignans. Flaxseed, nuts, beans, and soy also contain lignans as well as whole-grain cereals, oats, brassica and root vegetables, peppers, tomatoes, and many fruits and berries. Olives are rich in lignans and are just part of the variety of polyphenols found in extra-virgin olive oil. In many cultures, the regular consumption of coffee provides a rich source of lignan polyphenols.

Polyphenols in a chemical class called the secoiridoids called *oleuropein* and *oleocanthal* are being extensively researched because of their likely contribution to the anti-inflammatory and antioxidant benefits of extra-virgin olive oil. Like many polyphenols they can be recognized by the bitter and pungent taste. Oleocanthal in extra-virgin olive oil can result in a mild irritation to the throat and occasional cough similar to an effect also seen with some forms of the anti-inflammatory medicine ibuprofen.

Another group of polyphenols present in extra-virgin olive oil are the phenolic alcohols called *tyrosol, hydroxytyrosol,* and related compounds. There is confidence that these polyphenols act as antioxidants. Evidence of the ability of hydroxytyrosol and its derivatives in extra-virgin olive oil to reduce the damaging oxidation of LDL cholesterol has been used by the European Health Safety Authority to permit a regulated health claim on oils that have a minimum level of these polyphenols. The inability of the average consumer to understand such a statement makes it of limited use to most people.

Extra-virgin olive oil, the "fresh fruit juice" of the olive, contains at least 36 polyphenols. Olives carefully harvested for extra-virgin olive oil early in the season from trees that have been cultivated without excessive fertilization or irrigation are rich in protective polyphenols. These oils have a pleasant bitterness and peppery or pungent flavor, which is valued by people who enjoy the taste of extra-virgin olive oil. If bottled and stored correctly — away from heat, light, and oxygen to avoid the loss of antioxidant capacity — extra-virgin olive oil makes an important contribution to the antioxidant and anti-inflammatory effects of the Mediterranean diet. The pressing of the olives results in a food that is less bitter than the original olive in its natural state and has concentrated polyphenols. No other single food plays such a central role in any other diet. It is the main source of fat and the only oil used for cooking. In traditional diets of Greece, each person consumes an average of 35 to 70 milliliters per day — that's 1 to 2 liters per month!

A study from Bordeaux University published in 2011 in the journal *Neurology* showed a 78 percent reduction in rates of stroke in people who consumed a high quantity of extra-virgin olive oil when compared with those who consumed the lowest levels. Researchers from the European Prospective Investigation into Cancer and Nutrition (EPIC) reported the risk of heart disease to be halved and all-cause death rates reduced by 26 percent in participants who consumed 20 milliliters of extra-virgin olive oil per day. The polyphenols in extra-virgin olive oil have been shown to have beneficial effects on oxidative stress, inflammation, clotting, blood vessel function, the immune system, the gut microbiome, blood pressure, and cancer cells. The importance of extra-virgin olive oil's role as part of the Mediterranean diet associated with much lower rates of many chronic diseases, is being further explored.

Phenolic acids such as caffeic acid (present in coffee and many other fruits), vanillic acid, and rosemarinic acid, are also often found alongside numerous other types of polyphenols in herbs. Coumaric acid is another phenolic acid found in beans, tomatoes, basil, and garlic, as well as in fruits, cereals, and honey.

Enjoying the Taste of Bioactives

Bioactive compounds are produced to protect the plant from environmental oxidative stress including the effects of oxygen, heat, and UV light. They may have antimicrobial actions and many are bitter, peppery, or even poisonous to protect the plant from being eaten. Some species that depend on animals or birds to spread the mature seed send signals through changes in color and sweetness when a fruit is ready to be eaten and the seed deposited intact and wrapped in a helpful coat of fertilizer.

Bioactive compounds are responsible for the pigment and taste development as a fruit ripens. Plants that rely on animals and birds are so well evolved that it has been suggested that they appeal to the tastes of their preferred carrier. It may be that it is advantageous for an olive or chili parent plant to produce polyphenols that in their natural state are pungent enough to discourage mammals from eating the fruit, but appeal to birds that are unaffected by the taste, allowing the dispersal of seeds farther away so that the new plants do not compete for resources with their parent.

Bioactive compounds with their potentially protective effects often present us with interesting tastes. As infants and children, we are appropriately suspicious of very bitter or spicy foods, which may signify a plant to be poisonous (although there are genetic differences in how sensitive we are). Gradually we accept and learn to enjoy those flavors as we see from our parents what is safe and healthy to eat. We are certainly not unique in this capacity to develop our taste for nourishing foods. Researchers have observed chimpanzees consuming small amounts of plants with potentially medicinal effects when they are sick, and teaching others the same behavior.

REMEMBER

In a food environment where we are increasingly exposed to processed products that focus on appealing to our innate desire for sweetness evolved from periods of evolution when energy from food may have been scarce, it is important that we celebrate the diverse range of flavors and sensations of many bioactive compounds. Bitterness, spiciness, pungency, and pepperiness, especially when combined with other ingredients, can add interest, pleasure, and health to our diet.

How to Recognize Foods with Bioactives

Foods that are rich in bioactive compounds are often easy to spot. We know that carotenoids and polyphenols often give the colors to plants and the advice to "eat a rainbow" is a good suggestion. Plants tend to concentrate their protective bioactive compounds on the most exposed surfaces, and so much of the polyphenol content of a fruit or vegetable may be in the skin or outer layers. We get less benefit from potatoes if we peel them, and many of the polyphenols from almonds are lost if they are blanched with skins removed. Many spices that have high concentrations of polyphenol compounds (though we generally add them in small amounts for seasoning) are produced from the bark or outer layers of plants.

REMEMBER

Protective polyphenols increase in concentration when a plant exists in a challenging environment. Modern farming practices are not conducive to maximizing the amounts of polyphenols for a number of reasons. If a crop is irrigated heavily or where there is widespread use of insecticides, the result is a higher yield but risks a reduction in bioactive compounds. A loss of diversity also threatens and reduces the presence of species that have historically provided higher levels of polyphenols. An example of this is modern wheat when compared with heritage cultivars like spelt and rye.

It is sometimes all too convenient for food producers to suggest that consumers do not like foods that are bitter. Unfortunately, "taste literacy" may be diminishing as a result of the increase in sugar, fat, and salt in processed foods in our diet. Taste is learned and we may be "unlearning" our interest in bitter or pungent flavors. The good news is that we can gradually wean ourselves away from the sugary hit of low-cocoa chocolate toward a higher cocoa percentage, more bitter, and satisfying chocolate just as it is possible to enjoy the complex flavors of coffee without the cream and sugar.

The big olive oil producers have been shown to be correct in their assertion that most consumers prefer a bland tasting olive oil, which is what they have come to expect. Research even shows that people who have become accustomed to unwittingly buying rancid oil get to prefer what is familiar, much to the horror of producers of healthy, high-quality, fruity yet slightly bitter high-polyphenol extra-virgin olive oil so prized by enlightened customers.

Recognizing the variety of bioactive compounds in plants is one way to make sure we enjoy delicious foods that may well have the capacity to promote healing and good health. Research is just beginning to inform us of the potential benefits of eating a diet rich in carotenoids, glucosinolates, polyphenols, and other extraordinary bioactive compounds.

Chapter **9**

Equipping Yourself for Success

The importance of healthy eating when diabetes is part of your life can't be overstated. Managing what goes into your mouth is an essential part of diabetes self-management, and you are the chief security officer — no food goes in without your approval. Food gets intimate access to your most sensitive inner workings, so reviewing its resume and checking out trusted references are steps every good security chief should take.

And, after you're satisfied with the qualifications, be prepared to take full advantage of everything healthy food has to offer. Ultimately, enjoying food that's satisfying and flavorful goes a long way toward keeping your willingness willing.

Stocking Your Kitchen

Preparation for diabetes meal planning and nutrition starts with a very minor, but very important, makeover of your kitchen. You want your kitchen set up for ease of food preparation, and that includes everything from measuring cups and scales to the right ingredients.

REMEMBER
You should have healthier staple foods on hand. It's fun and can be easy to throw together a spontaneous breakfast, lunch, dinner, or snack that fits your diabetes meal plan perfectly by having the best food choices close at hand. These include frozen fruits and vegetables, dried or low-sodium canned beans, frozen lean meats or tempeh, whole grains like oatmeal, brown rice, or quinoa, and low-fat milk or yogurt.

Measuring your food is a necessity — not just for recipes, but also for eating. This is a difficult habit to adopt for many, but the portion size of any food is what determines the nutrient and, importantly, carbohydrate content. Getting the appropriate serving size of different foods that contain 15 grams of carbohydrate — one carb choice — is the foundation of healthy eating for blood glucose control.

TIP
Pour your normal bowl of dry breakfast cereal and then measure what you've poured. A 15-gram carb choice for most unsweetened cereals is ¾ cup — how'd you do?

Gathering tools and gadgets

It takes very little time and money to set yourself up for success in the kitchen. Measuring tools are the most essential devices for healthy eating. Americans suffer from what nutrition professionals call *portion distortion*, where years of super-sizing and ever-larger dinner plates have contributed to eating the wrong amounts of the wrong foods. It's simply necessary to measure the weight or volume of the food going into your mouth. You measure what goes into a recipe so the final product is what you want. Think of your meals as a recipe for the blood glucose levels you want.

Later in this chapter you discover some estimating tricks, but when you're at home, estimating shouldn't be necessary. The following sections describe what you really must have in your kitchen.

Kitchen scale

A kitchen scale is how you weigh appropriate portions of protein foods like fish or chicken, and carbohydrate foods, like potatoes, that don't fit into a measuring cup. Kitchen scales don't directly measure grams of protein or carbohydrate in a particular food, although there is at least one model that allows the user to enter a specific code assigned by the manufacturer to produce a nutrition facts label for any of the coded foods. Instead, you learn that a 3-ounce piece of white potato is one carbohydrate choice, giving you 15 grams carbohydrate. It's the 3 ounces of a white potato that needs to be weighed.

Kitchen scales range from less than $10 to more than $50. Some are simply mechanical and have a dial; but the battery-operated scales have an electronic or digital display. Whichever scale fits best into your budget or decor is perfect — managing diabetes with diet only requires some sort of kitchen scale.

TIP

Another great way to ensure that you eat just one serving is to get a kitchen scale with a tare feature. You put your bowl on the scale and press the tare button. The scale returns to zero and you can measure your one serving.

Measuring cups, scoops, and spoons

Measuring cups are essential tools that you probably already have in your kitchen. If not, you may want to read *Cooking Basics For Dummies* (Wiley). Measuring cups enable you to portion cooked grains like rice, starchy vegetables like peas and corn (you have liberated from its cob with your corn zipper), and dairy products such as milk or yogurt.

Measuring scoops are more convenient, and less messy, for getting to foods in a larger container like oatmeal or dry cereal. Measuring scoops have a handle just like regular scoops, but they're sized to scoop a specific measure.

Of course, a set of measuring spoons is a must have, too, although you'll be glad to know that very few food portions are measured by the spoonful.

Other tools

A few kitchen utensils just make healthy eating more convenient. These aren't must-haves for diabetes self-management like measuring devices, but there's a lot to be said for convenience. Here's a sampling:

>> **Sharp knives:** You don't need an expensive set of cutlery to do basic food preparation, but a few knives, kept sharp, can make a huge difference in the work involved. A 10-inch, curved-blade chef's knife is best for chopping, mincing, and slicing through tough foods, and the one knife where spending a little extra money and purchasing a sharpener can pay off. A small paring knife gets the assignment for smaller or finer work, like peeling fruit or trimming the extra fat from cuts of meat. You can top off your knife collection with a long serrated knife, perfect for slicing bread and for vegetables like tomatoes that bruise easily.

>> **Salad spinner:** A salad greens spinner is the most efficient way to wash and dry salad fixings. Chopped greens go into a slotted bowl, and you can run water liberally over the mixture. Then, the slotted bowl fits into a gear in a larger, closed bowl equipped with a lawn-mower-like rope pull that spins excess water off of the greens.

>> **Food and cheese graters:** A variety of graters come in handy for adding shredded cheese or vegetables to dishes. And, a microplane grater is great for fabulous flavor additions like fresh ginger, aged cheeses, or lemon zest.

>> **Steamer baskets:** Using either a stovetop or microwave steamer basket is the quickest and most flavor-preserving way to prepare fresh or frozen vegetables. Steaming your vegetables, as opposed to boiling them, preserves more of the nutrients because steaming uses less water. Microwave cooking had been under suspicion in this regard after a 2003 study found flavonoids depleted in microwave-cooked broccoli, but more recent results from Spain showed baking and microwave cooking preserves more nutrients than water-based cooking.

>> **Vegetable peeler:** A good vegetable peeler takes the work out of preparing fresh vegetables and fruits. Vegetable peelers come in a variety of space age designs, but the truth is the old fashioned metal one with a slightly pointed end for digging out potato eyes has never been topped.

TIP

Do consider when it is good to give the peeler a break. Many vegetables can be cooked unpeeled and many of the bioactive compounds may be concentrated there.

>> **Food thermometer:** Every kitchen should have a metal-stem food thermometer on hand for food safety. The U.S. Centers for Disease Control and Prevention estimate that 48 million Americans are sickened every year by food. Cooking *potentially hazardous foods,* like meat products, to the proper temperature can help reduce your risk for illness.

>> **Food processor:** While not absolutely necessary, a good food processor can help you make smooth and creamy soups, pesto sauce, hummus, and other purees in just a few minutes. It also allows you to shred vegetables into different sizes in minutes.

>> **Blender:** Blenders are great for making smoothies and transforming chunky vegetables into velvety soups and sauces in no time.

Planning a pantry

One trick to eating healthier is keeping healthier choices around — how simple is that? The truth is that even the most detailed plans, including your menu, need to be adjusted sometimes, even if it's only because you don't feel like preparing what's on today's plan. You can fight the urge to hit the fast-food drive-through or cooking processed ready meals and whip up a convenient and healthy breakfast, lunch, dinner, or snack if you keep the right foods handy. Your list of healthy items to keep on hand should include all six food groups, and the following sections offer suggestions for keeping healthy foods at arm's reach.

Grains and starchy vegetables

Grains and starchy vegetables are excellent sources of carbohydrate and fiber. Keep 100 percent whole wheat or other whole-grain pita or bread, and whole-grain crackers around for sandwiches, rollups, or spreads. Whole-grain pasta, brown rice, basmati rice, farro, soba noodles, and potatoes or sweet potatoes are common staple starches, and consider trying quinoa and amaranth, seeds that include protein.

Whole-grain dry cereal or oatmeal make a super breakfast, and for healthy snacking keep some plain yogurt, nuts, and fresh fruit and vegetable sticks around, but watch your portion sizes. Some fresh starchy vegetables keep well — potatoes, sweet potatoes, and hard-shell squashes are good examples — and frozen vegetables can be ready for the table in a jiffy.

Nonstarchy veggies

Nonstarchy vegetables are the foundation for healthy eating and should occupy half of your plate. Again, fresh, frozen, or canned are equally good for you, but watch for added fat and especially sodium. Frozen or canned vegetables like green beans, carrots, broccoli, cauliflower, Brussels sprouts, and stir-fry mixtures can be scooped up when on sale so you always have a selection ready at a moment's notice. Always keep salad greens on hand for a quick and healthy meal and for some fun with your salad spinner.

Fruits

Fruits are the healthiest way to enjoy sweetness, and fresh, frozen, or canned are equally nutritious as long as there is no added sugar. Keeping fresh fruit in plain sight can go a long way toward changing your snacking habits for the better. Just remember, all fruit includes carbohydrate, and the 15-carbohydrate-gram portion size varies somewhat from fruit to fruit. The portion size for dried fruit like raisins is only two tablespoons, for instance. You can find a comprehensive list of fruit portion sizes in Appendix A.

Healthy proteins

Healthy protein choices should include canned tuna or salmon (canned in water), peanut or almond butter, low-fat cheeses and cottage cheese, eggs, tofu or other meat substitutes like tempeh, frozen fish fillets (not breaded), and low-fat meats and ground meats like 96 percent lean ground beef, ground turkey, pork tenderloin, and beef filet or flank steak.

Dairy

Single servings of milk, full-fat Greek yogurt, cottage cheese, goat cheese, and aged cheeses can add protein, carbs, and fat into your diet. Remember that milk products include carbohydrate, and adding fruit to yogurt increases the carb content.

Healthy fats

Healthy fats are an important part of a healthy diet, protecting your organs, insulating nerves, transporting some vitamins, and forming cell membranes. Healthy fats include healthy oils like extra-virgin olive oil, nuts, seeds, and avocados. The objective is to limit saturated fats and to avoid *trans fat*. You can find that information on the nutrition facts label, which is discussed in the section "Understanding Nutrition Facts Labels."

Beans and legumes

Beans and legumes contain fiber, protein, and complex carbohydrates. They can help to fill you up, balance blood glucose and insulin, and enable you to build muscle and lose weight. It is recommended that you eat at least one serving per day. Stock chickpeas, brown and red lentils, cannellini beans, and Egyptian fuul medammes on hand to make the recipes in this book.

Spices, aromatics, and seasonings

Spices and seasonings are not a food group, but using a variety of flavorings not only enhances your eating pleasure while adding powerful antioxidant and anti-inflammatory bioactive compounds, but also can help you avoid adding salt. Garlic, onions, cinnamon, oregano, cardamom, za'atar, rosemary, thyme, cumin, and pure vanilla along with quality vinegars add flavor and nutrients to your food.

Understanding Nutrition Facts Labels

In the United States as well as in many other countries, nutrition facts labels are required on all packaged foods, and this is a good thing. The information included on the nutrition facts labels tells you everything you need to know about the labeled food product. To be honest, the label also tells you a lot that you don't really need to worry about too much. In fact, the information you don't really need to worry over can look so complicated that it may scare you away from using this valuable resource altogether. Understanding nutrition facts labels for diabetes meal planning and nutrition starts with ignoring some of the information. A typical nutrition facts label is illustrated in Figure 9-1.

Nutrition labels, such as "traffic light" warnings, are not without controversy. They often put an emphasis on macronutrients such as fats, rather than making distinctions between the different types, and they fail to take into account potentially harmful ingredients in ultra-processed foods, or celebrate the bioactive compounds that are understood to have health benefits. We recommend looking beyond nutrition labels to see how many unrecognizable ingredients are listed in the manufacturer's small print and, as a general rule, avoid products with unnatural-sounding additives.

For starters, don't worry too much about those values with a percent (%) mark, which are all related to the percentage of daily recommended values for certain nutrients in a 2,000-calories-per-day diet. (On some labels this becomes even more complicated than on the label illustrated.) Generalities are always too broad, but the issue here is that each label refers to only one serving of only one food. So, unless you're anxious to keep a detailed account of every serving of every food you eat each day (or are living on nothing but linguine salad), this information is more confusing than helpful.

Nutrition Facts

Serving Size 1/2 cup (140g)

Amount Per Serving

Calories 240	Calories From Fat 130

	% Daily Value *
Total Fat 15g	23%
Saturated Fat 2g	11%
Trans Fat 0g	
Cholesterol 0mg	0%
Sodium 530mg	22%
Total Carbohydrate 24g	8%
Dietary Fiber 1g	5%
Sugars 5g	
Protein 3g	

Vitamin A 15%	•	Vitamin C 60%
Calcium 2%	•	Iron 6%

* Percent Daily Values are based on a 2,000 calorie diet.

FIGURE 9-1: Nutrition facts label for prepackaged linguine and tomato salad.

The information to look for that is most important to managing your diabetes is serving size, calories, fat (total, saturated, and trans fat especially), total carbohydrate, dietary fiber, sugar alcohols, and sodium. Notice sugar isn't singled out as something that needs your special attention, even though sugar, dietary fiber, and sugar alcohols are listed as subcategories of total carbohydrate on the labels. That's because total carbohydrate includes carbs from sugar, carbs from fiber, and carbs from sugar alcohols.

REMEMBER

Total carbohydrate is the number that impacts blood glucose, and both fiber and sugar alcohol may deserve your attention because any time these exceed 5 grams you can subtract one half of the amount from total carbohydrate. Both fiber and sugar alcohol digest more slowly (or not at all), so glucose absorption from those is less efficient. These adjustments are mostly important when calculating insulin doses related to foods containing a lot of fiber or sugar alcohols.

Calories

Calories are the units used to describe the energy stored in food, and it's a word used in the sciences as a unit of heat. The term *calorie* as commonly applied to food is actually 1,000 of the heat units — a *kilocalorie*. Calorie has taken on the meaning of kilocalorie when speaking of food.

FROM THE AUTHORS

Many nutrition experts are advising that we move away from calorie counting. This is because it is becoming clear that the measurement of the energy of a food does not necessarily describe how it is handled by our bodies. The way we combine our foods together may change the way we absorb and transfer a meal into energy. The extent to which a calorie-rich food increases our sense of fullness may mean that we eat smaller portions overall. Bioactive compounds in foods influence the way our individual gut microbes process a meal and affect the conversion to energy. So, all calories in all foods in all people may well not be necessarily equal. Calories are still used widely and the following section can help you to understand what this means, but choice of foods and portion sizes may be a more meaningful way to approach weight management.

TECHNICAL STUFF

The calorie as a unit of heat is the amount of heat necessary to raise the temperature of 1 gram of water by one degree Celsius. It has been replaced in the International System of Units by the *joule*. One calorie is equal to 4.184 joules. How would a 7,113-joules-per-day diet plan sound to you?

You need food in part because you need the calories of stored energy to keep your body operating, and the more active you are the more calories you need. Calories in excess of what you need result in weight gain because your body stores the excess as body fat to provide energy in times of calorie shortages. Fat is the most efficient way to store calories, which explains why dietary fat gives you more than twice the calories in your food as the same measure of either protein or carbohydrate. Fat stores 9 calories of energy per gram, but protein and carbohydrates store only 4 calories per gram. Alcohol, by the way, stores 7 calories per gram.

Your calories can come from sources that provide no significant amount of other nutrients, like calories from sugars or alcohol. These calories are called *empty* calories. Your calories can also come from foods that provide nutrients along with energy. Calories coming from foods that also provide other nutritional benefits are called *nutrient-dense* calories. Healthy eating seeks to maximize nutrient-dense calories.

Losing excess body fat means reducing the calories you get from food to fewer calories than you use each day, so you are drawing from calories stored as excess fat. Many people with diabetes, especially type 2 diabetes, need to lose excess weight by reducing calories. Excess body weight, and particularly fat accumulating around vital organs, is at least partially responsible for the insulin resistance that characterizes type 2 diabetes. If you need to lose weight and you have diabetes, see a nutrition professional. It's possible to calculate your daily energy needs and reduce your calorie intake to less than your requirements on your own. Check out *Nutrition For Dummies* (Wiley) to find the equations for calculating your daily energy needs.

But are you willing to add the 240 calories you got from ½ cup linguine salad to the calorie content of every other food you consume every day? And, do you know how much you should reduce your calorie consumption, or how to be certain you aren't eliminating foods beneficial to diabetes management?

REMEMBER

You are far better off getting a personalized meal plan from a nutrition professional who can competently account for the requirements of diabetes and weight control, and incorporate medical nutrition therapy for other medical conditions you may have. As a general rule, your diabetes meal plan provides about 50 percent of your calorie needs from nutrient-dense carbohydrates, 20 percent from lean protein, and 30 percent from mostly healthy fats. It's just too important to not get it right.

Grams and milligrams

Food nutrition information is given in metric weight measures, grams, and milligrams, and if you're from the United States, unless you're a scientist, you may have no idea how a gram compares to measures you're more familiar with. There are 28.3495 grams in 1 ounce, and there are 1,000 milligrams in a gram (28,349.5 milligrams per ounce). But don't get your calculator out.

In some ways it's not that important. You don't have to understand grams and milligrams as related to units you know, but only that your diet should include certain amounts of various nutrients which are measured in these units. A 3-ounce portion of white potato contains 15 grams carbohydrate, 3 grams protein, and no fat. The 18 grams of nutrient weight is only slightly more than 20 percent of the total 3-ounce potato weight, however. And, weighing another carbohydrate food gives you a different percentage between total weight and carbohydrate grams — math doesn't always work here.

Instead, you can rely on memory, nutrition facts labels when available, a reference book, a cheat sheet, a website or app, or your personal assistant to find the grams of the nutrients in different foods. It's not as difficult as it sounds (especially if you actually have a personal assistant). Your main focus should be on carbohydrates, and the one number you may eventually be seeing in your sleep is 15 grams.

REMEMBER

The best foods don't have labels. Choose fresh, whole ingredients as much as possible.

Serving sizes

The serving size listed on a nutrition facts label is the weight or volume of the specific food that contains the nutrients listed. For the linguine salad label in Figure 9-1, the stated serving size is ½ cup, and ½ cup of the salad contains 240 calories, 15 grams total fat, 24 grams total carbohydrate, and so on. Nutrition facts label serving sizes vary significantly by product, from 1 tablespoon for vegetable oil to 1 cup for macaroni and cheese, as examples.

A food's stated serving size is not necessarily the appropriate portion size for healthy eating or for blood glucose control. The value of knowing the serving size related to nutrient content is that it usually gives you enough information to calculate or estimate the right portion size for you.

TIP

Recipes usually provide the serving size information as "makes 4 servings" or "yield is 8 servings." Just as with nutrition facts labels, the nutrition information applies to one serving of that recipe.

Calculating Food Choices

Remember when math class had you muttering to yourself, "When will I ever need to use this?" Well, the time has come, but don't worry. This math is simple, the answers don't have to be exact, and you can always fall back on your personal assistant for help. In all seriousness, there is more than one way to come up with the correct portion sizes for your meal plan. The real obstacle is convincing yourself to think about food in an analytical way before you start eating. After all, that's what meal planning is all about.

Sizing up your food: Portion sizes

Most foods are a mixture of the macronutrients — carbohydrates, fat, and protein — and you should choose the best types of these three macronutrients when making complete meals. Lean meats contain 7 to 9 grams of protein per ounce, but also contain fat. One cup of two-percent milk contains 12 grams carbohydrate, 8 grams protein, and 5 grams fat. You get the picture.

For diabetes-related nutrition the emphasis is on 15-gram portions of total carbohydrate, also known as a *carb choice,* or a starch, milk, or fruit exchange. Carbohydrates have a direct effect on blood glucose levels, and your intake of carbohydrates affects how well your diabetes medication works, too. Your meal plan specifies how many carb choices — how many grams of carbohydrate — you should have at each meal, which is usually three to five carb choices (45 to 75 grams) depending on your calorie requirements. From there you can easily put together the carbohydrate portion of your meals.

You can estimate/calculate a 15-gram-carbohydrate choice from nutrition facts labels by manipulating the label's serving size into a 15-carbohydrate-grams portion size. The linguine salad in Figure 9-1 has 24 grams carbohydrate in the ½-cup serving size. Estimating, you could say that if ½ cup is 24 grams then ¼ cup is 12 grams, and 15 grams is slightly more than ¼ cup. Calculating, you can multiply 24 grams by 2 to find the total carbohydrate in a 1 cup serving is 48 grams. Dividing 48 grams by 15 grams equals 3.2 carb choices (about 3) per cup, so ⅓ cup would be very close. In fact, 48 grams per cup divided by 3 equals 16 grams carbohydrate per ⅓-cup portion. The label *serving size* is ½ cup, but the 15-gram carb portion is about ⅓ cup. You may be glad to know that ¼ cup works just as well. Items such as nuts, seeds, celery, and cucumbers, nut butter, and tomato salsa don't have many carbohydrates but are satisfying snacks.

If your head hurts you'll be glad to know that measuring appropriate portions of carbohydrate is really easier, but it does require knowing what measure of which food equals 15 carbohydrate grams. Here's where memory, reference books, cheat sheets, experience, or that personal assistant come in handy. One tablespoon of pure maple syrup is considered one carb choice, but you can measure about three full cups of raw, nonstarchy vegetables (cucumbers, broccoli, bell peppers, green beans, and so on) before you get one 15-gram-carb choice (that's why healthy eating includes lots of vegetables). Table 9-1 shows a quick guide to common carbohydrate-containing foods to get you started.

TABLE 9-1

One Carbohydrate Choice for Common Foods

Food Description	Measure
Sugar or concentrated syrups	1 tablespoon
Oatmeal, dry	¼ cup
Grains (rice, barley, etc.), cooked	⅓ cup
Pasta, cooked	⅓ cup
Beans and peas (starchy vegetables)	½ cup
Fresh fruits	½ to 1¼ cup
White potato	½ cup or 3 ounces
Bread	1 slice
Milk	1 cup
Yogurt	¾ cup
Nonstarchy vegetables cooked	1½ cups

TIP

Common carbohydrate foods like those in Table 9-1 are easy to remember with experience, but a nutrition facts label or a pocket-sized carbohydrate reference book is an absolute must for deciphering food like the linguine salad in Figure 9-1 if you intend to manage diabetes well.

Portion sizes for protein and fat share one thing in common. Both should be smaller than what most Americans picture. A healthy meal plan for diabetes management may recommend 4 to 6 ounces of protein food (lean meat, tofu, cheese, nuts, and eggs) per day, equaling about one-half of the daily protein recommendation (85 grams for the 1,700-calories-per-day plan). The rest of your daily protein comes from low-fat dairy (milk and yogurt) and from carbohydrate foods containing protein.

You're also likely to get much of your recommended fat from other foods, including meat, nuts, low-fat dairy, cheese, and carbohydrate foods. Some of this dietary fat is the unhealthier saturated variety, but a healthy diet focuses on sources of healthier *unsaturated* fat. Sources of fat not included in another food group include oils, butter and margarine, and salad dressings. In general, choose low-fat versions of food, and use oils sparingly.

Estimating tricks

When you don't have access to nutrition facts labels or your measuring tools, you have to estimate portion sizes. Estimating is not a replacement for more accurate determinations of portion size, but all in all it works pretty well. The broadest estimating trick looks at how you fill your whole plate. You should allocate a quarter of your plate to a lean protein and half of your plate to nutritious nonstarchy vegetables, which you remember are very low in carbohydrate. The final quarter of your plate is reserved for your meal plan's three to five carb choices. (See Chapter 13 for the diabetes version of the USDA's MyPlate.)

You can estimate portion sizes by using your hand and your imagination. One ounce of cheese is the size of a domino, 3 ounces of meat matches a deck of cards, 1 tablespoon of margarine resembles half of your thumb, 1 cup of vegetables makes a fist, and a medium apple is equal to a baseball.

Referencing the Right Resources

Healthy eating to manage blood glucose and the risks for diabetes-related complications requires some thinking and preparation. Fortunately, there are credible resources that can help immensely. A pocket-sized reference book can be your best pal, but other resources work just as well.

Searching websites and apps

It may be debatable whether there is too much information available on the web, and now even on your mobile phone or tablet, but it's hard to deny that these technologies can be very handy. An Internet search for "carb counting" returns more than one million results, and there are literally hundreds of websites and apps where the nutrition information for specific foods is available.

For individual food items the American Diabetes Association currently offers searchable nutrition information on reading labels and planning meals at https://diabetes.org/healthy-living/recipes-nutrition.

Other websites have similar functions, many of which also include commercial raw products and restaurant items. Nutrition apps for mobile devices are plentiful as well, and some even scan a product's bar code and display the nutrition facts label.

WARNING

Be cautious about websites or apps that offer dietary advice or promote specific diets or products. It's much better that you learn for yourself what healthy eating and effective diabetes self-management requires. That way, you can take advantage of the valuable information and pass on the advice.

Collecting recipes

Enjoying food is absolutely essential, and if you're going to eat more often at home so you have better control of your diabetes — and we did agree that you are — you want wonderful recipes to draw from. Of course, with a market exceeding 20 million people in the United States alone, there are many diabetes cookbooks available. But, you don't have to get your recipes from diabetes cookbooks when you know what to eat. All you need are recipes that include nutrition information and serving size (number of servings the recipe yields).

TIP

Look for recipes that are based on whole foods and full of fresh vegetables and ingredients that are healthful for those with diabetes. They should be relatively low in fat, especially saturated fat, low in sodium, have a generous serving size so you're satisfied, and don't send you beyond your meal's carb recommendations. Search especially for vegetable recipes, like salads or roasted vegetables with spices, so you can really enjoy the food group that should make up the majority of your diet.

Converting recipes

There's no rule that your collection of recipes that don't include nutrition information have to go into the trash. You can take advantage of the nutrition resources on the Internet to calculate the nutrition information yourself.

Simply research the nutrition data for each ingredient — calories, total fat, saturated fat, total carbohydrate, fiber, protein, and sodium for a good start — and add it all up. Divide the totals by the number of servings you believe the dish should make, and check the result against what you've learned qualifies as a healthy and diabetes-friendly dish. If one of your old standards doesn't seem to make the cut (maybe the cup of lard couldn't pass muster), check Chapter 12 for some potential ingredient substitutions.

Considering Exchanges

Most dietitians and certified diabetes educators use the carbohydrate counting method for teaching nutrition to people with diabetes — counting carb choices. The Diabetic Exchange System was developed over 40 years ago as the best method for teaching healthy eating for diabetes at that time, and the Exchange System still holds some value for explaining healthy eating. The basics of the Exchange System is that all food we eat falls into one of, or a combination of, six categories — starches, fruits, milk, nonstarchy vegetables, meat and meat substitutes, or fats. Foods are placed into a group based on the nutrient makeup of the food item, and the portion size is already specified.

The Exchange System comes with a few benefits. Exchanges guide heart-healthy eating by subdividing meats into lean, medium fat, and high fat meats, and the fat category into monounsaturated, polyunsaturated, and saturated subgroups; exchanges aid in weight management by placing food into the groups based on caloric content; exchanges encourage consuming a variety of foods instead of just focusing on familiar carbohydrates; and carbohydrate counting can be used in combination with the Exchange System.

The Exchange System works by promoting the equal exchange of foods within the same category. For instance, if your nutrition professional gives you three servings of the starch group at breakfast, you can choose either three slices of bread, two slices of bread and ½ cup cooked oatmeal, or 1½ cups cooked oatmeal with no bread at that meal. The choices for how you can mix and match foods from the same food group are endless, and some people find choosing from actual foods easier than strictly carb counting. In any case, looking over the exchange list shows you that healthy eating and effective diabetes self-management don't limit the variety of available food choices. For a complete list of the exchanges, see Appendix A.

3

Eating for Pleasure and Better Health

IN THIS PART . . .

Understand the triggers and cues that cause mindless eating and how your eating behavior can be influenced by food descriptions and container shape and size.

Identify the forces that work against you and your best intentions for healthier eating, and discover how to create an environment that minimizes food-related temptation.

Explore simple eating habits that can help you improve blood glucose control.

Find out how to choose the best foods when shopping to help keep you on track.

Chapter **10**

Exposing Barriers to Healthy Eating

E ven though eating healthfully can be easy, inexpensive, and delicious, there is a widespread belief in the United States and many Westernized countries that it is difficult and expensive. What makes healthy eating so difficult for people? Many factors. The first is a lack of knowledge about how to nourish the body. If you were to ask the average person to name the three macronutrients (which make up the base of complete meals), they probably couldn't tell you. Couple that with decades of savvy advertising that distorts nutritional information and social media influencers who may use posts to sway opinion, and most people are left not knowing where to begin. Toss in busy schedules, a lack of cooking and shopping skills, and limited resources to the mix and a basic human skill that has kept us alive for millennia has been forgotten.

Most people have access to healthy food choices, and healthy food can be just as filling and tasty as unhealthy food. In modern societies, fresh produce often takes a back seat to more popular meat-based protein, and potatoes have become the most consumed vegetable (in the form of French fries). According to the Centers for Disease Control and Prevention only one in ten American adults reported getting enough fruits and vegetables daily as reported in 2023.

Many people also believe that eating healthily is expensive. The evidence for this has been mixed, with the conclusions of some studies contradicting others. It is complicated by the fact that many supermarkets or manufacturers offer specials that tempt consumers to buy discounted processed foods. However, when it comes to the Mediterranean diet, which we consider to be the gold standard of healthy diets, a study published in 2015 by the Miriam Hospital and Rhode Island Food Bank concluded that following a mostly plant-based Mediterranean-style diet (the "plant-based olive oil diet") was significantly cheaper than following the United States Department of Agriculture (USDA)–recommended "MyPlate" guidelines. Further research from Australia in the same year concluded that people with depressive illnesses on a "standard Western diet," which the authors considered to be typical of the general population, could save $22 (AUD) per week by switching to a Mediterranean diet. It has also been noted that if people spend time preparing fresh ingredients from scratch, costs can be reduced across the board.

So, what accounts for this confusion? With two thirds of the population either overweight or obese and type 2 diabetes rates skyrocketing, it's fair to say that healthy eating habits are not the norm. Is all the confusion about healthy eating and the difficulty most people seem to have adopting healthier eating habits all in the mind? In fact, in some significant ways it is.

This chapter explores how brain signals, culture, emotion, and the modern food environment all conspire to distort your concept of healthy eating and sabotage your sincere intentions to eat healthier. Fortunately, because thriving with diabetes means coming to grips with healthy eating, you can find some simple solutions that put you in the driver's seat on the road to better health.

Tracing Changes in the Food Environment

Just thinking of food can have physical effects on humans. But other images and impressions can have virtually the same effect and can keep you thinking about food even when you don't know you're thinking about food.

You may already be familiar with the story of Pavlov's dogs. Ivan Pavlov, a physiologist, was studying how dogs salivate when presented with food — a natural, *unconditioned* response in preparation for eating. But, when Pavlov began ringing a bell each time he brought food to the dogs, he noticed that their salivating could be stimulated by ringing the bell, even if no food was involved. The salivation in response to a bell was an unnatural, *conditioned* response — anticipation.

Your days and nights are now swamped with images and sounds designed to condition a certain response to a particular franchise or brand of food. Even if you've never tasted the food, chances are you have been conditioned to think about it in a certain way — to eat with your eyes. Of course, there's nothing new about advertising. What's new is the intensity of the sights and sounds and the absolute saturation of media. It hasn't always been this way, but there's no changing it now. Commercial food, whether at restaurants or snack-type foods, may not be your only less healthy eating habit, but chances are it has a starring role.

WARNING

The food industry spends as much as $10 billion a year to influence consumers to a brand, and the effectiveness of advertising is a science itself. Don't underestimate the power of advertising — keep your eyes wide open, and your brain on duty.

Surviving scarcity

In this book about meal planning it would be nice to pinpoint its beginnings, but that's not really possible. Human populations began growing plants and domesticating animals with purpose before they were leaving written records. Whatever the date, these ancient attempts to better control the availability of food are the beginnings of meal planning. Some 7,500 years ago, the Sumerians were systematically planting, harvesting, and storing excess food. Agriculture, where the work of a few people can feed many, made large communities possible and helped to fill basic needs for sustenance and security.

But, in spite of this long, long history of attempts to control food supply, scarcity has always been common. And, severe scarcity in localized regions has decimated populations throughout recorded time. In the 20th century alone it's estimated that 70 million people died as a result of food shortages caused by political intention or incompetence, overpopulation, weather patterns, crop destruction by floods or insects, or shortages during war. The great Irish potato famine, caused by a plant disease, is well known in the United States for triggering a wave of immigration from Ireland, but this blight also resulted in more than one million deaths.

Food storage is as important as food production, and archeologists have found grain storage structures that predate agricultural production — ancients were storing foods they collected in the wild. Storing food protects it from spoilage and theft by other animals, protects humans from disease, and greatly increases the security of adequate food. Dry storage, root cellars, meat curing or dehydration, canning, and, of course, refrigeration have contributed mightily to fulfilling this basic human need.

Still, throughout most of history, humans have been forced to carefully plan for the production, acquisition, storage, and preparation of food. Even in the relatively wealthy 20th century United States, family budgeting demanded careful planning for adequate food and sufficient nutrition. Selections were limited by transportation challenges, and the cost of some foods was significantly higher than now in relation to income during much of the 1900s. In 1920, average Americans worked for nearly 3 hours to buy a 3-pound chicken, but today they earn the same chicken in less than 15 minutes. In very real ways, only the wealthy had access to excess calories.

In the 1920s, food expenses represented 25 percent of the average American family's disposable income, and only 14 percent of those food expenditures went for food away from home. By the early 1980s, the cost of food had declined to 12.5 percent of disposable income, but nearly 35 percent of food expenses went for food away from home. The cost of food in 2011 had declined further as a percentage of disposable income, to less than 10 percent, but away-from-home food now accounts for 42 percent of the food budget.

TIP

Numerous studies have shown that we consume more calories when we eat out rather than when we eat at home. One simple way to cut back on your calories is to enjoy more of your meals in your own dining room. And by eating at home, you save money, too!

The rise in the percentage of a family food budget spent away from home tells part of the story of the American diet. But quantity is one thing, quality is another. Entire books have been written about the economic and political forces that make foods packed with fat and added sugar more accessible, and often less costly, than healthier whole food. The important point, however, is that the trend in eating away from home means meal planning, even when a serious condition like diabetes puts long-term health at risk, is too often left to the influence of advertising, rather than the thoughtful consideration of a health-minded consumer.

Being overwhelmed by food

Every nation has its own culinary history, and in many modernized places, a turning point occurred when some of the food-production integrity and freshness was compromised in order to mass-produce shelf-stable foods.

In the United States, many factors influenced our mass-produced food chain. In order for the railroads to deliver food across the nation, food had to be shelf-stable. This need especially grew during World War II, when it was impossible for women to cook because they had to work in factories doing the men's work. Food started to become packaged and sold in cans, and chemical "mixes" replaced homemade cakes, bread, and everything in between. To market and sell the new prepared foods, convincing advertisements told future consumers why those products were more intelligent, healthful, and more hygienic options than their homemade counterparts. Using processed food was portrayed as being savvy and cosmopolitan. Because of this and many other factors, little by little, people stopped cooking homemade meals. And because the changes happened gradually, people adapted to them, without noticing the detriment that they would face to our wellbeing.

To create packaged foods and make them shelf-stable and flavorful, excess salt, sugar, chemical additives, and other ingredients were added. Little by little people forgot both how to cook and how to properly nourish themselves. Advertisements now promote "meals" that have nothing to do with what is nutritionally balanced, but with what products they are trying to sell.

Consider how you're physically surrounded by food constantly — bright-colored restaurants line the main streets, and every convenience store or gas station hides the brake fluid behind rows of candy and snack chips. But, it's not unique signs or colorful packaging that subconsciously invites you to eat freely — it's advertising. Pavlov strikes again.

The following are two important points to keep in mind in regard to the advertising of convenience-food restaurants and snack foods:

>> **Eating away from home is generally significantly less healthy than eating at home.** Study after study, some using data from the Continuing Survey of Food Intake by Individuals (CSFII), has shown that eating away from home, especially quick-service food, results in more calories, more fat, more saturated fat, more sodium, less fiber, less vitamins A and C, less calcium, less magnesium, and fewer fruits and vegetables.

>> **Even if you are absolutely certain that advertising and atmosphere have no influence on you, it's almost certain that you're wrong.** Studies of eating behavior consistently show that humans are influenced by subconscious *cues* and *triggers* on where to eat, what to eat, and how much to eat. One study showed that matched groups of adults who were asked to evaluate the same TV program, but were shown different commercials, ate significantly more of the unhealthy snacks provided if their group was shown commercials for different unhealthy snacks. Participants in eating behavior experiments never believe they have been influenced by subconscious messages, and they're almost always wrong. Advertising has a powerful influence on your behavior.

So, what's the extent of your exposure to the advertising that subconsciously influences you to make unhealthier choices? Data for adults is difficult to find, but adolescents aged 13 to 17 are exposed to more than 6,000 food ads per year, equaling about 40 hours total. Their exposure to ads about nutrition, by contrast, is less than 30 minutes. That's an 80-fold advantage for the poorer choices. The story is, of course, the same for adults. When did you last see advertising for broccoli or any other natural food? The truth is that you are overwhelmed by food-related advertising, virtually none of which represents better choices for your health.

Recognizing Emotional Attachments to Food

The phrase *emotional eating* has come to represent a psychological state where food becomes a means for coping with feelings of anger, sadness, loneliness, or even happiness. Eating in excess as a response to feelings can be emotionally and physically unhealthy, but responding emotionally to eating is something altogether different — it's truly part of your chemistry. Remember that cookie your mother gave you when you scraped your knee? Or that ice cream cone you got when you brought home good grades in second grade? Don't blame your mother. She got the same messages when she was a little girl.

REMEMBER

If you only eat an ice cream cone on occasion, it won't have negative effects on your overall health. It's what we do the majority of the time that matters most.

While we often associate emotional eating with a negative connotation, it doesn't have to be that way. We can use our innate cravings and triggers to both soothe ourselves and eat nutritious foods. This is the basis of the discipline of *culinary medicine*.

TIP

To help identify your emotional triggers to food, make a list of the recipes or foods that you crave often. Then, try to figure out why. If those foods are good for you, such as homemade fresh tomato sauce, for example, then you can continue to enjoy them. If however, they're not healthful, you can identify what it is about them that you enjoy so much, and look for a better-fitting replacement.

It is believed that creamy foods are most comforting when we are stressed or scared. In this case, Greek yogurt, avocados, sugar-free frozen yogurt, and pureed vegetable soups such as cauliflower could be a great swap for unhealthful foods and could help keep your glucose in check.

You may find that at times you crave sweet foods. As humans, milk is our first taste in infancy. The sweetness of the milk triggers the sweet receptors in our brain, which in turn makes us associate sweet flavors with reward, empowerment, and good feelings throughout our lives. It's important to recognize that we are all conditioned this way, and how, as adults we can incorporate healthful, natural sweet flavors into our diets without the harmful effects of sugar or chemical sweeteners.

If you like salty snacks, a light sprinkling of unrefined sea salt on healthful fruits and vegetables drizzled with extra-virgin olive oil is your best bet. The minerals in baby dill also give salty and herbal flavor to food without the negative effects of salt. You can even chop it and add it into things like mashed potatoes. Munching on celery can also cure salt cravings while having a hydrating effect on the body.

You may crave crunchy foods from time to time. Some say this is when we are bored or lack adventure. Kids also love crunchy foods as a rule. Apple slices, unsalted almonds, homemade baked kale or sweet potato chips, carrot, celery, and pepper sticks are great ways to satisfy this urge and increase your nutrient intake without suffering the consequences of unhealthy crunchy foods.

Identifying with a particular culture

Genealogy has become more and more popular, in part because the research tools for tracing your family roots through generations past are now at your fingertips. Sixteenth-century French author and gastronome Jean Anthelme Brillat-Savarin famously said, "Tell me what you eat, and I will tell you who you are."

Just as language, customs, music, and art arise with a cultural identity, so does food. And, as families, ethnicities, and cultures mix, new connections between food and cultural identity form. Your cultural connection with food may be through certain holidays or celebrations, heirloom recipes, a favorite grandmother, your extended families, or your entire community. The important point is that your experience with food as something connecting you with others who are much like you is very deep, even representing, in some measure, who you are in a fundamental way. Food is love.

TIP

One of the ways in which we recommend people celebrate their culinary culture along with practicing healthful eating is to restrict the heavier, less healthful celebratory dishes to holidays. You can still indulge in those emblematic foods a few times a year, but just not on a daily basis. Next, we recommend making a regular habit of enjoying the healthiest ingredients from your own particular culture(s) as often as possible. For example, fresh tomatoes and green vegetables, garlic, chili peppers, and extra-virgin olive oil are both nutritious and symbolic of the Italian kitchen. While lasagna is a dish that is very rich and traditionally served only a few times a year on holidays like Easter in Italy, the previously mentioned ingredients are enjoyed by many people daily along with seafood, vegetables, and nutritious pasta dishes.

REMEMBER

Each and every national cuisine has elements to it that are worth celebrating for both their flavor and their health-promoting compounds; it's up to us to find them.

Making the social connection

Food is likely to be a centerpiece of your social connections, too, and social connections are another aspect of emotional security — you belong somewhere. Whether it's drinking a cup of coffee or tea with friends, cooking hot dogs on a stick over a campfire, monitoring an important business transaction, or planning an elaborate affair like a wedding, food (or drink) is almost always prominent.

Sharing food, for most of history a valuable commodity, has always been a symbolic offer of peace or friendship; the preparation of food for guests or friends demonstrates caring and intimacy. In the most basic sense, sharing food is helping others survive. Even in modern times, enjoying meals with others has many psychological, emotional, and physical health benefits. Eating with others helps us to digest our food better, make healthier food choices, and promotes a sense of wellbeing. If your health is a priority, make it a point to seek out others to eat with on a regular basis. Even school children have been shown to get better grades when they eat at least one meal with their families at home per day.

REMEMBER

It doesn't matter which meal you choose to eat with others. Tailor eating together to your schedule. If breakfast is the only time your family has, that's better than not eating with others when possible.

Food as a gift is common in every society, and how many romantic relationships begin with a shared meal? Restaurants and drinking establishments strive to create a certain ambiance to match different social interactions, from peaceful and quiet to loud and celebratory — an atmosphere for every occasion and mood.

All in all, food is woven intricately into society and into your social connections. Once again, the point is to simply understand that food has a larger role in your life than strictly sustenance and nutrition. When it comes to making conscious choices about your diet, it's important to look deeply into how food connects you to others.

Seeking the pleasure response

While your cerebral cortex is busy calculating away, something has to make sure you remember to drink, sleep, eat, form relationships, and reproduce. Your working brain is on the job, sending and receiving chemical messages here and there to keep essential behaviors humming along.

TECHNICAL
STUFF

Take appetite, for example. Appetite isn't quite this simple, but in a simplified context the hormones *ghrelin* and *leptin* are fairly straightforward. Ghrelin is released by stomach cells to signal your working brain that you are hungry. As you eat, stored fat cells release the hormone leptin, signaling your brain you have had enough food — your hunger is satisfied. Because eating is a behavior that is absolutely essential to your survival, however, another part of your working brain wants to personally thank you for eating, and helps you create a fond memory so you remember that eating is good the next time you encounter food.

Your reward is a dose of the *neurotransmitter* dopamine, and dopamine is the ultimate feel-good chemical. Dopamine is so powerful that addictive drugs such as cocaine, heroin, and amphetamines, are addictive to some extent because they stimulate dopamine release. Dopamine keeps you coming back.

This *reward pathway,* which also can include other neurotransmitters like *serotonin* and *endorphins,* reinforces learning through reward, and is a factor in motivating the essential survival behaviors of all higher order animals. Your working brain rewards you for eating whenever you have food available. Your working brain does not understand that you always have food available, or that you really don't need special memories or rewards for eating whenever food is available. This particular responsibility assigned to your working brain is outdated in an advanced and affluent human society, but there's no off switch.

Without proper supervision, the wonderful, chemically induced feelings that are intended to reinforce essential survival behavior can make overconsumption difficult to control. Recent research employing powerful brain scans suggests that some foods activate the same areas of the brain as commonly abused drugs. And, just as decreasing sensitivity to dopamine keeps drug users increasing drug dosage for the same dopamine reward, recent research is finding that obese people may eat more food for similar reasons. Obese people, it seems, have fewer dopamine receptors than normal-weight people, and may not get the same reward.

The reinforcing role of the reward pathway also involves the creation of fond memories, as mentioned earlier. To the working brain it's important that when you encounter a hamburger you recall that previous hamburgers have been good. But this response isn't limited to encountering an actual hamburger — the reward pathway is stimulated by images of hamburgers or by thoughts of hamburgers, too. In this regard, you are Pavlov's dog, and advertising is the bell. Advertising images trigger a conditioned response to food through your outdated reward pathway.

Lastly, overeating for the sheer delight of dopamine and other pleasure stimulating neurotransmitters might not be much of a concern if broccoli triggered the same response as donuts; however, this part of your working brain is all about survival and scarcity, and, therefore, favors energy-dense food. Fat, with

9 calories per gram, is more than double the energy density of either carbohydrate or protein, and brain research shows that both fat and sugar activate the reward pathway. Some contend that a combination of fat, sugar, and salt is actually addictive. The bottom line is that a marvelous biological system, which is essential for survival when food is scarce, contributes to excessive eating when food is plentiful, and even stimulates addictive-like behavior when food and food images are inescapable.

TIP

The good news is that there are other ways to increase dopamine in the body than just eating addictive foods. Exercising regularly in a way that you enjoy most, getting physical activity of any form, eating quality protein, taking care of your gut health, listening to a song you like, looking at something beautiful such as flowers or art, sleeping enough, meditating, basking in the sunlight, and getting fresh air are other great ways to boost dopamine without having to sacrifice your blood sugar levels. Actually, the items just mentioned can actually help to lower blood glucose levels and stress as well.

Losing logic to impulse from stress

Your thinking brain has the power and the authority to override your more primitive survival instincts related to food. In fact, your ability to imagine and understand future consequences helps keep all sorts of impulsive behaviors in check every day. As long as your cerebral cortex is on duty, it has the final say. About the only time this chain of command gets short-circuited is when you are threatened.

TECHNICAL
STUFF

The primitive threat response is often called the *fight or flight* response, and the decision between fighting or fleeing has no time allowance for the sort of expert deliberative consideration your thinking brain is so good with. Instead, your working brain takes control in an emergency response to heighten senses, make energy resources available, and supercharge strength for fighting or fleeing by dumping adrenaline and other chemicals into your system. This intense response to threat puts your *sympathetic* nervous system in charge, and input from your thinking brain is irrelevant. The stress stimulated by a threat is all about reflex, impulse, and reaction — no thinking is required.

Fortunately, most of you are not subjected to real threats on a regular basis, and in a more controlled circumstance — a carnival ride or skydiving — you might even seek out the intense physical thrill of the threat response. In modern societies, however, researchers are beginning to identify potential consequences to health of chronic, low-level stress.

WARNING

Low levels of constant stress from long work hours, too little physical activity, balancing relationships, financial worries, or health concerns like diabetes seems to have a distinctly negative impact on health. Chronic stress may also inhibit your capacity to make wise decisions about food.

Some researchers believe that chronic stress levels keep the sympathetic nervous system turned on, literally reducing your willpower and making impulsive eating more likely. Stated simply, your difficulties sticking with a healthy eating plan, when you clearly understand the long-term advantages of healthier eating, may be in part because a threat-like response to low-level stress turns down the volume of your thinking brain.

Other stress-increasing situations are directly associated with eating behavior as well. Moderate sleep deprivation, certainly not uncommon, disrupts the appetite hormones by increasing levels of the hunger hormone ghrelin and reducing levels of the satiety hormone leptin. Ultimately, stress is not only unhealthy by itself, but may very well inhibit your capacity to make logical decisions about your lifestyle.

TIP

The average adults needs seven to nine hours sleep every night — those who sleep consistently less don't perform as well on complex mental tests. Worse, studies show that adults who get less, or even much more, than seven hours of sleep each night have a higher mortality rate and a higher body mass index than adults who get seven to nine hours of sleep regularly.

Uncovering the mindless subconscious

Adults are not very gullible. It may take a hard lesson or two along the way, but eventually you can spot a load of manure a mile off. But, the truth is you are fooled every single day when it comes to food, and in some cases you're both the fooler and the fooled. And if you don't believe it, that's exactly what the research says you would think. Virtually everyone who's fooled in a food study swears they won't be.

Dr. Brian Wansink is a leading researcher into eating behavior, especially what he calls *mindless eating.* His carefully disguised experiments at the University of Illinois and Cornell University have demonstrated how your eating behavior can be significantly influenced by food descriptions, container size, whether your food waste is removed from your sight, and especially your surroundings.

Controlled experiments on eating behavior demonstrate something you probably already know — it's a little unnatural to think about food. The truth is that this lack of awareness makes you a potential sucker for being tricked into overeating — but who's doing the tricking? A restaurant owner who's trying to maximize profit may be doing you a favor by tricking you into eating less. However, that is not normally the case. In order to stay profitable in the United States, most restaurateurs offer large amounts of lesser quality foods. Most American diners like to feel that they are getting a lot of "bang for their buck" but this leads to "portion distortion" — meaning that those same diners then tend to no longer realize what an actual portion is when dining at home.

You eat less, studies show, if you eat off of a smaller plate. That may explain why single-price buffets often put out smaller plates, but the owners could increase their profits even more if they put the buffet out of sight. Mindless eating doesn't always work to your disadvantage, but more often than not it does.

REMEMBER

Ultimately, you are more often your own worst enemy. Scan your kitchen or office, and note what kinds of foods are in plain sight, ready to be scooped up when you begin grazing. It's very likely that you don't apply the "out of sight, out of mind" strategy to foods that are best eaten in moderation. How often do you purchase the larger size snack because it seems like a better deal, even though the actual cost is greater? Is supersizing your convenience food meals irresistible as a financial investment to you? Do you always assume the salad is the healthier choice without ever bothering to actually find out?

Early in this chapter this question was left unanswered — is the difficulty most people seem to have adopting healthier eating habits all in the mind? You can see now that much of the difficulty is all in the mind — in the brain, to be precise. But, if you took the phrase *all in the mind* as hinting at some weakness in character, maybe you can see now how wrong that assumption would be.

Food is a fundamental need, and having an adequate supply of food is a biological mission for every human. Food is such a key to survival that it's woven into your emotional identity as a member of a family, a culture, or a society. In modern, affluent societies, however, you are surrounded by convenience foods. The formulations of these unhealthy, high-fat, high-sugar convenience foods are especially effective at triggering your brain's natural reward feedback loop, where the release of neurotransmitters like dopamine creates a biological urge to have more. Images and advertisements for these foods, which saturate your environment, stimulate the same urges as having the actual food. In a significant way, the interplay between human biology and the modern food environment is expressed in skyrocketing rates of obesity and type 2 diabetes, and this unhealthy cycle of stimulus and reward may be a frustrating part of your life, too. There are, however, solutions.

Eating Healthier Forever

It would be going too far to say that you are completely powerless to resist the subconscious influence of unhealthy food, and helpless to win the battle for control of your working brain against focused and well-financed advertisers. But, whereas awareness of what's responsible for your history of less-than-healthy eating habits improves your understanding, it's still true that if you keep doing what you've always done, you keep getting what you've always gotten. Something needs to change.

Obviously, eating healthier foods is the simple answer, but it probably hasn't been simple so far, and now you know how some of the influences on your eating behavior go much deeper than simply deciding to eat differently. With diabetes and your health so closely associated with the eating behaviors, however, the stakes are greater than ever. Fortunately, you have one amazing asset on your side — your cerebral cortex, the most incredible thinking brain in the history of the world.

And the secret to eating healthy in this modern, affluent society, where unhealthy options exert so much influence, is to let your thinking brain do what it does best — plan. Planning is how individuals and organizations stay on track when surrounded by distractions and temptations — well thought-out, guiding decisions, made with a clear, long-term vision, can be more powerful than all distractions and temptations. Setting a new course for thriving with diabetes starts with minimizing the distractions and temptations in your life, and lets your thinking brain do the planning that keeps you on track.

Creating the right environment

Establishing an environment that minimizes the food-related temptations, which are reinforced by your working brain's chemical stew, could start by moving to the far reaches of Alaska or Wyoming and declining TV, telephone, or internet service. That may make getting important regular medical care for your diabetes more challenging, however. A better alternative might be to simply modify your own food environment to whatever extent you can. Although it may sound overly simple, the benefits can be amazing.

The previous section explained how *cues* and *triggers* in the media, your community, and your immediate environment influence unhealthy eating habits, but this is only a problem because the huge majority of cues and triggers are associated with unhealthy choices. It's unlikely you see many influences toward healthier foods in media advertising, but you can build an environment in your home and office that turns mindless behavior in your favor. You can fool yourself to be healthier. Always remember that "health is wealth" and that by choosing delicious and nutritious foods you can triumph over diabetes.

TIP

Take inventory of your home and anyplace else you hang out, like your office. What kinds of food have you stockpiled? Is there anything healthy, like fresh fruit, or some low-carbohydrate vegetables? Check to see if your less-healthy choices are the ones right out in plain view, begging you to grab a bite every time you glance up or walk by? Nobody says you can never snack, even on something that won't make anyone's list of healthy foods, but give yourself the chance to make better choices, or to forget you have cheese curls in the house.

Make some decisions about what foods you must have now and then, like chocolate, and eliminate stuff that just happens to be lying around. Choose the best options for snacks, like dark chocolate instead of milk chocolate, and hide it away so you're not reminded constantly. Display healthier foods, like fresh fruit, in plain view so cues and triggers to eat work in your favor (and you remember to count the carbohydrates in foods like fruit).

And, when it comes to actually eating, try the following tricks:

>> **Eat with others whenever possible.** This improves digestion, our mental state, and causes us to eat less, among many other things.

>> **Never eat snacks directly from the container.** Take an actual serving according to the label, and put the container completely away. This habit allows your thinking brain to ask you hard questions when you consider retrieving the container for another serving.

>> **You eat less if you eat off of smaller plates.** If you're not in the market for new dishware, practice putting much less food on your plate, and leave the second helping across the room instead of in a serving bowl that's sitting right in front of you. A trip across the room can really discourage additional eating in a mindless way.

>> **Incorporate a healthy, vegetable-forward appetizer.** Start with a salad of colorful vegetables with a good-quality extra-virgin olive oil and lemon juice or vinegar into your meals, and give the first course time to communicate with your brain before you gobble down the main course. It takes 20 minutes for your brain to get the all-full signal.

>> **Chew your food thoroughly.** In fact, chew it beyond what it normally takes for you to swallow. Time is your friend in healthier eating habits.

>> **Don't eat in front of the television.** Anything that takes your attention away from your food and your level of satisfaction and satiety opens the door for mindless overeating.

>> **Change your habits.** If you always sit down at 10 p.m. with a bowl of ice cream, try swapping out ½ cup of full-fat plain Greek yogurt with a few berries or a drizzle of olive oil. This helps to keep your blood sugar levels balanced during the night while giving you the snack you crave.

Asking for help when needed

If this chapter seems overwhelming to you, or you have tried to change your eating habits without luck in the past, you may want to seek out additional help. Nowadays there are so many qualified professionals to help with diabetes-friendly diets and nutrition, that it might be more challenging to select the person right for you than it is to find someone qualified.

Before reaching out for help, examine what you need most. Are you trying to transform negative habits? If so, a certified health coach or nutritionist may help. Sometimes habits have deeper routes that require mental counseling and psychological therapies to overcome. Or, you may have a challenging life situation that keeps you from eating well. In that case, seeking out help to cope with that particular crisis not only helps you to feel better, it also has an impact on your blood sugar and eating habits.

Planning: Deciding what to eat in advance

Your incredible thinking brain is a planner, and if you give it room to make your most important decisions, like how to improve your eating habits for diabetes, it will shine. If you call on your thinking brain to rescue you when you're stressed and surrounded by tempting, unhealthy food choices, it may ask you to call back later after it's had time to think about the issues for a while. When it comes to food, impulse often wins the spur-of-the-moment decisions. Impulse has a lot of support from that part of your brain, with its chemical reward system, that wants you to eat everything you see for survival in times of shortage.

The solution is actually simpler than you think, but it's something too many people in our society don't do anymore — decide what you're going to eat in advance. Making food-related decisions ahead of time, when you're not directly confronted with the cues and triggers that lead you down the wrong path, can disarm those influences that sabotage your best intentions, including your working brain. And, in some ways, facing the responsibility to manage your diabetes can be the final push that motivates you to begin thinking more about the foods you eat.

Planning ahead starts with a making a menu for your week's meals (or your month's meals, if planning is easy for you). Your diabetes meal plan provides a template for choosing food groups, especially your daily carbohydrate choices, but you fill in the actual foods and recipes. Chapter 17 gives you a sample menu and tells how to prepare it. But, you can also plan a menu yourself after you accept that thinking about food is simply necessary, no matter how unnatural it seems at first. Chapter 13 gives you step-by-step instructions.

Your second assignment is to make a shopping list, and because you're making wise decisions in advance with the assistance of your marvelous thinking brain, load your list with wise choices for healthy eating. And, if you make your list carefully, you can float right by all of the temptations that impulse might have had you reaching for in the past. Chapter 12 takes you on a grocery tour, and explains how to make wiser choices and where you'll find them.

Your final assignment is to learn to plan ahead when you're eating out. Frankly, this couldn't be simpler now that restaurants post their menus and nutrition information online. By scanning the choices and making your decisions before you're bathed in ambiance and check out what was just delivered at the next table, impulse doesn't rule the day again. Eating out is challenging, but Chapter 15 guides you in making the better choices for your diabetes.

IN THIS CHAPTER

» Accepting key personal and family commitments to health

» Learning simple eating habits that can improve blood glucose control

» Setting yourself up for success

» Getting help when you need it

» Patting yourself on the back

Chapter **11**

Setting Priorities and Staying on Track

I f you read almost any of the previous chapters you may have been surprised, or even shocked, to learn that you have so much power in affecting your own health. It's your new management job — diabetes self-management. Even though you never filled out an application and almost certainly weren't prepared or fully qualified for the job, you were put in charge of your own long-term health as soon as you were first diagnosed with diabetes. The truth is, all of us are always responsible for our health and longevity, but the modern medical paradigm is often focused on sickness, which means people tend to take their health for granted until they are no longer well. Taking good care of yourself is the most important job you have, and if you do it well, the payback is enormous.

You may have this eating-healthy-for-diabetes thing mastered already, but are looking for additional ways to increase the flavor in your foods and enjoy positive lifestyle changes. For many, probably most, though, eating appropriately now represents significant lifestyle changes. Lasting lifestyle changes are simply not easy to make, and anyone who has tried to lose weight can back that statement up. New behaviors are necessary, but before action comes attitude. And a new attitude can make all the difference.

In this chapter, we show you the importance of acknowledging the challenges of lifestyle change, how to stay committed to a healthier lifestyle, and some expert tips for staying on track.

Committing to Your Future

The future can be hard to think about. After all, for most people the demands on time and attention today and tomorrow are enough to keep them completely occupied. If you have type 1 diabetes, the daily contest to balance eating with your insulin injections probably puts the immediate dangers of very low and very high blood glucose in the front of your mind. Advances in continuous glucose monitoring with the technology to automatically dispense the insulin required are enabling people with type 1 diabetes to understand and control blood glucose levels much better. But, for many with type 2 diabetes, there aren't any daily reminders that diabetes needs more attention than taking a pill. A common response from patients to doctor or educator concerns about high A1Cs is, "But I feel fine."

The most serious threats to health for people with diabetes are in the future, something from the list of health effects we have innocently called complications. But, there is nothing innocent about diabetes complications. Some complications are life changing without being life threatening, like sexual dysfunction, but others are disabling or deadly, like kidney failure or heart attack. Two things all diabetes complications have in common, however, is they take time to develop — they are in the future — and they are much easier to prevent than to "fix" once they begin. Healthy eating for diabetes is about preventing complications later. The exception to this was the experience of people with type 2 diabetes during the COVID-19 pandemic. There is evidence that those with poorly controlled type 2 diabetes were at significantly increased risk of more severe illness.

The process of changing your lifestyle today needs a commitment from you, a commitment to your future, whatever you want that to be. Experts suggest visualizing, and most of us do that already when we daydream or imagine what we would like our future to include. Maybe you look forward to grandchildren, or maybe your dream is playing professional basketball. Visualizing is simply serious imagining — really feeling the details of what that perfect future will be like. Visualizing is positive and optimistic, and your vision of your future should not include having your life derailed by serious diabetes complications.

Adhering to a new philosophy

Behavior change experts recommend making your visualizations more real by writing them down and by collecting photos or objects that relate to your goals.

Having your own personal take on "eating healthfully" can also help to keep you on track. There has to be a buy-in for people to be successful with change. For some people, eating and living better to avoid future complications is motivation enough; others need spiritual reasoning or scientific logic in order to really make the new lifestyle be significant to them.

Making a personal commitment to managing diabetes well and eating healthy can keep diabetes squeezed down into the smallest possible part of your perfect future. Even if you don't quite have a grasp on exactly what you need to do (we're getting to that part), making this decision now is easy. It's all about attitude.

TIP

Once you've written down your goals, you can compile them into a new story for yourself. Write down, in present tense, a dream scenario of your health and life, if you choose to do so. Describe, in present tense, how great you feel when you wake up in the morning, the wonderful things that you smell, taste, touch, and feel during your day. Write down what you love most as if you are doing it, for example, "I love going for walks with my best friend" and "It feels great to spend so much time with family." Describe your ideal day and health with as much sentiment and description of how you want to feel.

Make this your new story and read it to yourself daily, morning and night, or whenever you are feeling stressed. Next, extract ten affirmations from the story and write them down in the notebook. For example, "I am happy and healthy" and "I feel great all of the time" are wonderful additions. Use them as a mantra and repeat them over and over as much as possible. This visualizing, writing down, and affirming helps pave the groundwork to make it easier for you to stay committed and achieve your goals.

TIP

Many people like to create vision boards that represent the way they would like to look and feel to gaze at for inspiration every day. It's also important to celebrate every victory, no matter how small. If you give yourself credit for the simple things such as drinking more water, walking a bit extra, or taking the stairs instead of the elevator, you are much more likely to stay on track with your new philosophy. It's also a great idea to set an intention each week and morning with goals for yourself. Think of creative ways to overcome any barriers in advance so that you can be better prepared to deal with them when they come up.

Making time for healthy eating

In the 1970s, as the potential for new technologies to improve worker productivity were becoming a reality, social scientists speculated that people in the 21st century would be challenged with how to spend an over-abundance of leisure time. Things haven't exactly turned out that way. Ironically, the years since then have seen the appearance of convenience stores, fast-food restaurants,

ATMs, and all sorts of technologies and services marketed to save time (for some reason mobile dog grooming comes to mind).

Because time is limited to 24 hours each day, you choose how you spend the time you have. It may seem like there aren't choices involved, but how you spend time represents how you prioritize time. Setting priorities always involves choices, and making a commitment to your future health may include reprioritizing how you spend some of your time.

Healthy eating involves time to plan, shop, prepare food, and keep yourself motivated. When you commit to healthy eating, the time spent on this commitment becomes, by definition, important. When an activity is accepted as an essential part of your schedule, the stresses of feeling like time is wasted are removed, and you can give yourself permission to actually enjoy the time. Healthy eating can be special family time or an adventure.

REMEMBER

You don't have to be a chef to learn to love cooking, and you will improve and get faster with time. A meal that takes you a while to prepare in the beginning will get faster with time as you continue to practice cooking.

Wondering where you'll find the time? Get out your pad and pen again (you will use more paper later, so bring extra). It's always revealing to write down where all of that time goes, and even more interesting to see what can be adjusted without missing anything. When you consider the importance of a healthy lifestyle to yourself and your family, you may discover that it isn't difficult to find a few minutes to improve your eating habits.

Enjoying the process

Conscious eating is a term used to describe the act of slowing down and enjoying the food we eat. It's important to remember that food was created for both pleasure and health. By setting aside time to make a meal special, taking time to appreciate its aroma and the way it looks, savoring it slowly, and being grateful go a long way to improve our mental and physical health.

Studies have shown that if we smell food being cooked prior to eating it, or hear it described in detail, we actually digest the food more slowly and feel full quicker. In the courts of the Abbasid Caliphate in Medieval Baghdad, poems were recited to dinner guests prior to eating food. While that sounds extreme by today's standards, it was a very advanced practice for its time. In addition to offering pleasing words to diners, the poems made for a more healthful dining experience. Saying positive affirmations, listening to beautiful music, and talking about pleasant things while eating also make the experience more pleasurable.

REMEMBER

Inconvenience, like beauty, is in the eye of the beholder. The intent of this chapter's discussion about fully committing to diabetes self-management and healthy eating is to elevate the importance of this task among your many priorities. When tasks are seen as important, the effort required can be accepted as an investment, not an inconvenience. You may find, for instance, that when you accept the importance of preparing healthy meals at home, you begin to enjoy cooking.

The truth is that no matter how committed you become, some aspects of diabetes self-management are simply inconvenient. People with type 1 diabetes understand this all too well. There's really no case to make that sticking your finger for a blood glucose test eight or ten times a day should be enjoyable. Nor can lugging around syringes, insulin, a meter, and test strips; or dealing with low blood glucose in an important meeting; or getting an alarm from an insulin pump while waiting in line at the department of motor vehicles.

People with type 2 diabetes don't usually share the same kind of frustration that comes with type 1, where it's impossible to "escape" for more than a few hours. Still, each person is different, and what comes easily to one person may be extraordinarily frustrating and inconvenient for another.

The bottom line is that dealing with a certain amount of genuine inconvenience is necessary if you're going to manage diabetes well and eat healthy. This book is filled with advice and tips that help make your diabetes meal planning easier, but accepting the unavoidable inconveniences with a smile is the only solution in some cases.

Learning new things

You may have noticed there is crucial but very simple information you need to know about food, such as which foods contain carbohydrate. Other necessary knowledge is somewhat more challenging — translating nutrition facts label information into a carb-counting format, for instance. Calculating insulin-to-carbohydrate ratios is another step beyond for those taking fast-acting insulin injections with meals, in part because being accurate is so important. We discuss calculating insulin rations in greater detail in *Diabetes For Dummies*, 6th Edition (Wiley).

Nevertheless, it's all too common to find otherwise extremely intelligent people who seemingly can't understand and apply the simplest facts about diabetes and nutrition. The issue isn't a shortage of brain power, but a refusal to think analytically about food. For some it's a rebellion against the unfairness of this demand, as if refusing to acknowledge diabetes can make it go away. For others, it's simply the view that eating should not require thinking.

Your new task as your own diabetes manager — that job you did not ask for — requires that you use your brain some. The thinking required is well within the range of most any adult who is willing to learn and, like any skill, gets easier as time passes. But no matter what your age, a commitment to your future health includes engaging your brain for healthy eating. In this case eating does not require thinking, but everything else until your plate is loaded does.

WARNING

Some personalities are virtually the opposite, absorbing every detail about diabetes and healthy eating like a mad scientist. Knowing the information without applying it, however, accomplishes no more than not knowing in the first place.

Standing your ground

After you make a commitment to your future health, reprioritize your time, accept the inconveniences of managing diabetes, and engage your brain for learning new things, one unexpected stumbling block may remain. You may find a lack of support from family and/or friends. It may take the form of whining from the family about changes in food options, or of friends urging you to stop being a party pooper. In most cases there's no intentional effort to sabotage your commitment to healthy eating, and a serious discussion about your reasons may resolve the stress. If the conflict continues, something more confrontational may be required, including an option for family counseling or finding new friends.

REMEMBER

A healthful diet for diabetes is a healthy diet for everyone. Targeted at heart health and weight management, the focus on carbohydrates is the only part of a healthful diabetes eating plan that's unique to people with diabetes. The changes you bring to your family's diet are most likely appropriate and beneficial to everyone. The dietary advice in this book is great for anyone who is aspiring to living a long and healthy life as well as for those who want an enjoyable and tasty menu.

Adopting Better Habits

So much of healthy behaviors, or not healthy behaviors, are simply the result of habits. The Merriam-Webster online dictionary defines *habit* as "an acquired mode of behavior that has become nearly or completely involuntary." Habits are learned, and old habits can be replaced by new ones. Many habits are helpful to improving blood glucose control, heart health, and weight management, but two are especially relevant to meal planning.

Eating at home more often

You only need to browse the nutrition information provided on the websites of your favorite restaurants to get an idea of how difficult it can be to eat healthy when eating out. Just scan the sodium content to keep your search simple, remembering that the population with diabetes falls into the "special" category with a daily sodium recommendation of 1,500 milligrams per day.

REMEMBER

Sugar and unhealthy fats are the easiest way to add flavor to food, and as a result, many restaurants rely on them for inexpensive additions. When you cook at home, or even assemble a few fresh ingredients, you can avoid this pitfall.

A report from the Keystone Forum on Away-From-Home Foods, commissioned by the U.S. Food and Drug Administration cited research that showed the following:

» Eating out more frequently is associated with obesity, higher body fatness, and higher body mass index.

» Women who eat out more often (more than five times per week) consume about 290 more calories on average each day than women who eat out less often.

» Eating more fast-food meals is linked to eating more calories, more saturated fat, fewer fruits and vegetables, and less milk.

So, does this all mean you should never eat away from home? Of course not. One key to success in eating healthy for diabetes is to avoid feelings of being deprived, and eating away from home is often associated with important social connections. Skipping these social occasions would certainly lead to frustration. And, people with diabetes who travel for work or pleasure must eat away from home for all practical purposes. For these reasons Chapter 15 is dedicated to helping you learn to eat away from home wisely. But make no mistake about it, eating a healthy diet away from home is challenging and the more often one eats out, the more important it becomes to plan carefully.

Eating more often at home not only makes it easier to know exactly what you are eating as it relates to diabetes management, it actually allows you to control what you are eating. Ask yourself if eating away from home as often as you do has simply become an ill-advised habit. If the answer is yes, it's time for a better habit.

Timing is everything

To say that timing is everything may apply better to stock market trades or hitting a baseball than to eating with diabetes, but the timing of your meals and snacks and medication can be important in several ways.

The most direct timing relationship, and the most important, is the timing between injecting or bolusing with rapid or short-acting insulin and eating carbohydrate food. These insulin varieties are formulated to take effect lowering blood glucose relatively quickly (5 minutes to 1 hour) and reach peak activity relatively soon (30 minutes to 3 hours). Unless taken specifically to lower high blood glucose levels, this insulin is intended to be followed by ingestion of a certain number of carbohydrate grams. A lapse in proper timing here can result in dangerously low blood glucose levels.

Timing is less critical, but still important for long-acting insulin and for some oral diabetes medications where low blood glucose is a potential side effect. Overall, eating on a regular schedule, following your dietitian's meal plan recommendations by spreading carbohydrates throughout the day, and not skipping meals can improve blood glucose control, especially after meals.

WARNING

Meal skipping, especially skipping breakfast, can sabotage one other important mission for a statistical majority of people with type 2 diabetes weight loss. We have already discussed why weight management is so important and how even a modest loss of body weight can have profound benefits to blood sugar control. Although it may seem logical that skipping the calories from an entire meal would promote weight loss, that logic doesn't hold up. On the other hand, breakfast is not a magic meal where you eat anything you want and watch the weight fall off. Breakfast — breaking the overnight fast — should include carbohydrates for energy and protein for feeling full enough to pass on the donuts you find at the office or the bank — or the donut shop.

For many, skipping breakfast is not a misplaced weight-loss strategy, but rather is an issue of time. Mornings can be frantic, and waiting a few minutes for a bowl of oatmeal can simply seem difficult. But, a healthy breakfast is too important, and this problem of timing is too easy to resolve. Breakfast is a priority, and therefore gets its necessary time.

The National Weight Control Registry is a database of individuals who qualify by having lost at least 30 pounds and by keeping lost weight off for a minimum of one year. The group is a valuable source of information to define weight-loss strategies that have proven successful. When it comes to eating breakfast, 78 percent of this group report eating breakfast every day, and 90 percent report eating breakfast at least five days per week. That is a strong hint that breakfast is a key part of reaching weight-loss goals.

TIP

When traveling across several time zones, talk to your doctor about how to adjust your medication, including insulin. Going by local time at your destination can result in taking doses too close together or too far apart, depending upon which direction you travel.

Staying on Track

Your dedicated change in diabetes health behaviors sparked by a newly found commitment to your future health comes with one ironclad guarantee — detours. Other labels like setback, failure, falling off the wagon, relapse, collapse, defeat, or breakdown may be commonly used, but those labels don't apply if you stay committed. *Detour* is the word. Detours are diversions that not only find the way straight back to the intended route, but also make forward progress along the way. Staying on track includes the detours.

Discovering delicious solutions

If a new focus on healthy eating for diabetes management is going to take root and grow, then feeling deprived of delicious food that satisfies your taste buds or an adequate amount of food can't be part of the plan. Even though you may be working to transition from too many calories and too much fat, there is a distinct difference between feeling unfamiliar with a new habit and feeling deprived. Finding a reasonably acceptable balance is key.

Balancing starts with flavor. There's much empty space available between your mother's recipe for cheese and bacon broccoli casserole (with cracker topping) and a plain, steamed broccoli stalk, but this sort of drastic leap from one to the other is common. And, it's commonly not successful. For some people this feels like the right approach because they expect suffering to be key part of a better eating plan. Suffering and deprivation can motivate action, but the action is fueled by defiance and is simply not sustainable. Luckily, there are tasty, health-promoting ways to enjoy our favorite foods. Tossing the broccoli in extra-virgin olive oil with garlic and chilies is a great way to enhance the flavor and antioxidant compounds, for example.

So, how can you find delicious recipes that are still okay for diabetes? You look for them — they are everywhere. Worldwide, 415 million people are currently living with diabetes, and the U.S. market for diabetes is currently estimated at 37.3 million individuals, so you might expect to find recipe options targeted at a market that size, and you can. We suggest you begin with a book that describes both the medical aspect of diabetes and offers great recipes, too, such as *Diabetes For Dummies* (Wiley). Ultimately, you can easily adapt virtually any recipe that's generally healthy to be "diabetes friendly."

REMEMBER

Just don't settle for food that's less than delicious and satisfying. The challenges that naturally come with any effort to change habits are challenge enough. There's no rule that forbids enjoying yourself along the way.

Embracing imperfection

Want to know the surest and quickest way to become completely disenchanted with your diabetes management efforts? Simply expect perfection and wait a day or two.

Starting any lifestyle change with unreasonable expectations is a certain path to disappointment. Unreasonable expectations can apply to both the anticipated results like an extreme weight loss or lofty goal to improve A1C, or your own capacity to carry out an overly ambitious plan. Going from a mostly sedentary lifestyle to running five miles every day, for example, is likely to be discouraging starting on day one.

But, even if you have kept your expectations reasonable, sometimes things just don't go the way they should. Religiously cutting 500 calories per day for a week to lose one pound, according to the standard formula, may not work precisely for you the first week. Covering 45 grams of carbohydrate with your mathematically perfect and proven five units of insulin won't keep your blood sugar levels perfect every time. There are simply too many variables for perfection.

The real risk with unmet expectations is that constant disappointment and frustration can lead you to stop trying. Wandering away from your meal plan one time shouldn't trigger weeks of unmanaged binge eating, but that's an all too common response among dieters. Likewise, an unexplainable glitch now and then with your insulin/carbohydrate equation is no reason to stop pre-meal blood glucose testing in favor of guessing.

TIP

Embrace imperfection because imperfection is reality. Focus on the big picture: adopting healthier behaviors. Weight loss is about eating fewer calories on average and increasing physical activity slowly but surely. Glycemic control comes when you are more often in a normal blood glucose range than a higher than normal range. It's simple arithmetic that three steps forward and two steps back equals one step forward — and that's progress. If we reject expectations of perfection, accepting detours as reality, success is infinitely easier to find.

A survey of more than 2,000 members of the website https://sparkamerica.com looked to identify keys to successful weight loss. Among the common characteristics of strong starters, who lost five times more weight than false starters, was listing their number one goal as "building a strong foundation of healthy habits." On the other hand, false starters tended to list a number, like lose 4 pounds in two weeks, as their main goal. Two-thirds of false starters lost momentum in two weeks, 18 percent after just three days.

Ignoring fads and quick fixes

A study by researchers at Oregon State University looked at available evidence for hundreds of weight-loss supplements and concluded that no research evidence exists that any single product results in significant weight loss — and many have detrimental health benefits. The magic pill doesn't exist, yet Americans spend an estimated $2.4 billion each year on the promises of a shortcut. The language sounds legitimate — guaranteed, scientific breakthrough, money back if not satisfied. And most have personal testimonies, complete with before and after photos to prove the point. Don't believe it.

REMEMBER

Dietary supplements are not approved by the FDA, nor are they tested for effectiveness or safety. Even invasive treatments like injections claiming to dissolve fat are not regulated in the way you might expect. And the FDA's case files support the Oregon State University study's statement that weight-loss supplements can be dangerous.

By the way, the history of weight-loss drugs that have been approved by the FDA is not a glowing success story. Drug after drug approved for weight loss has been pulled from use after side effects proved to be more dangerous than the extra weight. Fenfluramine with phentermine (fen-phen), dexfenfluramine (Redux), and sibutramine (Meridia) are a few examples. The search for safe and effective weight-loss medication continues.

ASK THE DOCTOR

Some medications for type 2 diabetes have been shown to help people lose weight. For example, the weekly semaglutide injection (brand name Ozempic), which can be used as an appetite suppressant as well as to stimulate insulin release, has been licensed for weight loss in patients without diabetes who are considered to be obese and have very high BMIs. Such medications are also used in some countries by people who are not obese and who don't have type 2 diabetes. While this may be useful for a small number of people who are morbidly obese and under a doctor's supervision, Dr. Simon Poole cautions against reliance on this kind of injection for weight loss alone unless recommended by your doctor, particularly because of the possibility of regaining weight after a course of treatment as well as the risk of side effects and of it being a shortcut to weight reduction without the benefits of a healthful diet and lifestyle.

Claims for a diabetes cure are common also, often promoted with the ominous "what your doctor won't tell you" accusation or "the best kept secret" revelation. The story here is much the same; if it sounds too good to be true, it probably is. Ironically, reading the fine print of some diabetes-cure claims often reveal a program focused on a new healthy diet and plenty of physical activity, as if this approach was a secret.

The scientific consensus is that diabetes can't be cured, but it is certainly possible for type 2 diabetes to be put into remission through the proper lifestyle changes. Researchers focused on type 1 diabetes have done transplants of the insulin-producing pancreatic islet cells with some limited success. Other type 1 research aims at stopping the renegade immune system attack on islet cells or developing an "artificial pancreas." For type 2 diabetes, certain bariatric surgical procedures (gastric bypass) have proven effective at bringing blood glucose levels back into normal range even without medication. The success of these surgeries is generally not labeled as a cure, but rather a remission.

The artificial pancreas is actually a closed-loop information exchange between a continuous blood glucose sensor and an insulin pump. Many people already use sensors and pumps, and in 2023, the FDA approved a combination of the two that is fully automated to keep blood glucose at a normal level without the participation of the patient.

REMEMBER

In many cases the high blood glucose levels that define type 2 diabetes can be effectively kept in the normal range by practicing diabetes self-management. Learning about meal planning and nutrition gives you valuable tools for managing blood glucose with diet, and we've touched on other aspects of self-management, too.

The bottom line here is that promises of miracle weight-loss formulas or a secret cure for your diabetes only serve to divert your attention away from what actually does work, where your attention and your commitment are necessary. Put your faith in what's tried and true, your effort into developing new healthier habits, and your money into a savings account.

Achieving Your Goals

This chapter emphasizes how your attitude and willingness to participate in improving your own health are so important to adopting and staying with healthier habits. Your overall goal is to live a long and active life in spite of diabetes, but your doctor and dietitian may have defined individual goals for you. Weight loss is a common assignment because studies show that shedding even a little weight can greatly improve blood glucose control. An A1C less than 7 percent is recommended by the American Diabetes Association, and that organization sets ideal goals for blood pressure and cholesterol known all together as the diabetes ABCs.

Whatever your goals, healthy eating certainly plays a role in achieving them. And, a final few words of wisdom can keep you accountable, informed, and confident.

Writing it all down

Recording what you eat, what time you ate it, what your blood glucose readings are at what time, when you take your medication, how much activity you got, if you are ill, and even your mood can provide a wealth of important information to evaluate.

Study after study shows this same connection between recordkeeping and success with lifestyle changes. Writing it down gets your brain involved and knowing you intend to write it down keeps you accountable to doing the right thing. Having the data is almost an extra bonus; the bigger motivation is simply the act of consciously writing down your diabetes-related activities.

TIP

If you're comfortable with technology, there are websites or phone/tablet apps where you can record the relevant information in a database. If you're more a pen and paper person, use pen and paper. Just write it down. The time and effort is negligible, but the benefit is incredible.

Using blood glucose readings

Having the capacity to get an accurate reading of your own blood glucose level in a few seconds, at home, was a significant advance in diabetes care, and undoubtedly has literally saved lives among people with type 1 diabetes. But, the tremendous increase in cases of type 2 and the associated costs in medical care has some questioning whether the cost of testing supplies for type 2 diabetes should be reimbursed. Please work carefully with your healthcare provider to ensure that you can get the best technology for your lifestyle and budget.

Learning to use blood glucose test information gives you important insights into what effects your blood glucose levels negatively and allows you to make changes. The information gained from targeted testing is especially useful if your diabetes is not in good control. If you test after meals, for example, you can identify specific foods that spike your blood glucose and what spikes yours may not affect others the same way.

If your type 2 diabetes is not under good control or you want to better understand how stress, specific meals or foods, exercise, and sleep or lack of it can affect your personal glucose levels, you might have a period where you have continuous glucose monitoring. Continuous glucose monitoring is now routine for type I diabetes. This test involves you wearing a small sensor that reads blood glucose levels every few minutes over the course of an entire day. This is transforming the way we are understanding our individual response to foods and other aspects of our lifestyle.

IN THIS CHAPTER

» **Preparing in advance for your shopping trip**

» **Selecting the best quality foods**

» **Getting the goods on food additives and preservatives**

» **Touring the store with a new purpose**

» **Using nutrition labels to make the better choices**

Chapter **12**

Choosing the Best Food When Shopping

There is surely no doubt that most people want to preserve their health, and for some, a diagnosis of type 2 diabetes offers a surge of motivation to change their ways. Maybe this describes you right now. Or, maybe you've already passed that point and still haven't figured out which of your ways you can change to really impact your diabetes for the better. One common denominator among all people, diabetes or not, is the pursuit of food that tastes great. Our mission is to equip you with the knowledge and strategies needed to shop with both taste and health in mind.

While it's not fair to assume that you eat out too often, the numbers hint that it's a good possibility. Currently, the average American household spends more than 49 percent of its food budget on food eaten away from home. It's not impossible to eat away from home and eat healthy — it's just very difficult. (Check out Chapter 15 for some tips on how to do diabetes meal planning when eating away from home.) But overall, making the best choices for the foods you prepare and eat at home, and eating these foods at home more often, may just be the most important change you can make. This chapter helps you discover what foods to select and where you can find them.

Starting Healthy Meal Planning

Meal planning for diabetes starts by developing your menu and collecting the foods that make up your meals, and there is a wide range of possible destinations that offer everything you need. While this is often the most daunting aspect of starting a meal plan for most people, it needn't be that way. Chef Amy began planning diabetes-friendly meals for her family at age 15 when her mother was diagnosed with diabetes. Her mentality is that if she could do it as a teenager, in a time when there were much fewer resources both in terms of recipes and in terms of actual ingredients available, anyone can do it. Instead of viewing meal planning and list making as chores, Chef Amy learned to embrace the opportunity to create the most nutrient-dense and delicious dinners she could for her mother and family.

TIP

No one wants to cook separate meals for separate people's tastes and dining habits, so it's important, we believe, to create lists of nutritious foods that you and anyone else dining with you enjoys eating. Keep lists of nonstarchy vegetables, good-quality complex carbohydrates, and lean proteins together at all times. When planning meals, start with these lists and mix and match ingredients using the modified MyPlate Method we describe in Chapter 13 and the recipes in Chapter 18.

TIP

One of the great public health concerns is the lack of conveniently available, affordable, and healthy food in less-affluent and underserved neighborhoods, where rates of diabetes are often highest. Access to healthy food can be compromised by transportation difficulties, personal safety concerns, and crime rates that discourage retailers. In the United States, several new initiatives are aimed at improving the situation via food co-ops, mobile food markets, and bus stop farmers' markets, and through organizations such as Feeding America. If you live in the United States, you may want to reach out to one of these services to donate, volunteer, or take advantage of their services if you need them.

Making Your Menus

Prior to purchasing groceries, it is important to create solid menus that account for all of the food — three meals per day plus snacks — you need until your next shopping trip. We always recommend having a well-stocked pantry and freezer full of high-quality complex carbohydrates, lean protein, and vegetables to help you stretch the time between your trips to the store.

Online grocery delivery services can be a valuable time-saver when needed.

You need to take a few things along on your food shopping expeditions, but first things first — making time to go. Like it or not, managing your diabetes effectively can be inconvenient at times, and one category of inconveniences is making the effort to gather and prepare food at home. Once again, it's a matter of perspective and priority.

If you accept the reality that food and your health are tied together, you clearly see the value in the time and effort you devote to planning your meals, and to gathering and preparing food yourself. Now, for a plan.

Compiling a list

You wouldn't dream of building a bookshelf, packing a suitcase, planting a tree, or jumping into just about anything else without some kind of forethought. If you have launched into a project or a trip with no plan, it's likely the outcome was less than ideal. By the same token, there's no doubt that you can visit a grocery and come home with a lot of food, but without a plan the outcome may be less than ideal. Your plan is your shopping list.

Plans are the nuts and bolts of a vision, and the vision that inspires your shopping list is your menu — the breakfasts, lunches, dinners, and snacks that will help keep your blood glucose levels steady, work to manage your weight, and protect your cardiovascular system. Here is key advice for making and using your shopping list:

>> Keep a running list so you can add replacement items as soon as you notice your supply is low.

>> Organize your list according to the general plan of the grocery (pantry, produce, seafood, dairy, meat sections). Even if you're going to a store you're not familiar with, the foods are usually grouped in the same way, even if not in the same place.

>> Make your list specific, and don't get anything that isn't on your list unless you stumble across a particularly delicious and healthy ingredient or food offer that completely fits with your meal planning

That last point may sound a little extreme, and it's okay, of course, to grab something you actually need. But, planning your meals and making a specific list has a purpose beyond saving you trips. Making a plan and then sticking to the plan is an effective way to resist impulse.

Stretching your money

The proportion of disposable income we spend on food and the choices we make depend on many factors, but don't forget that a healthy diet need not necessarily be more expensive. It is important to spend a little more on a staple ingredient like extra-virgin olive oil where quality, price, and health benefits may be linked, and perhaps less on ready meals or dining out. Substituting sodas with drinking safe and clean water and replacing meat with beans are other examples of improving health and reducing costs.

Here are some more great ways to save on groceries:

>> Look for coupons and sales on foods that work with your diabetes meal plan. Canned tuna or salmon are great examples of foods you can grab at a bargain.

>> Register for every store's preferred customer plan, because some deals apply only to registered customers.

>> Shop for fresh produce that's in season because it's likely to be less expensive. You may also find better deals at farmers' markets or stores that specialize in produce.

>> Check frozen and canned fruits and vegetables. As long as there's not added salt or sugar, frozen and canned food is as nutritious as fresh, sometimes even retaining more nutrients than fresh.

>> Try generic foods, which are always less expensive than brand names. You may notice a difference in some specific products, but most of the time generic brands are virtually identical in nutrient content and taste.

>> Buy foods in bulk. That doesn't mean a 50-pound sack of potatoes, but simply buying something like yogurt in a larger container saves significant money when compared to single-serving containers.

>> Do your major shopping alone, if possible. It's important that you take time to read labels and ingredient listings and compare prices. It's easy to feel hurried if an uninterested companion or children are tagging along.

>> Look on high and low shelves. The food at eye level is sometimes higher priced than foods stocked in less-convenient spots.

>> Avoid buying prepared food that you can easily fix yourself.

>> Explore famers' markets if they are available in your area.

>> Consider growing a little of your own food, even if it is just some herbs on a window shelf. Not only is the food the best tasting and the freshest, but the satisfaction derived from seeing your seeds or plants turn into food at the table is enormous.

TIP

Another way to save money at the grocery is to make sure you know what you already have on hand. Perfectly good food can get pushed to the back of the pantry or freezer, never again to see the light of day. Take a look in the way back of your freezer or cupboards every now and then, do an inventory, and make a point of using older items nearing their expiration date. Most fresh food that you may not be able to eat before its expiration date is able to be frozen, sometimes in its original state or sometimes after cooking. It is possible never to throw food away, which is good for your pocket and good for the planet.

REMEMBER

There is food that's clearly beneficial to your health, and there's food that's better avoided. Getting a great deal on food you should best avoid isn't such a great deal after all. Don't let a few dollars, or the thrill of victory from that great deal, steal your attention away from your health.

Avoiding temptation

Making your shopping list into an ironclad agreement with yourself is a surprisingly simple way to avoid impulse buying and assure that the foods you have at home are those that work to improve your health. But, in many groceries it's possible to eat enough food for an entire day one toothpick at a time — free samples.

Temptation is everywhere, and when it comes to food, it's hard to connect what you choose to do today and tomorrow with the state of your health in five or ten years. If you follow the advice in this book, you may find that your taste shifts from convenience, processed foods to fresh, healthy, and sustainable ones.

Assessing the Quality of Your Food

We talk about the quality of macronutrients in Chapter 6 to help you make distinctions between whole grain and refined carbohydrates, unsaturated and saturated fats, and proteins derived from unhealthy, processed meats and those from plants. In addition to choosing foods based on macronutrient quality, you can also choose foods that are better for the planet, better for the animal being raised for food, and better for the environment in which the food is produced.

Sometimes higher-quality foods cost more to produce and that may be reflected in the price. It is difficult to define what makes a food high or low quality, and there are certainly no widely accepted terms or standards, but here are a few tips:

>> Foods that are highly processed may have a long list of added ingredients that are often there to preserve what are essentially low-quality foods.

>> The nutritional quality of meat from animals that have access to a wide variety of natural foods has been shown to be higher and contain healthier fats.

>> Plants that are grown in soil rich in minerals show higher levels of micronutrients than crops raised on overexploited land.

>> Food raised organically has more nutrient density and plants have more bioactives than nonorganically raised food.

>> Polyphenol levels may be higher in produce that is less intensively farmed. Intensive farming techniques involve the widespread use of fertilizers, pesticides, and breeding plants for higher yields, often at the expense of diversity and quality. For example, higher levels of the bioactive carotenoid lycopene is present in tomatoes grown in natural sunshine and with less irrigation than in those grown in large glass houses with automatic watering systems to increase yield. Olives harvested earlier from trees that grow in challenging environments are higher in polyphenols. Old-grain cereals such as spelt, millet, teff, and Khorasan wheat are less easy to manage with standardized modern machinery but are a better source of polyphenols and often have lower glycemic profiles than common wheat.

>> Intensive farming of crops and animals increases the need for pesticides and antibiotics, which may be harmful for human health. Not only are these practices detrimental to the animals' well-being, but also the stress induced and the pressure for quick growth may produce changes to the nutritional quality of the meat.

Unraveling Food Terminology

Food is always the subject of much debate in popular culture, but there are a few terms that can be confusing, especially when there's so much passion on either side of the discussion. For you to make the best decisions, it's important to sort through some of the terminology clutter so you fully understand what you're buying and why.

Prepackaged food

Prepackaged food simply means food that is packaged before sale. If you think about it, that covers most everything in the grocery, whether it comes in cans, bags, boxes, bottles, jars, vacuum packed, or plastic wrap. So, how is it that prepackaged food has a bad reputation in some circles? Is prepackaged food getting a bad rap (pun intended)?

Well, the devil's in the details, as the saying goes. There are really two considerations when it comes to prepackaged food — the food itself, and anything else that may have been added to the food.

The story of the food itself is told to some extent by the nutrition facts label, where you find the amount of protein, fat, carbohydrate, and sodium for the specified serving size. Total fat is further divided into unsaturated fat, saturated fat, and trans fat. Total carbohydrates are divided into sugars, fiber, and sugar alcohols.

The ingredients list tells the rest of the story. Ingredients are listed in descending order, from the most to the least. The ingredients list allows you to see that a bag of frozen vegetables contains only vegetables, and that packaged blueberry muffins contain more sugar than any other ingredient, including flour. Because most recipes for homemade blueberry muffins call for two or three times more flour than sugar, the prepackaged muffins illustrate perfectly how some prepackaged foods include ingredients you're better off not having, like lots of added sugar.

The prepackaged muffins also include guar gum, sodium acid pyropophosphate, monocalcium phosphate, potassium sorbate, and sodium stearoyl lactylate — additives and preservatives. Food additives and preservatives are other ingredients or chemicals added to prepackaged foods to improve quality, shelf life, flavor, appearance, safety, or very occasionally to add nutritional value. These other ingredients can be familiar to you, like salt or iron, or can seem like a chemistry lab experiment — disodium ethylenediaminetetraacetate or neohesperidin dihydrochalcone. There are, literally, thousands of additives or preservatives classified by the U.S. Food and Drug Administration as generally recognized as safe. And, whereas the muffins wouldn't be recommended for your diabetes eating plan simply because of the added sugar, there are foods that may be considered healthy that still include the chemistry experiment near the bottom of the ingredients list. That leaves the choice up to you.

ASK THE DOCTOR

It may take many years for the effects of additives and preservatives to be fully understood. Some experts are calling for greater investigation into the possible harms of commonly used preservatives such as sodium nitrite. Aspartame, still commonly used as a sweetener and promoted as a "calorie-free" way to avoid sugar in sodas and other foods, not only fails to support weight loss, but has also been listed by the World Health Organization as a possible cancer-causing chemical. We agree with the author Michael Pollan who so wisely said, "Don't eat anything your great-grandmother would not recognize as food."

The bottom line on prepackaged foods is to make your judgments based upon blood glucose control and general health first; then consider whether you want to make these additives and preservatives part of your diet, too. Remember, some prepackaged foods, like most frozen vegetables, don't include any added ingredients.

TIP

There's just no way around developing an understanding of and an appreciation for nutrition facts labels (you may have noticed). Managing carbohydrate, fat, and sodium in your diet are the keys to blood glucose control and heart health. If the discussion of nutrition facts labels in Chapter 9 didn't click, try reading *Nutrition For Dummies* (Wiley). Better yet, meet with a registered dietitian. Remember, the information is not difficult — it's a subconscious reluctance to think too much about food that keeps the light bulb from lighting up. Just don't give up.

Processed foods

The phrase *processed food* is another hot potato, generally viewed in an even more negative context than prepackaged food. But, processed foods are just foods that have been altered from their natural state and can include freezing, canning, cooking, dehydrating, or even pasteurizing milk for safety. You probably wouldn't consider the processing of a grape into a raisin as some horrible insult to a formerly healthy food. To judge whether a food has been processed for your benefit or to your detriment, you have to consider what processing does to the nutritional value of the food.

Whole grains, such as wheat and rice, provide good examples of how processing can reduce nutritional value. To make white flour, for example, both the germ and the bran of the original whole-grain wheat are discarded. The same holds true for white rice. It wouldn't be accurate to say that white bread and white rice are unhealthy, but neither offers the health benefits of the natural whole-grain versions.

The hydrogenation of liquid fats to create a solid *trans fat,* however, is processing with clear negative effects on health. Trans fats raise bad LDL cholesterol levels and lower good HDL cholesterol levels, increasing the risk for heart disease. Consuming red meat processed into hot dogs and lunch meats appears to increase the risk for diabetes significantly beyond the risk of red meat alone, according to data from long-term observational health studies. Processed meat is mechanically manipulated, but also usually includes the addition of preservatives like sodium nitrite. These two examples illustrate processing that has a distinctly negative effect on your health.

Notice that hydrogenation and the addition of nitrites refer back to additives and preservatives, discussed previously as related to packaging. Much processing of food is to improve the quality, shelf life, flavor, appearance, safety, or nutritional value of the food products. Many cereals and breads are enriched with added vitamins, for instance, and the processing of milk by pasteurization reduces the risk for disease.

REMEMBER

Once again, your focus should be on the nutritional benefits of food to blood glucose control and the risk for heart disease instead of on the popular idea that processed equals bad — in some cases that's true, but in some cases it's just the opposite. Knowing how the foods you choose can minimize the impact of diabetes on your long-term health and adopting those healthy eating habits is what's really important.

Frozen and canned foods

In most cases, fresh, in-season, freshly picked and prepared foods are the best choices to consume. Frozen vegetables along with chicken breasts and fish fillets can also offer a lot of nutrients and help to cut down on trips to the store. Be sure to choose the best quality possible for maximum benefits.

Frozen foods come in a wide variety of options, too, but plain frozen vegetables are particularly handy for healthy eating. Frozen vegetables are generally blanched with steam and frozen within hours of harvest. Because freezing temperatures inhibit microorganism growth, further processing or preservatives are not required.

Like most everything discussed in this chapter, the plainer the food, the more likely the food is to be healthier. Frozen vegetables also come in butter sauce, cheese sauce, and with other seasonings. Often, these varieties have — you guessed it — added fat, salt, and sugar. Once again, grab your reading glasses, and check the nutrition facts labels.

The same goes for carbohydrate-containing vegetables and fruits — great options for convenient meals, as long as you count the carbohydrate and avoid added fat, salt, or sugar. Look for fruit with no sugar added — the nutrition facts label always shows sugar content because fruit has natural sugar, but if you see sugar in the ingredients, make a different selection.

Considering frozen entrees brings you back to the discussion earlier in this chapter about prepackaged and processed foods. Don't be surprised to find that the ingredients list reads like a chemistry lab stock room and the sodium content very high. Even low-calorie entrees with names that include lean or healthy can pack 600 to 800 milligrams of sodium into a frozen dinner. Frozen entrees demonstrate the importance of knowing the meaning of nutrition facts. Again, these aren't forbidden, and there are healthier choices, but don't put on the healthy halo — evaluate the information yourself.

Canning food dates back to the early 1800s, and the general idea is to kill microorganisms that can spoil food or cause illness by heating and sealing the food in an airtight enclosure to prevent contamination. Most foods are canned under pressure to achieve temperatures high enough to kill the spores of the organism that causes botulism. *Clostridium botulinum* is an organism that lives naturally in soil, but can grow in environments with no oxygen, like a sealed can, and produces a powerful toxin. Botulism intoxication from commercially canned foods is extremely rare, but always reject cans with dents in the seams or bulging ends.

You can get just about any vegetable canned, but don't forget canned fruits, soups, and canned meats and fish, especially tuna and salmon. The key to selecting the healthiest canned goods is to read the labels and ingredients, a common theme in shopping for food (by now you may be glad you got the advice about reading glasses). Many canned goods include added salt or sugar. They may also include large amounts of sodium and/or chemical preservatives, and sometimes contain hidden sugars and fat for flavor as well. So compare labels to get the least added sodium, always buy canned fruit packed in its own juice, and buy canned fish packed in water or olive oil.

TIP

In recent years, preserving food in jars has become fashionable again. Many people have rediscovered the art of preserving vegetables, tomatoes, and jams in cans. This is a great strategy for those with diabetes, because canning your own food isn't only fun, it's also better for you because you can determine which foods you'd like or not like to include. You can combine your own flavors and make items perfect for your personal taste.

Organic foods

If prepackaged and processed foods are generally viewed in a negative light, then organic foods have the opposite reputation. But what does *organic* actually mean when referring to food? It turns out that laws and regulations are involved.

In general terms, organic foods are produced and processed with minimal input of chemicals, including fertilizers, pesticides, ripening agents, antibiotics, and growth hormones. And, producers must follow strict guidelines to claim the organic label. The objective of organic food production is not only to minimize the input of manufactured chemicals into food, but also to promote recycling of resources, facilitate ecological balance, and conserve biodiversity. It's not possible to say anything bad about organic food production, and organic foods are the fastest-growing segment of the food industry. Organic foods also generally cost more than conventionally produced foods.

So, how can eating organic foods improve blood glucose control, reduce your risk for heart disease, and improve your nutrition? Producing food organically does not alter the macronutrient content in any appreciable way. Studies have shown differences in micronutrients and certain bioactive compounds like polyphenols, which may mean an increase in antioxidant potential, but the evidence of benefits to health is not yet conclusive.

WARNING

Studies have found that the consumption of organic foods is subject to the *healthy halo* effect, where people make unfounded health assumptions. One study found that university students inferred that organic cookies were lower in calories than conventional cookies, even when the nutrition labels showed the calorie content to be identical.

The questions about synthetic chemicals in your diet are unsettled. Conventionally produced foods probably expose you to more pesticide residues than organic foods, but the levels are very small and are considered safe by the regulatory agencies. That said, there are differences in official standards from country to country, and sometimes evidence emerges that suggests a link with human disease, eventually resulting in the revision of guidance or withdrawal of a commercially available chemical used in agriculture. Ultimately, if choosing organic foods is the right choice for you, there is no down side — that is, as long as you choose foods that promote good health.

Choosing the Best Foods

So, you've chosen a store, scoped out sales and coupons, made a detailed list of foods to buy from your week's menu plan, promised yourself you won't give in to impulse purchases (or food samples) — now what?

Picking produce: The colorful base of your diet

Your goal in the produce aisle should be to choose the freshest, in-season fruits and vegetables in a rainbow of colors so that you get the most vitamins and minerals out of them. Start with nonstarchy vegetables. These nutrient-packed foods should make up half of your plate every meal, and this pattern is especially important with diabetes. Why? Because nonstarchy vegetables are very low in carbohydrates. So, with a variety of textures and colors you get a full stomach plus calcium, iron, magnesium, potassium, vitamin A, vitamin C, vitamin K, folate, fiber, antioxidants, and phytonutrients like beta-carotene, lycopene, lutein, anthocyanidins, and isoflavones — all with minimal impact on blood glucose. Nonstarchy vegetables include lettuce, spinach, kale, collards, broccoli, cauliflower, carrots, turnips, cabbage, tomatoes, cucumber, soft-shell squashes (think zucchini), peppers, asparagus, beets, Brussels sprouts, onions, green beans, eggplant, okra, and more. Nonstarchy vegetables are the foundation for healthy eating, and don't forget you can grow your own or get fabulous in-season vegetables at farmers' markets. Select nonstarchy vegetables that are colorful and crisp.

Starchy vegetables like potatoes, sweet potatoes, corn, peas, and hard-shell squashes shouldn't be shunned. These foods are carbohydrate foods that you need to account for in your diabetes meal plan, but don't forget that carbohydrates should account for about half of your daily calories. Starchy vegetables offer many of the same nutrients as nonstarchy vegetables, and what would summer be without corn on the cob? Just be aware of serving sizes, and count the carbohydrates.

Fresh fruits are carbohydrate foods, too, but what a fine way to get your carbs and satisfy your sweet tooth. Today's food transportation efficiencies allow you to choose from an incredible variety of fruits from around the world, like papaya, mango, and kiwi, in addition to U.S.–grown oranges, apples, grapes, peaches, pears, grapefruit, cherries, blueberries, melons, apricots, and strawberries. Too numerous to mention all, eating a variety of fruits gives you a variety of vitamins, antioxidants, and powerful phytonutrients, as well as healthy fiber. Select fruits that are bright, free from blemish, and the appropriate firmness. Eat the skin of fruits with an edible skin, like apples, grapes, peaches, and pears, because it's rich in fiber and that is where many of the bioactive compounds are found in greatest concentration (see Chapter 8), and remember to count the carbohydrate.

TIP

Tropical fruits are often sweeter and have higher glycemic index values and, depending on where you live, may well have had farther to travel, so for reasons of glucose control and sustainability, try to choose a higher proportion of locally grown fruits.

Often, the produce section of your store includes bulk nuts in their shell. Nuts are not carbohydrate foods, so they can make an excellent and healthy snack if eaten in moderation, and nuts offer a variety of healthy unsaturated fats. One benefit to buying nuts in the shell is you can generally get them without added salt.

You may also find soy foods in the produce section, such as tofu, tempeh, or soy processed into chicken-like or beef-like strips. Soy is a complete protein, and has been shown to help reduce bad LDL cholesterol and lower blood pressure. It's easy to add soy to your diet by trying these options with a vegetable stir-fry.

Incorporating whole grains

You may not think of bread, cereal, and crackers as grains, but of course the primary ingredient in these products is grain, or grain refined into flour. Like grains, bread, cereal, and crackers are carbohydrate foods — one slice of bread equals one carb choice, or 15 grams carbohydrate.

Whole grains that contain the bran, germ, and endosperm are the healthier choice, and that goes for bread, cereal, and crackers, too. Going for whole-grain options does not change the carbohydrate content, but may slow the impact on blood glucose levels. More important, whole grains help lower cholesterol levels, work to reduce blood pressure, and provide nutrients lost in the refining process.

Oats, barley, millet, quinoa, farro, wheat berries, cracked wheat, rice, rye, buckwheat, and amaranth are all nutritious, high-quality complex carbs that you can feel comfortable preparing to your tastes and adding to your meals. Just ½ cup (cooked) of one of them along with a portion of low-fat protein, a serving or two of nonstarchy vegetables, and a drizzling of good-quality extra-virgin olive oil and citrus juice are the perfect foundation for a wonderful meal. Making your own cereals, breads, pilafs, and salads with these ingredients are the perfect way to add complex carbs to your meals.

The processed grains in bread, cereal, and crackers, however, include added ingredients — fat, salt, or sugar, in particular. Cereals are infamous for added sugar, but many healthy-looking granola cereals can have 6 or more grams of fat in a ½-cup serving. And, crackers would be the obvious place to watch for excess sodium from salt.

Fortunately, these items almost always have a nutrition facts label, and you have your reading glasses. Check the serving size and total carbohydrate content first; then look at the grams of sugar under total carbohydrate, and finally for sodium. It's common to see some sugar in all of these products, but when the sugar portion of total carbohydrate exceeds 30 percent, it becomes a sweetened product.

There's definitely room to work bread, cereal, and crackers into your eating plan. It's worth noting that many of these products are fortified with vitamins — bread in the United States has been fortified with niacin since the late 1930s, and it's common to see vitamin C, vitamin D, folic acid, and several B vitamins including vitamin B12, which is often missing in vegetarian diets.

TIP

Thinly sliced, whole-grain bread is great for sandwiches because you can get two slices for 20 grams, more or less, of carbohydrate. A sandwich needs two slices of bread, after all. Choose sourdough and the least-processed breads.

Adding beans and legumes

Beans and legumes provide the main sources of daily protein in many heritage diets around the globe. Particularly beneficial to those with diabetes, beans and legumes are rich in fiber and they can help to slow down digestion and prevent huge swings in blood sugar — a major plus. Legumes and nuts contain large amounts of vitamins B12 and B6, protein, iron, magnesium, zinc, thiamin, niacin, phosphorous, and magnesium. Beans are similar to animal proteins in that they are a good source of protein, but unlike the animal proteins, they are fat-free. It is important to note that a little goes a long way when it comes to legumes. Serving sizes of legumes and nuts differ from animal sources. Only ¼ cup of cooked beans is considered a full serving.

Enjoying nuts and seeds

Nuts and seeds are an easy and flavorful way to add taste, texture, and nutrients to your meals. Nuts are often avoided by health-conscious people because of their high caloric content. Remember, though, that because they are high in heart-healthy monounsaturated fat, the quality of calories they provide is very high, making them an extremely satisfying food. They also contain high amounts of copper, magnesium, protein, fiber, selenium, vitamin E, and antioxidants. Various studies have shown that people, including those who were already following a Mediterranean diet, were able to decrease their LDL (bad) cholesterol and total cholesterol simply by increasing the amounts of pistachios, almonds, and walnuts they ate. In fact, adding 3 ounces of almonds to the daily diet was shown to drop total cholesterol by 9 percent in just nine weeks.

Increasing flavor with spices, herbs, and alums

Adding flavor and nutrients instead of fat, sugar, and salt doesn't come easily to many cooks. Those trained in making classical European cuisine have relied on sugar, butter, and salt to enhance the taste of their dishes in an inexpensive way. Unfortunately, those are all items we should be cutting down on or eliminating. Take the fat, sugar, and salt out of many modern meals and you'll be left with flavorless food.

FROM THE AUTHORS

Our favorite way to add taste is to use copious amounts of fresh herbs along with anti-inflammatory spices, and alums such as garlic, onions, and shallots to heighten the flavor profiles in dishes while increasing their health-boosting properties. See Chapter 18 for recipes and ideas.

Dressing dishes with extra-virgin olive oil

As we mention throughout the book, a good-quality extra-virgin olive oil is a perfect condiment for those with diabetes for many reasons. Olives are rich in beta-carotene, calcium, iron, dietary fiber, antioxidant nutrients (vitamins A and E, and polyphenols), and monounsaturated fatty acids. Further, various studies have shown that olive oil or an olive oil–rich diet may

>> protect against malignant tumors.

>> reduce the risk of breast, colon, and bowel cancer and the incidence of melanoma.

>> prevent the formation of blood clots and lowers the levels of total blood cholesterol (believed to be responsible for the low incidence of heart problems in countries where olive oil is the main cooking fat).

>> improve calcium absorption in the body and prevent osteoporosis.

>> prevent memory loss in healthy elderly people.

>> lead to less risk of developing rheumatoid arthritis.

Antioxidants such as vitamin E, carotenoids, and polyphenols (known for their anti-inflammatory and antibacterial effects) are found in extra-virgin olive oil. The body's overall ease in digestion and absorption of olive oil, as well as the need for its many nutrients, make it an ideal cooking ingredient and traditional medicinal.

Considering fats and oils

Plenty of different oils are on the market, and they vary significantly in their nutritional qualities. In recent decades, oils as a source of fat, either in their "raw" form or used in cooking, was promoted as an alternative to butter given that butter is high in saturated fat, and saturated fat has been associated with increased levels of "bad" LDL cholesterol, which is in turn has been linked with an increased risk of heart disease and stroke. *Unsaturated* fats are fats with a different chemical structure from saturated fats and do not have the same adverse effect on LDL cholesterol. Having said that, a little butter from time to time is not harmful, though if it is the only fat you cook or put on your food, you are missing out on some very healthy anti-inflammatory and antioxidant compounds found in extra-virgin olive oil, which is the foundation of the Mediterranean diet.

TECHNICAL
STUFF

Fats consist of chains of carbon, hydrogen, and oxygen atoms bound together. Saturated fats are chains of various lengths where all the carbon atoms are joined to another carbon atom or a hydrogen atom, and are therefore "saturated" with hydrogen atoms. Unsaturated fats have one (mono-) or more than one (poly-) double bond between the carbon atoms where a hydrogen atom might otherwise have been chemically bonded.

There is not only debate about the health of fats in terms of their effects on LDL cholesterol. There is some evidence that Western diets have an excess of polyunsaturated fats called omega-6 found in many vegetable oils such as sunflower oil, which might increase drivers of inflammation. Such a pro-inflammatory effect may prove to be just as harmful to health than any negative effects on LDL cholesterol though more research is needed. In terms of fat content, monounsaturated fats like olive oil or canola oil are probably the best, although the refining process to produce these oils strips out many of the important bioactive compounds. (For more information on bioactive compounds see Chapter 8.) *Extra-virgin* olive oil is "pressed" at low temperatures and is unrefined, maintaining its high level of polyphenols.

Another area of contention is the relative health of oils when used for cooking. At high temperatures the fats in oils can break down, become oxidized, and produce chemicals that may have the potential to cause cancers. In general, saturated fats have the greatest tolerance to heat, with monounsaturated fats somewhat less (though still in general higher than usual cooking temperatures) and with polyunsaturated fats being most likely to break down if heated at high temperatures. In practice it is not quite as simple as this. The chemical processes during heating include oxidation of fats, and therefore, oils that have naturally occurring antioxidants such as those in the fruit of the olive tree found in extra-virgin olive oil, are protective and preserve the oil, as well as the components of other foods during the cooking process.

There is a lot of talk about the "smoke point" of an oil, and producers of some seed oils like to compare different numbers if they feel this can help market their product and disadvantage their rivals. The process of breakdown is more complicated and more prolonged than imagining a change in an instant occurring at a single "point." The argument becomes particularly irrelevant between the heavily refined canola oils and extra-virgin olive oils (with canola oil said to be marginally higher) when you consider that the smoke points compared are above all usual cooking temperatures, and the acrid, unpleasant smell of burning oil is always a good reason to keep to sensible levels of heat. Research from Australia published in the journal *Acta Scientific* in 2018 measured the stability of different oils undergoing sustained heating at usual cooking temperatures. Extra-virgin olive oil was lowest in the formation of harmful trans fats and showed the highest retention of beneficial antioxidants.

TIP

For all these reasons we recommend extra-virgin olive oil as the first choice for cooking and adding to food as the healthiest oil. It is high in unsaturated fat, but most important, many extra-virgin olive oils contain antioxidant and anti-inflammatory polyphenols (described in Chapter 8). It is best to choose one from a specific region or grower rather than a "product of many countries," and many oils that appear to be Italian are in fact sourced from other countries. Such oils produced on an industrial scale are likely to be lower in polyphenols. Always look for a local product that tastes pleasantly bitter and a little pungent to know you are getting a good-quality extra-virgin olive oil.

Selecting condiments

Condiments include mayonnaise, ketchup, mustards, salad dressings, salsa, relish, or other sauces, and although the refrain may be getting old, check the nutrition facts labels. Ketchup and bar-b-que sauces often include added sugar, high-fructose corn syrup, or other sweeteners, and salt. The same goes for mustard as well as soy sauce — even the reduced-sodium blends are extremely high in sodium. Generally speaking, these products are used sparingly, and for the most part won't cause your healthy eating plan to crash and burn. Still, manage fat, sodium, and sugar with care.

TIP

Condiments such as balsamic and other vinegars slow the glycemic rise of a meal and may improve insulin sensitivity. Take care to choose a traditionally made balsamic vinegar, which is made only from grapes and cooked *must* — the squeezed skins and seeds of the grape that is able to ferment. Some vinegars that claim to be balsamic vinegars contain thickening agents and caramel and other artificial colorants.

Consuming yogurt, eggs, and dairy

Two additional sources of high-quality dietary protein are eggs and dairy, and both have seen their share of controversy. For a time, eggs were outcasts due to their relatively high levels of cholesterol. But eggs have gained favor again as an excellent source of high-quality protein, choline, riboflavin, folate, selenium, vitamin B12, and vitamin D. As much as one egg per day falls within current dietary cholesterol guidelines if dietary cholesterol from other sources is minimized. Egg substitutes, made from egg whites, are cholesterol-free because the yolk is not included, but whereas the protein content is the same, some of the egg's natural nutrients have to be added.

TIP

Egg substitutes, or using two egg whites as equal to one whole egg, can help moderate cholesterol intake and keep you enjoying eggs.

Dairy products such as milk, yogurt, sour cream, and cheese are a complex mixture of food options. And, dairy products contribute all three macronutrients to your diet — protein, fat, and carbohydrate — with some notable exceptions. One cup of whole milk, for instance, contains the three macronutrients in approximately the same proportion — 8 grams protein, 9 grams fat, and 12 grams carbohydrate. Cheese, however, does not retain significant amounts of carbohydrate.

The protein in dairy products is high-quality protein, easily absorbed by your body, and includes all of the essential amino acids that you can't manufacture. So, dairy products are a great way to start your day.

The fat in dairy products is mostly saturated fat, and a high intake of saturated fat has been linked with an increased risk of heart disease and stroke. However, a meta-analysis review published in the journal *Nutrients* in 2022 supported the increasing evidence that shows no increased risk from consuming up to 200 grams (7 ounces) of dairy foods per day. Foods are more than just their macronutrients. The specific saturated fatty acids, which are chemically shorter molecule chains in goat's and sheep's milk, may have less effect on "bad" LDL cholesterol levels than those from cow's milk. Fermented dairy such as yogurt and good-quality cheeses are likely to have beneficial probiotic effects (see Chapter 7). The regular consumption of dairy foods has been associated with improved insulin sensitivity and a lower risk of developing type 2 diabetes.

The carbohydrate in dairy is primarily *lactose,* or milk sugar, and a large percentage of adults can't properly digest this carbohydrate — they are *lactose intolerant.* For those who can, the carbohydrates in dairy products need to be accounted for in your daily eating, as the carbohydrate content of dairy products can vary significantly.

REMEMBER

There are differences between brands of yogurts and cheeses. Some yogurts may be promoted as low-fat options (which is not necessarily a benefit) and contain added sugars and other unwanted chemicals. A processed cheese like the slice of the rubbery stuff usually found between the bacon, patty, and bun of a burger may contain ingredients such as water, salt, artificial coloring, flavorings, lecithin, enzyme-modified cheese, dehydrated cream, anhydrous milk-fat, phosphoric acid, albumin from cheese whey, acetic acid, monosodium phosphate, potassium citrate, sodium tartrate, and potassium sorbate. In contrast, the artisanal production of traditional cheeses from free-roaming livestock produces a high-quality, very nutritious, and delicious food.

Choosing fish and seafood

High in protein and low in calories, fish is an excellent choice for anyone trying to gain muscle, lose weight, or increase brain function. Fish is full of omega-3 fatty acids, which the body requires to function, yet cannot produce on its own. They are known to lower triglycerides and blood pressure, and reduce blood clotting and risk of stroke and heart failure. Consuming fish as little as one time a week promotes total body wellness and can have positive health benefits. In addition to omega-3s, seafood also contains essential nutrients such as zinc (immune system support), potassium (heart health), selenium (anticancer protection), and iodine (necessary for thyroid function), along with vitamins A (vision, organ function, immune support) and D (bone strength, nutrient absorption, disease prevention).

TIP

To get up-to-date information on selecting the best quality fish in the United States, consult the Monterey Bay Aquarium Seafood Watch list (www. seafoodwatch.org), which gives consumer guides, seafood basics, and helps you search for sustainable seafood.

Looking at poultry

Chicken provides high-quality protein and a relatively low amount of fat. In addition, fat in chicken is mostly of the unsaturated type, which protects against heart disease. One 3-ounce serving contains just 1 gram of saturated fat and less than 4 grams of total fat, yet is packed with 31 grams of protein, which is more than half of the daily recommended allowance for adult females. Chicken meat contains a significant amount of B vitamins, which aid in metabolism, immune system, and blood sugar level maintenance; cell growth; and nerve cell and red blood cell maintenance. It also contains iron (oxygen transport and cell growth) and zinc (immune system functioning and DNA synthesis). For these reasons, chicken is a favorite among athletes, dieters, and the health-conscious alike. Single portions of both organic, unprocessed chicken and turkey breast can be part of a diabetes-friendly diet.

What you need to know about red meat

Red meat offers the highest quality, complete protein to your diet, but can also add unhealthy saturated fat that increases your risk for heart disease. Red meat, in particular, has also been associated with increased insulin resistance in large population studies. A healthy approach to meats is to rotate lean cuts of beef, pork, or lamb with skinless chicken or turkey, and fish or shellfish. Fish and shellfish are low in saturated fat and include healthy omega-3 fatty acids. All meats are cut today with less fat than years ago, but you can reduce fat and saturated fat even more in your diet by choosing the leanest cuts.

TIP

Choose USDA *select* cuts of meat, which are naturally lower in fat, and buy ground beef that's at least 90 percent lean when possible. You can further reduce saturated fat at home by trimming visible fat from meats and cooking without adding fat. Trimming visible fat can cut another 30 percent from your diet, and removing the skin from poultry (or buying skinless) reduces fat by as much as 50 percent.

Consider sandwich meats such as bologna or pastrami, bacon, sausages, and the like very carefully. This may be a difficult transition, but excess fat and sodium are not compatible with diabetes management, and we don't recommend eating them. One slice of bologna can account for 25 percent of your daily sodium recommendations.

Lamb, on occasion, can be an occasional indulgence on a diabetes-friendly diet. On average, a 3-ounce serving of lamb is lean — about 175 calories. Lean cuts include the leg, loin, and rack. Lamb provides vitamins and minerals and is an excellent source of protein, which helps keep hunger at bay, preserves lean body mass, and regulates blood sugar. A 3-ounce serving has 23 grams of protein — nearly half of the daily recommended needs. The same serving size also offers a good dose of heart-healthy monounsaturated fat and almost five times the amount of omega-3 fatty acids as found in beef.

4

Ready, Set, Plan

Discover how to customize your meal plans so that you can eat healthful foods and practice healthful eating habits.

Read about several popular diets that can be diabetes-friendly, including the Mediterranean diet, Dash, and WW.

Calculate amounts and modify ingredients to turn your favorite recipes into healthy diabetes-friendly dishes.

Discover tools to help you make good choices when eating out.

Give up snacks? No way! Find out which snacks and drinks are best for you.

IN THIS CHAPTER

» **Getting a personalized meal plan**

» **Modifying the USDA MyPlate for diabetes**

» **Assembling complete meals**

» **Figuring out the unknown foods**

» **Reclaiming heirloom recipes**

Chapter **13**

Customizing Your Meals

M eal planning can be one of the most challenging aspects of diabetes management, but it doesn't need to be that way. There has never been a better time to find helpful resources, wide varieties of fresh ingredients, and recipes that are both delicious and nutritious. It is our hope that you are inspired to find the joy in home cooking, and that you reap the full benefits of culinary therapy. But even in busy times, it's important to know that just a few handfuls of nutritious ingredients combined together can satisfy your taste buds and keep your blood sugar levels in check.

In this chapter, you uncover the nuts and bolts of meal planning for effective diabetes management. If you've never planned a meal before, don't be intimated. All you need to do is adopt a few basic principles and you'll be on your way. By keeping lots of fresh produce, high-quality carbohydrates and protein, as well as some additional foods that are especially beneficial to those with diabetes on hand, you'll be able to mix and match great meal options in no time. You also discover ways to fit your family's favorite heirloom recipes into a diabetes-friendly meal plan, too.

Laying the Foundation

It's really not possible to eat in a way that's best for your health if you don't even know what you should be doing. And, knowing what you should be doing means *knowing exactly what you should be doing* — having precise and personalized information that comes from a registered dietitian. Registered dietitians and certified nutrition specialists provide a service known as *medical nutrition therapy* when a metabolic disorder like diabetes is involved, and when diabetes is involved, food really is medicine. The drugs you're prescribed for diabetes can only do so much, even if you have type 1 diabetes and take insulin injections to directly control blood glucose levels. Preserving your health over the long run means addressing your lifestyle choices, especially the food you eat.

So, step number one in laying a strong foundation for managing diabetes effectively with food is to see a registered dietitian or a certified nutrition specialist — and you may need to request a referral from your doctor. There really is no shortcut to getting an effective eating plan — a meal plan tailored to your specific physical and medical needs is an integral part of your diabetes treatment, and you can't get that from a friend or off the Internet. And, if you want to impress a nutrition professional on your first visit, begin keeping a food journal before you go, recording everything you eat, the time of day you eat it, and your blood glucose level whenever you take one over several days or weeks.

Whereas a personalized meal plan may be the most valuable result of your visit, your nutrition professional can also explain why a meal plan is so important and work with you so that you can identify carbohydrates in your diet. Maybe most important, you can evaluate your food journal together and make adjustments — maybe only minor ones — to your normal eating pattern. If you have also kept a record of your blood glucose levels — and you should — you're able to see how certain food choices can have a greater impact than others. Don't let one visit with a nutrition professional be the end. Most insurers cover multiple visits, and your department of public health likely has dietetic services as well.

TECHNICAL STUFF

Certified nutrition specialists (CNSs) are nutrition experts who help clients or the public reach health-related goals by customizing meal plans. CNSs often work with clients who have been diagnosed with chronic conditions such as diabetes, heart disease, high cholesterol, high blood pressure, autoimmune diseases, and other chronic conditions. CNSs assess their clients' individual needs, and then promote positive dietary changes and additions using up-to-date nutritional research.

Knowing your personal meal plan

Your personalized meal plan, which guides your daily choices for managing your diabetes with food, isn't a menu, telling you exactly what to eat. Instead, it's a framework, like a house under construction where the various rooms have been established, but leaving you a world of options for how you're going to finish the decor. In general terms, your personalized meal plan will be based on the following criteria:

>> Your daily calorie requirements, which depend to some extent upon whether your health status would benefit by gaining weight, maintaining your current weight, or losing weight over time.

>> Your recommended carbohydrate consumption based upon your calorie budget, your diabetes-related health status, and your medications. Usually, your daily carbohydrate recommendation is expressed as a certain number of carbohydrate, or carb, *choices,* which is a food portion containing approximately 15 grams of carbohydrate.

>> Your health status related to possible conditions, and medications for conditions, other than diabetes.

REMEMBER

Your personal food preferences are always a consideration in developing your personalized meal plan.

Your daily calorie needs are based upon your current body mass index (BMI), activity level, age, gender, and a goal for reaching a weight that makes sense for you. It's no secret that most people with type 2 diabetes are overweight, and losing excess weight clearly promotes better blood glucose control. If you fall into that group, your meal plan helps you both manage blood glucose levels and lose weight at a healthy pace. Any effective diabetes management plan also addresses prevention of the most common diabetes complications and *comorbidities* — related health conditions caused by diabetes, or often occurring with diabetes. High blood pressure, high LDL cholesterol, low HDL cholesterol, and high blood triglycerides are all related, to some extent, to diet.

TIP

Your BMI is your mass (weight) in kilograms, divided by your height in meters squared. You can calculate your own BMI in English measures by dividing your weight in pounds by your height in inches squared, and multiplying that number by 703 to correct for using English measures. If, for instance, you weigh 190 pounds and are 5'7" tall (67 inches), the formula is $190 \div 67 \times 67 = 190 \div 4489 = .0423 \times 703 = 29.75$. A BMI higher than 25 is considered overweight, and higher than 30 is in the obese range. See Chapter 5 for more about the BMI scale.

Based upon your daily calorie needs, your meal plan divides those calories among the three macronutrients — protein, fat, and carbohydrates. You may expect to see the calories allotted as follows:

>> Calories from protein likely account for 20 percent of your daily calorie total. Each gram of protein stores 4 calories of energy. Some diabetes eating plans suggest that a higher percentage of calories come from protein, and in some cases, especially where kidney function is compromised, protein may be restricted.

>> Calories from fat likely account for about 30 percent of your daily calorie total. Each gram of fat stores 9 calories of energy, and your eating plan suggests that saturated fat make up only a modest percentage of your daily fat intake, with trans fat strictly limited.

>> Calories from carbohydrates often account for a full 50 percent of your daily calorie total. Like protein, carbohydrate stores 4 calories of energy per gram, and it's carbohydrate that has the greatest effect by far on your blood glucose levels. For that reason, carbohydrates deserve a lot of attention, and are the main focus of your meal plan.

REMEMBER

The key to understanding your meal plan, and to getting the benefits of following one, is learning the correct portion sizes for food. Even though your meal plan is set to provide a certain number of calories each day, you don't have to add up calories as you go along. Instead, with each meal you have set amounts of carbohydrate, fat, and protein, and the sum of the calories from those recommended amounts over the whole day should hit the correct calorie mark. Nobody, except maybe an accountant, likes keeping a running tally of their daily calories, so this approach is much more user friendly, and extremely effective as long as you eat the correct portions.

Portion sizes need to be specific. If someone told you the proper portion for an apple is the size of a ball, you wouldn't know whether they meant a golf ball, baseball, basketball, or a giant beach ball. And, the difference is obviously significant. With diabetes, knowing the correct portion sizes of carbohydrate-containing foods is essential — a baseball-sized apple would be the proper size for one carb choice (15 grams of carbohydrate), but only 1 tablespoon of maple syrup would give you the same amount of carbohydrate. In general, both portions have the same effect on blood glucose.

TIP

It's not necessary to learn every portion size of every food. The best strategy is to learn the correct portion size of the foods you most commonly eat, and refer to a carb-counting book or an exchange list for foods you haven't memorized. A comprehensive exchange list is included in Appendix A.

Be aware that you probably have a natural resistance to thinking too much about planning the food you should eat — it just seems that eating shouldn't require any advance planning. In reality, the more that you think about food, the better off you are. And not just for carbohydrates. Even though carbohydrates have the most direct impact on blood glucose, dietary fat contributes to excess body weight by piling on calories, and saturated fats contribute to unhealthy cholesterol and tri-glyceride levels. Your personalized meal plan, however, accounts for all of these issues, and minimizes the amount of thinking and calculating you have to do.

WARNING

Calorie requirement and BMI are both calculations that are useful, but they do have some limitations. Calories measure energy in a food, but this may not translate directly to weight gain or loss — many factors determine how foods are metabolized. And BMI may not accurately predict an unhealthy weight, for example, if much of the mass is muscle rather than stored fat. Our advice is to use these numbers as a general guide while enjoying a diet with sensible portions of healthy foods.

Making MyPlate into YourPlate

In 1992 the U.S. Department of Agriculture (USDA) published its first Food Guide Pyramid. The idea was to demonstrate how foods represented as the wider base of the pyramid — whole grains — should be consumed in greater quantities than the foods associated with the tiny tip of the pyramid — fats, oils, and sweets. The USDA pyramid was revised in 2005 to an image that represented the various food groups in colorful vertical sections, rather than stacked in layers, complete with a stairway and a stickman. Other pyramids, including one developed by the World Health Organization, have followed the original Swedish version put out in 1972. Pyramids have been created by other organizations to depict the Mediterranean, Nordic and African-American heritage diets for example.

In 2011, the USDA replaced its pyramid with MyPlate, a visual representation of relative portion sizes for different food groups in a dinner place setting, including a dinner plate and a separate section for dairy. Figure 13-1 is the current official icon representing the general categories of food that make up a healthy diet, showing recommended portions of protein, grain, fruit, vegetables, and dairy. One key take-home message is that vegetables and fruits should make up one half of your plate, more or less. Public health bodies in other countries have copied the dinner plate concept. The United Kingdom has its own version called the Eatwell Plate.

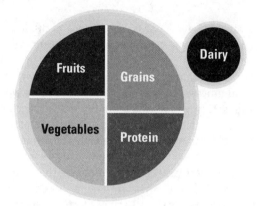

FIGURE 13-1:
The current USDA
MyPlate icon.

Unfortunately, the USDA MyPlate doesn't address the particulars of a diabetes eating plan, where identifying quality carbohydrate foods is the key to success. Although it's not completely obvious looking at the icon, the official MyPlate has carbohydrate foods spread through every single category, because beans are included in the protein group, and starchy vegetables like potatoes and corn are included in the vegetable group. Fruits, grains, and dairy, except for cheese, are always considered carbohydrates.

You can make a case that MyPlate encourages you to get your carbohydrates from a variety of different food groups, and that certainly fits in with a healthy diabetes eating plan. The importance of segregating carbohydrate foods and increasing your consumption of low-carbohydrate vegetables really justifies a special plate for people with diabetes.

Figure 13-2 is a variation of the USDA's MyPlate from the American Diabetes Association that has been adjusted for people with diabetes.

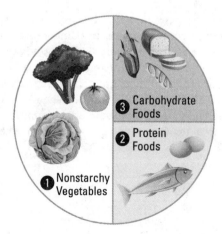

FIGURE 13-2:
MyPlate adjusted
for a healthy
diabetes eating
plan.

This representation of your plate emphasizes two important healthy eating strategies. Eat lots of nonstarchy vegetables such as artichokes, asparagus, green beans, beets, Brussels sprouts, broccoli, cabbage, carrots, cauliflower, celery, cucumber, eggplant, leafy greens, leeks, mushrooms, oats, onions, peppers, radishes, salad greens, sprouts, squash, Swiss chard, tomato, and turnips. Cover half of your plate with them. Nonstarchy vegetables are low-calorie, low-carbohydrate, packed with vitamins and essential nutrients, and keep you feeling full. Also, limit your protein portion to about one-quarter of your plate, usually about three ounces (no fair cutting your 16-ounce T-bone into pieces and stacking them high).

In addition, this plate gathers the carbohydrate foods together — grains, fruit, starchy vegetables and beans, and dairy (except for cheese). From this group you select the appropriate number of carb choices your meal plan recommends for each meal.

REMEMBER

The USDA MyPlate and the U.K.'s Eatwell Plate have focused on simplicity, and there is some virtue in simplicity. However, the Mediterranean diet pyramid and other heritage diet graphics are much more comprehensive, providing detailed descriptions of foods and their contribution to these healthy dietary patterns while moving away from focusing on macronutrients.

Understanding carb portions

Carbohydrates — sugars, starches, and fiber — liberate single molecules of glucose during digestion, which are promptly absorbed directly into the bloodstream. When blood glucose levels begin to rise, insulin is released from special cells in the pancreas to assist in getting glucose out of circulation, stored away inside of certain cells, bringing blood glucose levels back to normal. Carb loading is something athletes do before competition to make sure their body's storage capacity for glucose, your body's favorite and most efficient source of energy, is filled and ready for action. Diabetes, however, interferes with your body's ability to store glucose quickly and efficiently, so glucose that's loaded doesn't necessarily get stored.

The glitch in this systemic imbalance is an inadequate amount of insulin, a diminished response to insulin by those cells that should be storing glucose for later, or both. Glucose that can't be stored continues to circulate in the bloodstream, keeping blood glucose levels high. High blood glucose levels cause damage to cells over time, and lead to serious complications of diabetes like heart disease, vision loss, kidney damage, and more.

It's important to remember that not all carbohydrates are created equal. Quality carbohydrates are desirable and necessary in a healthy diet. The secret to eating healthy carbohydrates and keeping blood glucose levels in better balance is, in part, managing the amount, timing, and the quality of the carbohydrates you eat. That means knowing how much carbohydrate is in the food you're eating, spreading your carbohydrate consumption throughout the day, and choosing some of your carbohydrates from foods that don't get digested and absorbed as quickly. Think carb *trickling*, rather than carb *loading*. With technological advances now allowing for real-time blood glucose monitoring, it may be that we can add to our knowledge of the effects of carbohydrates on blood glucose levels by measuring our own individual response to particular foods. This kind of personalized approach has the potential to help each of us to understand the effects of our meals in the real world.

REMEMBER

Timing your carbohydrate consumption means don't skip meals, eat meals around the same time each day, and eat an approximately equal proportion of your daily carbohydrate budget at each meal. Your meal plan may even set aside one or two carbohydrate choices for between-meal snacks. Giving your body a lighter load of glucose at any one time helps blood glucose levels come down more efficiently.

Carbohydrates that digest and absorb slowly are usually *whole* foods, like unrefined grains, beans, and whole fruit. These foods have a low *glycemic index value*, meaning their impact on blood glucose levels is slower, giving your body extra time to find vacant storage for the excess glucose. Managing diabetes is partly about getting blood glucose levels to come down after eating carbohydrate foods. Carbohydrates make the blood glucose levels of people with normal glucose metabolism go higher, too, but a normal response between insulin and cells storing excess glucose brings blood glucose levels down significantly in a couple of hours. Managing the amount, timing, and quality of carbohydrate intake works to get blood glucose levels decreasing more efficiently in people with diabetes.

Knowing the amount of carbohydrate you're eating is a more complicated issue because the portion of a food that contains a set amount of carbohydrate — look for 15 grams, which is called one *carb choice* — is different for different carbohydrate-containing foods. You can get one carb choice, 15 grams of carbohydrate, all of the following ways:

>> One tablespoon of sugar or concentrated syrup

>> Two tablespoons of raisins or dried cherries

>> One-quarter cup granola

>> One-third cup cooked rice, barley, pasta, or plantain

>> One-half cup beans, corn, cooked oatmeal, mashed potatoes, parsnips, or applesauce

>> Three-quarter cup blackberries or canned grapefruit

>> Two-thirds cup yogurt

>> One cup canned pumpkin, papaya, honeydew, or acorn squash

>> One-and-a-quarter cups strawberries or watermelon

>> One-and-a-half cups of cooked nonstarchy vegetables

>> Three cups raw, nonstarchy vegetables or plain popcorn

The difficulty many people with diabetes have with modifying their eating habits for better management is with the staple grains and starches — potatoes, rice, pasta, and corn. It's obvious from the list earlier in this chapter that there are plenty of healthy carbohydrate foods with a generous portion size for one carb choice — see Appendix A for the long list. But ⅓ cup of rice or pasta, one corn tortilla, or the pointed end of a giant baked potato can seem drastically insignificant if you're used to eating these grains and starches by the pile or by the pound.

That makes managing these foods all the more important. You likely have a meal plan recommendation of between 9 and 15 carb choices per day — 3 to 5 per meal. That definitely leaves room for your favorite staple foods if you manage portion sizes, and include other carbohydrate foods in your diet. You might consider alternative recipes, like mashed potatoes and cauliflower, or a pasta that's processed to make some of the carbohydrate indigestible. You might even splurge on rice as your only carbohydrate for a meal — choose whole-grain brown rice, keep the number of servings you eat consistent with your carbohydrate budget for that meal, and get your carbs from different foods groups most of the time.

Finally, how can sweets fit into a diabetes management plan? There are really two different considerations when it comes to sweets — empty calories and portion size. Empty calories are calories that don't bring along any compensating nutritional value. With diabetes and sweets, the concept can be extended to include both empty calories and carbohydrates — a cost to your weight and blood glucose without any redeeming benefit. A 20-ounce sugar-sweetened soft drink crosses off more than four of your daily carb choices; for example, 65 grams of carbohydrate for a negligible amount of phosphorous from phosphoric acid. Getting your sweet calories and carbs from foods with real nutritional value, like fruits, is a better choice. But, in the big picture it's not necessary to avoid sweets or even sugar completely as long as you fit them responsibly into your diabetes eating plan.

Starting simple

Diving into anything without starting simple is a recipe for discouragement, and diabetes meal planning is no different. It's not that you can't prepare a five-star Russian Salmon Coulibiac — it's that figuring out the appropriate serving size of a complex fish and rice loaf baked in a pastry shell leaves much room for error. If you're just starting to get serious about managing your diabetes better by getting serious about food, it's important that you see positive results. And the less room you leave for error, the better the result.

Starting simple, therefore, means focusing on foods that contain predominantly only one of the macronutrients — carbohydrate, protein, or fat. In practice, that's not always completely possible, but you can get close. And it is feasible to actually eat this way, but that's not really the intent of this section. The intent is allow you to concentrate on one food at a time so that you can get the hang of where your macronutrients come from and understand how you can construct meals that manage carbohydrates, keep your eating habits heart healthy, and keep your appetite satisfied. It's like practicing with a paint-by-numbers project before you tackle your chapel ceiling.

Picking a perfect protein

About 20 percent of your daily calories should come from protein, although your personalized meal plan may vary somewhat. Nevertheless, protein is an important macronutrient for building and repairing tissue, to create enzymes that accelerate important biochemical reactions, and for constructing important hormones like insulin.

TECHNICAL STUFF

Proteins are assembled from amino acids, and your body needs 20 specific amino acids to build all the different proteins you need. The protein in your diet is broken down into its various amino acids during digestion, and your body recycles those amino acids to make your proteins from scratch. You can even make some amino acids by modifying other amino acids in some cases, but there are nine amino acids you must get intact from your diet — these nine are referred to as *essential* amino acids.

When considering which foods supply all essential amino acids in a useable form, and in sufficient quantity, there really are perfect proteins — they are called *complete* proteins. And, there are scoring systems, one of which is called the *protein digestibility corrected amino acid score*. By this scoring system, which measures both the essential amino acids and your ability to easily absorb them, the perfect proteins are egg white, soy protein, and the casein and whey proteins in milk. It's only fair to point out that meats score well on this scale, too.

Soy and milk both contain carbohydrates, and whole milk is a significant source of saturated fat (soy contains healthier unsaturated fats). Likewise, meats always include some saturated fat. So, contrary to the title of this section, for keeping meal planning simple there is no perfection in protein. But, for almost perfect you can consider the following options:

>> Organic soybeans (edamame) contain about the same amount of carbohydrate as protein, but when processed into tofu the carbohydrate content is significantly reduced compared to the remaining high-quality protein. Tofu does retain the fat content of the beans, but the fat in soy in primarily healthy unsaturated fat.

>> Trimming the visible fat from lean cuts of beef and pork, or removing the skin from poultry, can reduce the fat content profoundly. Removing the skin from a chicken breast, for example, can cut the fat to only about one gram. Or, start with a lean cut of beef like flank steak, round, or tenderloin, and you'll know you're on track.

The take-home lesson is that you can choose your protein in this manner without having to account for carbohydrates, too, and with some comfort that the included fat is either healthy unsaturated fat, or a minimal amount of saturated fat from lean meats.

Isolating carbohydrates

Carbohydrates account for approximately one-half of your daily calories, and carbohydrate foods are the foods that have a direct impact on your blood glucose levels. For that reason, choosing quality carbohydrates are the main focus of your eating plan. You can track carbohydrates bundled into 15-gram portions called a *carb choice*, and with type 1 diabetes especially you always look to match insulin injections with the carbohydrate content of your foods.

Anyone with diabetes considers, at some point, the prospect of eliminating carbohydrates from their diet. At first glance the logic makes sense — carbohydrates equal higher blood glucose levels, and higher blood glucose levels are unhealthy. In reality, however, that strategy can be compared to deciding you can walk everywhere on your hands to save wear and tear on your feet. Just like humans are made to walk upright, you're made to run on carbohydrate fuel. Plus, eliminating carbohydrates from your diet isn't really going to leave much for you to eat. It's natural to have that passing thought, but be sure it passes so you can get down to the business of managing carbohydrates in your daily eating.

TECHNICAL STUFF

Carbohydrates in your food come in the forms of sugars, starches, and fiber, going from the simplest sugar molecules with six to ten connected carbon atoms to the most complex, and often indigestible, fiber with thousands of carbon atoms in a chain. The simple sugar glucose is a frequent participant in building carbohydrate, and glucose is liberated from these complex molecules in digestion and absorbed directly into your bloodstream. A certain level of dissolved glucose circulating in your blood is essential — too little, or too much, has consequences.

Isolating carbohydrates in your diet is similar to isolating protein — many excellent sources of carbohydrate also come along with protein and fat; but like the previous search for the perfect protein, perfection isn't necessary for this simple lesson in meal planning. Here are a few relatively pure carbohydrate foods, and your meal plan might recommend three to five carb choices you can choose from the following:

>> Fruit is perhaps the purest carbohydrate, often without any protein or fat. Virtually every fruit has at least ten times more carbohydrate than protein, and if you discount a few outliers like avocado (which has so much fat and so little carbohydrate it's placed in the dietary fat group), fruit is mostly fat-free. A carb choice for fruit varies depending upon the fruit itself, and whether or not it's dried. Two tablespoons of raisins or 1 ¼ cups of watermelon are both one carb choice. Canned and frozen fruits are excellent as long as there is no added sugar, and whole fruit offers more nutritional value than fruit juice. Having fruit with every meal is a wise choice, and you'll always know to count the carbohydrate.

>> Brown rice, the whole-grain version of rice, contains protein and fat, but in negligible amounts. The same is true for most whole grains — even quinoa, a grain noted for its protein content, contains five times as much carbohydrate. A carb choice for whole grains, including pasta, is ⅓ cup cooked, and you can also get your whole grains from bread, where one slice of a whole-grain bread is equal to one carb choice.

>> Starchy vegetables (potatoes, corn, and peas, for example) contain significantly more carbohydrate than protein, and are nonfat foods unless fat is added. Peas have three times more carbohydrate than protein, and both corn and potatoes have an even higher ratio. One carb choice for a white potato is 3 ounces weight, and for peas and corn the correct volume is ½ cup.

These represent the simplest categories of healthy carbohydrate foods, and if you recognize other healthy carbohydrate foods that aren't included here (dairy products and beans) it's because they are not quite as simple. That doesn't mean they aren't extremely beneficial to your health and an essential element of your eating plan. I discuss dairy, beans, and other complicated foods in the next section.

Filling up on vegetables

Vegetables, specifically nonstarchy vegetables, are special to diabetes. Not only are they packed with vitamins, loaded with water to help keep you hydrated, and a source of dietary fiber, they are your best choice for the volume you need to feel full. Nonstarchy vegetables are your best choice because these foods are low in calories, low in carbohydrate, and nonfat — 1 whole cup of sliced cucumber, for example, has but 16 calories and 4 grams carbohydrate. A carb choice, 15 grams of carbohydrate, would be about 4 full cups.

The MyPlate representation adapted for diabetes suggests that one-half of your plate should be nonstarchy vegetables. In general, a carb choice for these foods is considered to be 3 cups raw, or 1½ cups cooked, but the foods do vary some. Nonstarchy vegetables include:

Artichoke	Chayote	Peppers (all varieties)
Artichoke hearts	Cucumber	Radishes
Asparagus	Daikon	Rutabaga
Baby corn	Eggplant	Salad greens (all types)
Bamboo shoots	Greens — collard, mustard, turnip	Sauerkraut
Beans — green, Italian, wax	Green onions or scallions	Soybean sprouts
Bean sprouts		Spinach
Beets	Kale	Sugar snap peas
Bok choy	Jicama	Soft-shell summer squash
Broccoli	Kohlrabi	Swiss chard
Brussels sprouts	Leeks	Tomato
Cabbage — Chinese and green	Mung bean sprouts	Turnips
Carrots	Mushrooms	Vegetable juice cocktail
Cauliflower	Okra	Water chestnuts
Celery	Onions	Zucchini
	Peapods	And more!

Nonstarchy vegetables can go into omelets, on sandwiches, make a colorful tossed salad, be used for dipping, become the featured ingredients in a stir-fry, be eaten as a snack without worrying about raising your blood glucose, or served as a side dish to any meal. The only caution is to watch for added fat or salt, and that means keeping an eye on yourself, too. When all is said and done, nonstarchy vegetables can be your most powerful weapon for controlling blood glucose, losing weight, and improving heart health.

Moving Beyond Simple

Like any true artist, after you paint by the numbers for a short time, you're ready for something more challenging. With diabetes and food, that's a good thing. There are excellent food choices waiting in the wings to join those simple foods reviewed in the previous section, and now that you've had a little practice it's time for some introductions.

Knowing the sneaky foods

Don't misunderstand the word sneaky here — there's nothing malicious about these foods. In fact, these are some great choices for your diabetes meal plan because they are complex, offering more than one of the macronutrients in addition to a host of other nutritional benefits. In general, the most significant issue with these foods comes if you fail to recognize them as carbohydrates, and it's possible you don't think of these foods as carbohydrates. But you will, because you are becoming a carbohydrate expert.

Beans

Beans are the sneakiest of sneaky. Beans are included in the protein section of the USDA's MyPlate, and with good reason. Soybeans, called edamame, are the only vegetable source of complete protein, a food containing all nine essential amino acids in an easily digestible form. Chickpeas (garbanzo beans), and other beans score well on that scale, too. Beans, like kidney beans and black beans, give you about 15 grams of high-quality protein per cup, and that protein comes with very little fat unless it's added. And, beans are an excellent source of fiber, including soluble fiber, which helps lower LDL unhealthy cholesterol.

Those beans are one healthy source for protein. But, that cup of beans also counts as two carb choices — about 40 grams of carbohydrate reduced by one-half of the 10 to 12 grams of fiber, leaving between 30 and 35 grams total carbohydrate per cup. So, what's that mean for your diabetes eating plan? It means eat lots of beans — beans of all kinds are very healthy little packages of nutrition. Just remember to count the carbohydrates and to consider the beans as a significant part of your mealtime protein.

Dairy

Dairy products bring to mind calcium, protein, and maybe even fat because you are probably familiar with the 2 percent, 1 percent, and nonfat skim milk options. Greek yogurt has gained popularity thanks to its higher concentration of protein than regular yogurt. But don't forget the carbohydrates in dairy products, thanks to lactose, commonly called milk sugar. One cup of milk is considered one carb choice, even though it's actually 12 grams of carbohydrate, and yogurt can vary remarkably in its carbohydrate content depending upon added sugar or fruit.

Plain Greek yogurt can supply almost 25 grams of protein per cup, but also contains as much as 8 grams of carbohydrate, and some fat, which means that it contains all three macronutrients. It also contains inulin, a substance shown to help balance blood sugar levels. A serving of plain Greek yogurt is an excellent snack for those with diabetes, and when eaten before bed, can help you balance your blood sugar levels. What does that mean for your diabetes eating plan? Dairy products can fit very well into your meal plan — just remember to count the carbohydrates.

WARNING

There's one other sneaky thing about dairy products — cheese. The carbohydrates in milk feed the microorganisms that turn milk into cheese, and these bugs are hungry. As a result, cheese contains very little of the original carbohydrate, but retains its protein, especially in the harder, well-aged varieties.

Sugar-free foods

Sugar free or *no sugar added* are labels that can grab the attention of anybody with diabetes. There's something about those phrases that can get mysteriously translated into *carbohydrate free,* but don't be misled. Although it's likely that a sugar-free food has less carbohydrate than its thoroughly sugared variety, all carbohydrates aren't from sugar. Baked items contain flour, for example, which includes the carbohydrate from the original grain. And *no sugar added* doesn't mean that the sugar naturally there, like the lactose in ice cream, was removed. Often it also means that sugar alcohols were added to sweeten the food, and sugar alcohols are included in total carbohydrate content separately from sugar. What's this mean for your diabetes eating plan? It means always read the label so you can always count the carbohydrates.

In fact, that's the best lesson for this section, because no matter what your preconceived notions about any food may be, the nutrition facts label always makes sure you get the real story before you eat.

Estimating mixed dishes and casseroles

A recipe for Salmon Coulibiac includes flour, cornstarch, rice, sour cream, butter, eggs, salmon, mushrooms, shortening, milk, white wine, shallots, bell peppers, and dill. What's the carbohydrate content you must count for your meal? Time's up.

Of course, you can't answer that question without knowing how much of each ingredient goes into the dish, the nutrition facts for each ingredient, and the number of servings. Even then, you're talking about a project to compile all of the information you collect. This recipe made 8 servings, and each serving was 1,130 calories, 62 grams of total fat (35 grams saturated fat), 28 grams protein, 1,750 milligrams of sodium, and 117 grams of carbohydrate. This particular recipe for Salmon Coulibiac does not fit well into your eating plan, but that doesn't mean there aren't fabulous mixed dishes that do.

Mixed dishes and casseroles often contain combinations of all three macronutrients and can seem overwhelming. These dishes commonly include foods that you know are dense carbohydrates, like potatoes, rice, or pasta, and can include flour or sauces you're not so familiar with. Even foods you've been enjoying for your whole life, like pizza, can be a varying mix of ingredients that are hard to decipher. But, it's not as complicated as it seems if you take an organized view of mixed dishes.

TIP

Have an idea of how your daily carbohydrate, fat, and protein recommendations divide out for each meal. You can find this information on your meal plan. For a 1,700-calorie meal plan, an approximate target for each meal would be 25 grams of protein, 19 grams of fat, and 70 grams of carbohydrate. It's also worth remembering that your daily recommendation for sodium is 1,500 milligrams, or about 500 milligrams per meal.

Compare these mealtime macronutrient recommendations with the per serving nutrition information for the dish in question. You can already see how the Salmon Coulibiac works well for your mealtime protein but is significantly higher for the other dietary concerns. There is, of course, room for adjustments, but that dish would require a profoundly smaller serving size. You can usually get the per serving nutrition information from the recipe, or from a restaurant website, and starting from scratch with an ingredients list is always an option. It's a much better option for dishes that have 4 ingredients than for dishes that have 12 ingredients, however. You can also adjust the serving size of a combined food if a smaller portion fits better into your meal plan. If the serving size that fits best seems too small, add a salad or nonstarchy vegetable side dish to your meal.

Evaluate recipes from a general health viewpoint, and consider modifying a recipe to improve its nutrition profile. You may want to avoid cured fatty meats, like bacon and sausage, as well as lard, shortening, or butter. If the dish fits well into your meal plan otherwise, substitute ingredients with less fat, like Canadian bacon or margarine.

If you don't have access to the nutrition information, consider carbohydrate-dense casseroles with rice, pasta, corn, or potatoes, as about 30 grams of carbohydrate per cup. You'll be surprisingly close, but it's always an excellent idea to check your blood glucose levels a couple of hours after eating.

TIP

Don't forget that a good, pocket-sized reference book or mobile app can be invaluable in getting relatively accurate nutrition information for all sorts of dishes. Appendix A is a fairly detailed list of exchanges.

Mixed dishes aren't as tricky as they seem if you've taken some time beforehand to understand what your meals should provide. After all, mixed dishes are just single foods joining together to give you a different flavor and texture — the single foods still have the same nutrition facts as before.

Knowing basic recipe formulas

Chapter 18 is full of recipes that are considered to be complete meals in order to help get you started preparing the proper foods for yourself. Among the main barriers to home cooking is not having the proper ingredients on hand, and not knowing how to prepare simple foods. Table 13-1 outlines simple recipe formulas that you can make straight from ingredients in your freezer. When made with the proper portions (see Appendix A), these formulas fit well into a diabetes-friendly diet. They also help to ensure that you are consuming quality carbohydrates and beans and legumes all while enjoying varied, homemade recipes.

TABLE 13-1   **Pantry Creations**

Dish	Ingredients
Hummus	Chickpeas + Tahini + EVOO* + Spices + Lemon juice
Middle Eastern Lentils with Rice	Lentils + Vegetable or Chicken Stock + Lentils
Falafel	Chickpeas + Spices + EVOO + Tahini
Risotto	Carnaroli rice + Stock + Saffron + Vegetable/Protein of your choice (optional)
Pasta with Beans	Beans + Rice + Tomato sauce + Stock
Pasta with Lentils	Pasta + Lentils + Garlic + Tomato sauce and/or Stock
Pasta with Tuna (or other fish)	Pasta + Tuna + EVOO + Olives and/or Tomato sauce
Rice Salad	Arborio rice + Olives + EVOO + Jarred vegetables + Beans
Pasta Salad	Short pasta + Olives + EVOO + Jarred vegetables + Beans
Chickpea Soup	Chickpeas + Stock + EVOO
Minestrone Soup	Beans and/or Lentils + EVOO + Pasta or rice or other grain + Tomato sauce + Stock + Dried porcini mushrooms + Vegetables

(continued)

TABLE 13-1 *(continued)*

Bean Soup	Beans + Stock + Tomato sauce + EVOO
Pasta and Beans	Pasta + Beans + Stock + Tomato sauce + EVOO
Lentil Soup	Lentils + Stock + Tomato sauce + EVOO + Vegetables
Rice Pudding	Rice + Milk + Dried fruits and nuts + Honey or sugar
Tuna Salad	Tuna + EVOO + Beans of your choice
Chickpea or Bean Salads	Quinoa + Chickpeas or beans + EVOO + Vegetables + Spices
Pasta with Tomato Sauce and Vegetables	Pasta + Garlic + EVOO + Chili paste + Tomato sauce + Vegetables
Risotto Croquettes	Carnaroli rice + Stock + Saffron + Vegetable/Protein of your choice (optional)
Spaghetti with Garlic, Oil, and Chilis	Spaghetti + EVOO + Chili paste + Garlic
Bean or Lentil Dip	Beans or Lentils + Stock + EVOO + Spices
Roasted Chickpeas	Chickpeas + Spices + EVOO
Lentil, Bean, and Vegetable Skillet	Lentils + Beans + Fresh Vegetables or Olives + EVOO + Spices
Date, Almond, and Sesame Balls	Dates + Almonds + Sesame Seeds
Barley Soup	Barley + Stock + Beans or Legumes
Rice Pilaf	Rice + Spices + EVOO + Chickpeas + Nuts
Lentil Croquettes	Lentils + Spices + Bread crumbs + Tomato Paste + EVOO

Extra-virgin olive oil

Pairing complete meals

Once you are familiar with basic recipe formulas, you can create complete meals that fit into your diabetes meal plan by mixing and matching foods from different categories. To tweak the MyPlate portion-sizing method mentioned earlier in this chapter to make it appropriate for diabetes, plan your meals around three main components: one quarter of the plate (or meal) would be dedicated to healthful carbohydrates, another quarter to lean protein, and the other half of the plate to nonstarchy vegetables, as shown earlier in Figure 13-2.

To get started, create three separate lists of high-quality carbohydrates, lean protein, and nonstarchy vegetables. Circle or highlight the foods in each list that you and those you cook for enjoy the most. From the highlighted items in your lists, you can now start planning meals that are not only good for you, but also that you will actually enjoy. Here are the steps:

1. **Cover all your bases.**

   Make sure you pick one item from the carbs list, one from the protein list, and two from the nonstarchy vegetables list.

2. **Make portions count.**

   Double-check the portion sizes in Appendix A and make sure they are appropriate for your needs.

3. **Mix and match.**

   Choose the protein, carbohydrate, and vegetables you enjoy the most.

4. **Decide on cooking methods.**

   Just because you are incorporating different foods to meet your nutritional needs doesn't mean preparing them has to be complicated. You may combine the carb portion of potatoes with the protein choice of chicken breast cubes, along with broccoli and asparagus in a quick skillet-type dish, or enjoy them roasted, or even in a stew. If you want to cook the potatoes separately, you can grill the chicken breast, serve the potato on the side with sauteed broccoli and asparagus (or you can serve the vegetables as a salad). There are many possibilities.

5. **Add in layers of flavor.**

   Decide which spices you want to season your food with. (ceylon cinnamon, ginger, cumin, and turmeric with a bit of freshly ground black pepper all have anti-inflammatory effects.) Load up on fresh herbs like parsley, dill, basil, rosemary, mint, and oregano. Drizzle good-quality extra-virgin olive oil and fresh lemon juice over top of your favorite foods and salads.

Planning breakfast and lunch

With diabetes, it's important to spread your food, especially your daily carbohydrates, over time. Spreading your carbohydrates minimizes blood glucose spikes and gives your body an opportunity to bring levels down. The same holds true for both type 1 and type 2 diabetes. Spreading your meals out also is associated with successful weight loss. That means, don't skip meals.

It also means that breakfast and lunch give you two new opportunities each day to incorporate foods into your eating habits that benefit your health. So, are you? Or are you hitting the drive-through in the morning for your driving entertainment and picking up a sandwich and chips for lunch? The truth is that breakfast and lunch can sabotage your best efforts at managing diabetes if you don't treat those meals with the same consideration as dinner.

TIP

The week of menus offered in Chapter 17 has seven different diabetes-friendly options for breakfasts and for lunches. Breakfast and lunch are the perfect times to work healthy dairy foods into your day, like low-fat milk or yogurt. And, what other time are you likely to enjoy the benefits of the soluble fiber in oatmeal? Canned fish, like tuna packed in water, and portable fruits are perfect to grab and go for lunch, and whole-wheat bread gives healthy grains a place to shine.

Breakfast and lunch do take some planning, but many people find they're perfectly happy to eat the same thing every day for these meals, or rotate a few favorites. If that's the case with you, the planning for these meals into the foreseeable future requires an incredibly small investment of your time. By the way, if you're thinking you can find a way to make takeout food work well for these meals, think again. Better yet, visit a few websites with your pen and pad handy, and read Chapter 15 for a look at typical restaurant food.

Swapping out popular condiments

A little more than two pounds of uranium-235 fueling electricity generation in a nuclear power plant has the potential to produce as much energy as 6.5 million pounds of coal. And, 1 tablespoon of soy sauce contains more sodium than 20 cups of shredded bok choy. The lesson is that it's possible to pack a lot into a small container. When you don't account for that small container, if that container happens to be a condiment going onto your healthy food, you may be symbolically pitching your healthy diabetes meal plan onto the considerable fire 6.5 million pounds of coal can make.

Not all condiments are a nutrition disaster, and in fairness to soy sauce the low-sodium versions reduce the 900 milligrams of sodium per tablespoon down to less than 600 milligrams — that is an improvement. Condiments are concentrated little doses of flavor, so you might expect the sources of those flavors to be high, and it's not always sodium that deserves attention. Whatever the case, it's to your advantage to check the nutrition facts for condiments you enjoy and look for alternative varieties that might have lower amounts of the item that's out of bounds. Here are a few tidbits, good and not so good, about your favorite condiments:

>> Soy sauce dates back to the second century, and it is made from healthy soybeans, and is fat-free without any carbohydrate. But, as mentioned earlier, the sodium is incredibly concentrated in the dark liquid, and even the low-sodium versions deserve a second look before you douse your food. Remember,

excess sodium is associated with high blood pressure, and high blood pressure increases your already increased risk for heart attack, stroke, and kidney failure. Use small amounts of low-sodium tamari in its place.

» Mayonnaise is a mixture of egg yolks, oil, and vinegar or lemon juice, and is a popular addition to sandwiches and creamy salads. The combination of oil and egg yolk gives mayo a load of fat, both saturated and unsaturated. One tablespoon of full-strength mayonnaise is about 100 calories with 11 grams of total fat. Consider low-fat or fat-free mayo, or try avocado for a really creamy texture and half the calories and fat. You can also use plain Greek yogurt with a bit of lemon juice and good quality extra-virgin olive oil instead.

» The National Mustard Museum is located in Middleton, Wisconsin, and displays more than 5,000 different mustards from around the world. Mustard is made with the ground seeds of the mustard plant mixed with vinegar, water, and secret spices — well, salt isn't really a secret. Obviously, mustard is a popular condiment with so many commercial varieties available, but it does tend to be high in sodium and sometimes contains additives and preservatives. Swap out low-sodium varieties of mustard, and if it's the kick you're looking for, you might consider horseradish, which has only about a third the sodium as regular mustards.

» Ketchup was originally known as table sauce, and it's made with pureed tomatoes, vinegar, spices, and a sweetener. Ketchup has more calories, almost as much sodium, and more carbohydrate than mustard. And, even though the carb content is only 4 grams per tablespoon, that can add up when you're shaking that bottle. Freshly sliced tomatoes are a better option — you can have a whole cup of chopped tomatoes for the same carbohydrate investment.

» Sour cream and butter are traditional baked potato toppings, and in some ways it's fortunate that the appropriate diabetes-friendly serving size for a baked potato doesn't resemble a football. Sour cream and butter are both relatively high in fat. Sour cream is the less-fat choice, with 23 calories and 2 grams of fat per tablespoon. Butter, by contrast, has 100 calories and 11 grams of fat for that same tablespoon. But, plain, nonfat Greek yogurt can give you the creaminess you desire at 8 calories, no fat, and a scant 6 milligrams of sodium per tablespoon.

» Salsa has become quite popular in the United States as a dipping sauce, and without any commentary on what food you might be dipping your salsa with, salsa is a pretty healthy condiment. Most salsa in a jar has no fat, only 4 or 5 calories, and 100 milligrams of sodium per tablespoon. You can make your own salsa, or *pico de gallo* (uncooked salsa from fresh ingredients), and cut the sodium way down.

>> Salad dressings deserve mention here, in part because there are so many varieties, and in part because they represent a clear and present threat to a healthy bowl of salad greens. A tablespoon of common salad dressings can have 85 calories, 9 grams of fat, and more than 100 milligrams of sodium. And, contrary to what you may be inclined to believe, it's not necessarily the creamy salad dressings that are highest in calories and fat, although the creamier dressing can include 3 grams of carbohydrate in that tablespoon. The potential issue with salad dressings is the tablespoon — who actually uses only one on their salad? It's better to swap out a bit of good-quality extra-virgin olive oil and your favorite vinegar or lemon juice instead.

Adding in snacks

Snacks are the simplest foods to prepare, but the ones that are often overlooked. Life is hectic and we often go too long in-between meals. Having appropriate snacks on hand can help keep us on track.

People with diabetes should be eating snacks that are balanced and complete (containing all three macronutrients) every five hours. That means if you have breakfast at 8 a.m. and lunch at 1 p.m., you should be okay. But, if you are traveling and can't have a full meal within that time, or your normally eat dinner after 6 p.m., eating a nourishing snack can help to keep your blood sugar levels even. The same goes for if you start to feel hungry in-between meals, or if you've just completed a workout. Chapter 16 discusses great snack options at length.

Salvaging Heirloom Recipes

Heirloom recipes are those that are passed down from generation to generation in our families. They are the recipes we anticipate the most at holiday times and associate with our sense of home and our affiliation with our particular culture. Unfortunately, many people think that these foods are off-limits completely for those with diabetes. Giving up certain foods completely is simply non-negotiable for many people because it feels like in doing so, we are giving up our roots.

Chapter 14 discusses heritage diets as popular meal plans. And, in fact, those diets are an excellent way of honoring one's own heritage while following a healthful diet plan. That's because no matter where you find yourself around the globe, there are nutritious options such as leafy greens, low-fat proteins such as beans and legumes, fish and chicken, and different types of high-quality proteins. The ways in which they are paired together, how they are seasoned, and the manner in which they are prepared and for what reasons, are the culturally-specific components to food that can still be honored.

As for the more indulgent recipes with higher fat, carb, and sugar contents, there are three ways to approach them. The first one is to use the swap-outs mentioned earlier in this chapter and in Chapter 21 to come up with a diabetes-friendly version of the same dish that you can enjoy more often. The other alternative, and this is the one that Chef Amy prefers, is to not alter the recipes, but to enjoy them in small portions only a few times a year. That way, you can still enjoy the same food and all of the same great memories and traditions associated with it without derailing your diet plan. The third option is to enjoy the healthier version more regularly and still keep the traditional version for special occasions in small portions. The good news is that you can still have your heirloom recipes and eat them, too!

IN THIS CHAPTER

» Discovering the many benefits of the Mediterranean diet

» Appreciating heritage diets

» Controlling blood pressure with DASH

» Harvesting the benefits of a plant-based diet

» Considering the pros and cons of low-carb diets

» Letting someone else do some of the planning

Chapter **14**

Analyzing Popular Diet Plans

O
n a National Geographic documentary film you might hear a biologist quietly whisper something like, "These mountain gorillas live primarily on a diet of tender leaves and stems." In everyday language, however, the word *diet* is rarely used to simply describe a general eating pattern. Instead, *diet* more often refers to a temporary, unwanted, and unpleasant assignment that you must tolerate in order to lose weight — "I need to go on a diet." For this book, and for a more enjoyable life, the National Geographic use of the word is a better way to think.

Our modern use of the word diet might be described as an acronym standing for "D-are I- E-at T-hat" because so often the advice about eating is all about restriction and avoidance of foods we might like. The aim of such diets is usually for weight reduction, sometimes with the aim of excessive weight loss to emulate a fashionable body shape, and they are almost always unachievable and unsustainable. For many people who are overweight, steady weight loss to a healthier target certainly reduces the risk of diabetes and many other chronic illnesses and is beneficial. However, it's important to remember that the foods we eat and the lifestyle we choose have more impact on our health, quality of life, and longevity than our weight alone. The word diet derives from the Greek word "diaita," which means way of life. We prefer this definition.

FROM THE AUTHORS

A healthy diet is definitely one that sustainably supports people to achieve and maintain a healthy weight, but it must also deliver reduced risks of many chronic diseases including the prevention or reversal or better management of type 2 diabetes. The advice in this book and in *Diabetes For Dummies* (Wiley) can help and support everyone to adopt the healthiest of lifestyles to add quality years to their life.

In this chapter, we review some popular diet plans, including a few commercial ones you may have seen advertised, to evaluate how they might fit with accepted diabetes management principles. We also take a look at the lure of fad diets and how you can modify some of your favorite recipes to make them diabetes-friendly.

Basking in the Mediterranean

The Mediterranean diet is a perfect example of a diet you can live with, not a diet you'll go on, as it is a general pattern of eating. The primary benefit of this eating pattern was first identified in the Seven Countries Study, which started following middle-aged men in 1958 across four different regions of the world to systematically look at the effects of lifestyle on health. This study contributed to current understandings about the health risks of high blood pressure, smoking, cholesterol, and obesity, and about the health benefits of physical activity and dietary fiber. But, researchers noted something odd in the data. Deaths from heart attacks were much higher in the United States and Northern Europe than in Southern Europe, even when statistics were adjusted to account for age, weight, physical activity, smoking, cholesterol, and blood pressure. The diet and lifestyle in this Mediterranean region seemed to be protecting the population.

REMEMBER

A diet for effective diabetes management controls blood glucose averages, helps you manage body weight, and reduces risk factors for heart disease like cholesterol and blood pressure.

The Mediterranean diet, as a contemporary eating plan with health distinct benefits, began gaining popularity in the mid-1990s, and the characteristic foods are modeled from the dietary patterns of Southern Italy, Greece, Crete, Morocco, and Spain in the 1960s. Literally thousands of studies have examined the health effects of the food and/or the Mediterranean lifestyle, which includes physical activity and stress reduction. Two studies published in 2013 added credibility to the Mediterranean diet's benefits to heart health, other chronic diseases, and diabetes.

>> In the PREDIMED Study, researchers in Spain followed more than 7,000 individuals at high risk for cardiovascular disease over nearly five years after placing one group on a low-fat diet and two groups on different Mediterranean eating patterns. The Mediterranean diet groups experienced 30 percent fewer major cardiovascular events (heart attack, stroke, or death) as well as significant reductions in type 2 diabetes.

>> A meta-analysis published in the January 2013 issue of the *American Journal of Clinical Nutrition* evaluated 20 different studies to determine the effectiveness of different dietary approaches for the management of type 2 diabetes. The analysis showed the Mediterranean diet improves average blood glucose levels (A1C), improves HDL (good) cholesterol, reduces blood triglycerides, and effectively promotes weight loss, all-important to reducing risks for diabetes-related complications.

TECHNICAL STUFF

A meta-analysis is essentially a study of the results of other studies. A meta-analysis evaluates whether the results from multiple independent studies looking at the same issue, more or less, gave statistically consistent results so that the data from those studies can be combined to strengthen a conclusion.

One interesting aspect of many studies involving the Mediterranean diet is that researchers often observe the eating pattern is easy to sustain over time. In the study from Spain, the group assigned to a low-fat diet dropped out of the study at a high rate and ultimately could not stick closely with their assigned diet. By contrast, participants assigned to either of the two Mediterranean diet groups showed a high level of adherence to their assigned plan. Because no healthy eating plan is effective if it can't be followed, the desirability of this eating plan is an important feature. *Mediterranean Lifestyle For Dummies* by Amy Riolo (Wiley) can help you really explore the possibilities of this healthy diet and lifestyle.

THE MEDITERRANEAN DIET AND MORTALITY

Most people worry about being overweight either for reasons of appearance (which is based on social norms and fashion — there have been times in history and regions of the world where it was considered attractive to be larger in size). We also might have justified concerns about the association between being overweight or obese and the risk of developing chronic diseases including heart disease and diabetes and of dying early. Research has shown that as we become older, it may actually be protective to have a BMI slightly above the target "healthy" zone, and a large cohort study published in the journal *PLOS Medicine* in 2020 showed that a healthy Mediterranean diet could mitigate significantly some risks associated with being overweight.

Obese individuals with high adherence to a Mediterranean-type diet did not experience the increased overall mortality otherwise associated with high BMI, although a higher level of cardiovascular risk did remain. On the other hand, having a lower BMI did not counter the higher mortality associated with a low adherence to a Mediterranean diet. These are not reasons for anyone to purposefully aim to be overweight, but it certainly shows the vital role a healthy diet can play in lowering risks of chronic diseases and early death whatever weight we are.

Balancing grains, legumes, and fruit

Dietary fiber is a key component of the Mediterranean diet, and the fiber comes along with carbohydrates and other key nutrients from unrefined grains, legumes (beans and peas), fresh fruits, and vegetables. One benefit of dietary fiber is simply making you feel full sooner and for a longer period between meals. That's called *satiety*. A satisfied appetite often leads to fewer calories, and consuming fewer calories leads to weight loss. But the health benefits of these foods don't stop with satiety.

Legumes — beans, chickpeas, peas, and lentils — are a key source of low-fat protein in a Mediterranean diet and are a rich source of soluble fiber. The different types of soluble fiber help reduce cholesterol, especially LDL (bad) cholesterol, a key risk factor for heart disease and, along with bioactive compounds, are prebiotic — food for our gut microbes. Consumption of whole grains is associated with lower blood pressure, even when consumed in relatively small amounts. High blood pressure along with diabetes is a double whammy for your kidneys, as well as a risk factor for heart disease and stroke.

Fruits and vegetables in the Mediterranean diet also contribute to satiety and add an assortment of vitamins, nutrients, and bioactive compounds including polyphenols to the mix. Fresh fruit is the dessert of choice, and the fruits and vegetables should be enjoyed without added sugar, fat, or salt (sodium). The dietary fiber from this fruit and vegetable part of the Mediterranean diet, as well as from legumes and grains, can benefit your health in another very important way — blood glucose control.

A typical Mediterranean diet gets about 50 percent of daily calories from carbohydrate, and the great majority of the carbs come from legumes, unrefined grains, and fruit. These sources tend to have a lower glycemic index than added sugars or refined grains because the liberation of glucose during digestion is slower. The glycemic index is discussed in more detail in Chapter 6, but the key issue is that the effect on blood glucose levels from low glycemic index foods is gradual. The Mediterranean diet has been shown as appropriate, even beneficial, to blood glucose control. And, while the glycemic index of the primary sources of carbohydrates surely is important, that fact alone doesn't seem to account for the total picture of this eating plan and diabetes. The meta-analysis, mentioned earlier in this section, found the Mediterranean diet reduced A1C more than any of the diets in the comparison, including, by the way, low glycemic index diets.

REMEMBER

If you have diabetes, type 1 or type 2, you need to account for your consumption of carbohydrates, even those from low glycemic index foods. These foods do elevate blood glucose at a slower rate than high glycemic index foods, but it's still your supply and response to insulin that brings your blood glucose levels back to normal.

TIP

If your idea of beans and grains is bland and blander, you're in for a surprise. Mediterranean cuisine livens up the main ingredients with vinegars, capers, rosemary, mushrooms, citrus, mint, garlic, honey, fennel, peppers, cumin, paprika, onions, saffron, thyme, tomatoes, sage, bay leaf, oregano, nuts, dill, yogurt — to name just a few.

Swapping meat for fish and extra-virgin olive oil

The predominant sources of protein and fat in the typical Mediterranean diet are what sets this eating plan apart from other patterns, especially from the eating patterns typical in the United States (sometimes called the Western diet). On balance, the protein component is relatively low (15 to 20 percent of daily calories), and the fat component relatively high (35 percent of daily calories). But, the specific foods providing the bulk of these macronutrients are somewhat unique to the Mediterranean diet.

Yogurt and cheese make up the dairy component of this eating plan, and these foods, even if eaten every day, are consumed in moderation. Likewise, poultry and eggs provide a portion of the diet's protein, but are eaten in moderation also. Poultry or eggs may be on the menu a few times each week.

The most distinctive trait of the Mediterranean diet, especially when contrasted with the Western diet, is the focus on red meat. More accurately, there is no focus on red meat in the Mediterranean diet — red meat is consumed very sparingly, and in small 2- to 4-ounce portions. Limiting meat consumption leads to a general reduction in unhealthier saturated fats, enhancing the cardiovascular benefits of a Mediterranean diet. But, red meat consumption, especially processed red meat products like hot dogs or salami, has recently gotten attention for its role in blood glucose imbalance, too.

Looking at more than 440,000 participants in the long-term Nurses' Health Study and similar groups, researchers at Harvard University's School of Public Health found a 2-ounce serving of processed red meat product per day increased the risk for developing type 2 diabetes by 50 percent. The ATTICA Study of men and women in Greece (carried out in the Greek province of Attica in Athens), all without cardiovascular disease or diabetes, showed that red meat consumption was associated with reduced insulin sensitivity and excess insulin secretion, typical of type 2 diabetes. Red meat consumption clearly has a negative effect on blood glucose balance. Any factor that accelerates the development of type 2 diabetes or promotes insulin resistance in healthy people is certain to make controlling blood glucose more difficult if you already have diabetes. Limiting red meat intake, therefore, likely accounts for some of the compatibility between the Mediterranean diet and improvements seen in A1C.

So, if cheese, poultry, eggs, and especially red meat are only a minor part of this eating plan, what are the remaining sources of protein and dietary fat? The answer is probably the key to what makes the Mediterranean diet easy to follow for the long term — fish and seafood, nuts, and olive oil.

Fish, seafood, and nuts not only supplement the dietary protein already provided by legumes, but also add healthy unsaturated fats, including omega-3 fatty acids, into the mix. Your Mediterranean diet might add a small serving of nuts every day and a serving of fish or seafood several times a week. Fresh fish, of course, was plentiful along the coast of the Mediterranean in the 1960s when the Seven Countries Study first noted the mysteriously low cardiovascular risk associated with living there.

REMEMBER

At the heart of the Mediterranean diet is extra-virgin olive oil. Extra-virgin olive oil contains mostly healthy monounsaturated fats (oleic acid), vitamin E, and natural polyphenols with healthy antioxidant properties. Clinical data suggests that extra-virgin olive oil has anti-inflammatory and antithrombotic (preventing blood clots) properties, and improves the flexibility of blood vessels. With respect to diabetes, a 2011 study actually looked at individual variations in the composition of a fat that is part of cell membranes, *phosphatidylcholine,* and found when oleic acid was a component of this complex molecule, insulin resistance was lower. Among the 360 participants in Spain, none with diabetes, every 1 percent increase in the oleic acid composition of phosphatidylcholine represented a 20 percent reduction in insulin resistance (prediabetes). Extra-virgin olive oil, therefore, may offer clear benefits for both cardiovascular health, and blood glucose control.

TIP

As a food, extra-virgin olive oil replaces the saturated fats other societies consume as butter, and adds flavor to vegetable dishes in particular. It can be used for cooking or can be drizzled directly into salads, vegetable dishes, onto bread, or in marinades.

Finally, the Mediterranean diet's combination of fats seems to strike a beneficial balance between omega-3 fatty acids and the less famous omega-6 fatty acids. You need both omega-3 and omega-6 fatty acids, and both are healthy fats. But when omega-6 consumption is much higher than omega-3 consumption, the imbalance in fats can lead to inflammation and atherosclerosis. The typical Western diet may favor omega-6 fatty acids by 20 to 1 or more, but in a typical Mediterranean diet the balance is closer to a healthy 4 to 1.

Understanding Heritage Diets

In 2010, UNESCO recognized the Mediterranean diet to be an "Intangible Cultural Heritage of Humanity" and characterized it as "a set of skills, knowledge, practices, and traditions ranging from the landscape to the table, including the crops, harvesting, fishing, conservation, processing, preparation, and, particularly, consumption of food."

The Mediterranean diet has been long established, deeply rooted in ancient ways of living, and has continued to evolve, embracing new flavors of herbs and spices from the Far East along early trade routes as well as chocolate and tomatoes from the New World and coffee from Africa. The dietary pattern has spread its influence beyond the Mediterranean Sea with the planting of olive groves, vineyards, and other crops emblematic of the Mediterranean in places with similar climates along the 40-degree parallels North and South such as California, Australia, South America, and Southern Africa.

It is increasingly recognized that there are other diets that are similarly based on traditional, natural, and plant-predominant patterns of eating, and are likely to be beneficial for health. It's perhaps just that they have not been studied so extensively. They share common features such as having low glycemic-index carbohydrates rich in fiber and proteins commonly sourced from legumes and nuts, with healthy unsaturated fats and foods good for the gut microbiome. Perhaps most important, they are low in refined carbohydrates, added sugars, and other additives and preservatives typically found in highly processed Western diets. They are also rich in the minerals and bioactive compounds such as polyphenols found in foods grown in traditional ways. A project called Blue Zones identified several regions in the world with exceptional numbers of people who thrive, living long and healthy lives. Diet is one factor and the areas span the globe from Costa Rica through the Mediterranean to Japan.

Oldways (https://oldwayspt.org) is a not-for-profit organization dedicated to improving public health by inspiring individuals and organizations to embrace the healthy, sustainable joys of the "old ways" of living. Having been early advocates of the Mediterranean diet, the organization now recognizes the importance of also respecting and championing food and culinary cultures from around the globe. There is an urgent need for further research to identify the components of these diets that are particularly healthy and to push back the advance of the processed, industrial foods that are bringing high rates of obesity and chronic diseases to countries previously unaffected by the epidemic of illnesses now seen in Western societies. Meanwhile, Oldways has led the way by illustrating African heritage, Asian, and Latin American diet pyramids and by describing the common features that are likely to confer good health.

Dining with DASH

High blood pressure, *hypertension*, is common among people with diabetes. By some estimates, two of every three people with diabetes have high blood pressure, too, in some measure because the risk factors for type 2 diabetes — overweight, lack of physical activity, and age — are also risk factors for high blood pressure. Having both high blood pressure and diabetes multiplies the risk for some serious complications, such as kidney failure, heart attack and stroke, and problems with the eyes.

DASH is an acronym for "dietary approaches to stop hypertension." DASH is an eating plan developed experimentally by the National Institutes of Health when that agency conducted clinical trials on three distinct diet plans through five medical centers between 1993 and 1997. The study clearly demonstrated a capacity to lower blood pressure with diet.

Controlling high blood pressure with diet

Blood pressure is a measure of the force of blood pushing on the walls of your arteries as your heart pumps blood throughout your body. High blood pressure can be caused by a loss of flexibility in blood vessels and arteries, by deposits that decrease the size of arteries and decrease the smoothness of blood flow, by changes in blood volume or thickness, or by unknown factors. Blood pressure measurements are expressed in millimeters of mercury (a measure of pressure) when the heart pumps (*systolic* pressure), and the pressure when the heart is resting between beats (*diastolic* pressure).

WARNING

A normal blood pressure is considered to be lower than 120/80. If you have either number higher than a systolic/diastolic 140/90, you are considered hypertensive.

The National Institutes of Health study found that a particular eating plan, now known as DASH, lowered blood pressure by an average of 5.5 systolic and 3.0 diastolic compared to the typical U.S. diet eaten by a matched group. The DASH plan lowered blood pressure even more among the African-American and other ethnic participants, who are at a statistically higher risk for hypertension. And, for participants with hypertension, systolic pressure dropped by an average of 11.4 and diastolic by an average of 5.5. The original DASH eating plan notably did not include a reduced sodium component.

Considering grains, fruit, and dairy

The DASH eating plan is typical of most healthy diet recommendations in its emphasis on more vegetables, fewer added sweets, and less saturated fat. The DASH plan is somewhat unique, however, in its strong emphasis on whole grains. A typical DASH eating plan also incorporates several servings of fruit and low-fat dairy into a daily menu, and taken together with the grains there are a lot of carbohydrate-containing foods you need to balance for blood glucose management.

Table 14-1 shows the recommended number of servings from the various food groups as they're divided in the DASH plan. For a 2,000-calorie diet, the plan could (emphasizing *could*) include up to 25 carb choices per day. A typical eating plan for diabetes management is more likely to include closer to 15 carb choices each day (remember that a carb choice is 15 grams of carbohydrate). This kind of variation can be significant in managing blood glucose effectively, but it's easy enough to adjust the daily carbohydrates and still follow the DASH plan.

Chapter 13 discusses how the United States Department of Agriculture's (USDA's) representation of a healthy and balanced diet with MyPlate spreads carbohydrates into more than one group. The DASH eating plan does this, too, so it's important to know where carbohydrates are hiding.

TABLE 14-1   **DASH Plan Recommended Servings***

DASH Plan Food Group	Number of Servings (Per Day Unless Noted)	Examples
Grains	6–8 servings	Whole wheat bread or rolls, whole-grain pasta, cereals, grits, brown rice, quinoa, popcorn, oatmeal, pretzels
Vegetables	4–5 servings	Broccoli, carrots, greens, squash, potatoes, sweet potatoes, tomatoes, peas, cucumbers, green beans
Fruit	4–5 servings	Fresh, frozen, dried, canned without syrup, or juices
Fat-free or low-fat dairy products	2–3 servings	Milk, buttermilk, cheese, yogurt
Lean meats and poultry	6 or fewer 1-ounce servings	Lean meats, trim fat, broil, roast fish, remove skin from poultry, limit eggs to four per week
Nuts, seeds, and legumes	4–5 servings per week	Almonds, walnuts, peanuts, sunflower seeds, peanut butter, beans, lentils
Fats and oils	2–3 servings	Margarine, oil, salad dressing
Sweets and sugars	less than 1 serving	Candy, syrup, jelly, sugar

*Based on a 2,000-calorie diet.

REMEMBER

All grains contain carbohydrate, so the DASH recommendation for six to eight servings per day is pretty clear — always count grains as carbohydrates. But, did you notice some starchy vegetables hiding in the vegetable category? Potatoes, sweet potatoes, peas, lima beans, and hard-shell squashes are carbohydrate foods, and you would need to account for them as carb choices. You know that everything in the fruit category should be counted as carbs, but while cheese has no carbohydrate, both milk and yogurt in the dairy group should be accounted for in your daily carbohydrate consumption. The sweets group is, of course, all carbohydrate, and there's no need to look for carbs in the fat and oils or in the lean meats groups. But, the nuts and seeds group also includes the legumes beans and lentils, and these legumes are candidates for carbohydrate counting.

TIP

When following the DASH eating plan you simply need to remember your diabetes meal plan's carbohydrate recommendations and know that carbohydrate foods are not completely segregated with grains, fruits and sweets, but also can be found in vegetables, dairy and nuts. If you, for instance, decide to go with the full eight servings of grain in a day, then you won't throw in five servings of fruit, two glasses of milk, a bean burrito, a baked potato, a mocha latte, and a frozen yogurt.

Finding potassium, magnesium, and calcium

The DASH eating plan has a focus on providing three substances that can help keep blood pressure levels lower — potassium, magnesium, and calcium. And, the plan focuses on getting these elements from food.

Tomato gardeners know that when their fertilizer says 18-18-21, it means 18 percent nitrogen, 18 percent phosphorus, and 21 percent potash. Potash is a potassium compound, and potassium (scientific symbol K) is essential for you and your tomatoes. Potassium is an *electrolyte* that plays a key role in important activities like helping your heart beat in rhythm, and many studies have shown that adequate levels of potassium help lower blood pressure. Fruits, vegetables, legumes, fish and dairy are all DASH sources of potassium, and the eating plan looks to provide 4,700 milligrams per day.

If you're familiar with milk of magnesia, you're familiar with magnesium. This common earth element has more important roles than bringing relief from constipation, however. Magnesium is involved in hundreds of biochemical processes in your body, including regulation of blood pressure and blood glucose. The DASH eating plan looks to increase your intake of magnesium by emphasizing whole grains, fruits and vegetables, nuts, seeds, and legumes. People with type 2 diabetes tend to have lower levels of magnesium. The DASH plan's goal for magnesium is 500 milligrams per day.

Calcium is known for its relationship to bone health. But calcium also plays a complex role in blood pressure. The first studies exploring the effects of dietary calcium on blood pressure were published in the early 1980s, and the benefit has become clearer since. The DASH plan aims to provide 1,250 milligrams per day from fat-free and low-fat dairy, green vegetables, fish, and beans.

Losing sodium is even better

The Centers for Disease Control and Prevention estimates the average American diet includes 3,436 milligrams of sodium per day, compared to your body's requirement of less than 500 milligrams. Excess sodium consumption is related to hypertension, and the DASH plan limits sodium intake to 2,300 milligrams per day. The dietary recommendation for people with diabetes, however, is no more than 1,500 milligrams of sodium per day. Interestingly, a follow-up to the original DASH study looked at the effect on high blood pressure of a lower sodium DASH eating plan — 1,500 milligrams per day. The lower sodium plan reduced blood pressure more than the original plan.

Don't think that throwing your salt shaker out the window automatically solves the challenges with reducing sodium. If your sodium intake is average, it's likely that 70 percent comes from foods, not that shaker. The most likely culprits are canned foods, cured meats, and restaurant food, and reducing sodium is so important you should really learn to look for it in your diet.

The DASH eating plan can be consistent with effective diabetes management, but you need to locate the carbohydrate foods to balance DASH with your meal plan. Talk with your doctor before you jump in, especially if there are concerns about kidney function.

WARNING

The DASH diet does have some limitations. First, it is a plan that evolved to control the specific issue of high blood pressure. While it may include many healthy foods, it does not specifically focus on the most beneficial nutrients and bioactive compounds (see Chapters 7 and 8). The emphasis on salt reduction may be helpful for some, but sensitivity to salt and its effects on blood pressure are by no means universal, and people may differ in their response. The value of counting calories has also been challenged by many researchers in nutrition citing evidence that it may be more useful to consider portion size and food combinations.

The evidence in favor of reducing saturated fat and in particular advocating low-fat dairy products is not without controversy. Full-fat fermented foods have not been convincingly associated with high blood pressure or heart disease and may even be protective against developing type 2 diabetes. Some versions of the DASH diet have recommended less healthy vegetable oils such as safflower and corn oils as well as "light" salad dressings and margarines, which usually contain numerous additives.

Preferring Plants: Vegetarian Diets

An impressive body of evidence demonstrates the effectiveness of a vegetarian diet in weight management, A1C improvement, increased insulin sensitivity, and cardiovascular health indicators. But, can you really get adequate nutrition from plants? According to the Academy of Nutrition and Dietetics, "appropriately planned vegetarian diets, including total vegetarian or vegan diets, are healthful, nutritionally adequate, and may provide health benefits in the prevention and treatment of certain diseases." Maybe this is worth a look.

The Vegetarian Society was founded in Manchester, England in 1847, and that event marks the beginning of what could be called the modern era of this approach to diet. Defining a vegetarian depends to some extent upon whom you ask. A *pollo-pescetarian* vegetarian, for instance, eats poultry and seafood. Most likely, only pollo-pescatarians can add the word vegetarian to that lineup with a straight face — a giant turkey leg with a shrimp cocktail appetizer may leave only limited space for the vegetarian part of their meals.

Many people around the world, however, fall under more accepted variations of vegetarianism, and it's reasonable to address the question of diabetes management as it applies to a couple of different views on plant-based eating. The truth is that most people should lean more toward vegetarian to add more vegetables and to cut down on red meat. But, there's one surprising nutrient most Americans could use a little more of — protein — and getting enough of this from plants while managing blood glucose levels takes a little thought.

In the broad picture, a surprising number of Americans are not getting enough protein relative to the recommendation that protein should account for 20 percent, more or less, of total calories. One challenge of a plant-based diet is finding nutrients, including protein, to replace what's lost when giving up meat and other animal products.

Adopting the ovo-lacto view

Movie credits often run the disclaimer, "no animals were harmed during the making of this film." Ovo-lacto vegetarians take a similar view, and include eggs and dairy products into their primarily plant-based diet because no animals are harmed in the making of those foods, although many people might agree that it is harmful to raise any animal intensively in an environment where they are unable to flourish. Adding eggs and dairy provides additional options for dietary protein — the best dietary source of calcium and better access to vitamin B12 (more on that next). But, it isn't that these nutrients aren't available from plant foods.

Eating protein is all about getting the *amino acids.* Protein is built from amino acids, and your body uses about 20 different amino acids to build everything it needs for good health. Of the 20, a specific 9 are called essential amino acids because your body cannot produce them from scratch — these must be in your diet. Protein is readily available from plants like beans, nuts and seeds, and grains, but whereas most animal sources of protein include all nine essential amino acids, single sources of plant protein are often missing a few. In practice, that simply means that vegetarians should eat a wide variety of protein foods. Adding eggs and dairy, however, does provide a couple of one-stop shops for essential amino acids, but soy protein is of equal quality. All in all, concerns about inadequate protein in a vegetarian diet are irrelevant as long as a variety of foods are included and adequate protein consumption is a focus.

Adequate calcium is only slightly more a concern in a vegetarian diet. Calcium is available in dark greens like collards or kale, green soybeans (edamame) and soy, and sesame seeds, to name a few, but calcium in plants may not be as available for absorption as calcium in dairy or fish. And, dairy is the richest source of calcium.

Consuming dairy products as part of a plant-based diet, therefore, adds some distinct benefit. In the big picture, eggs and dairy in the diets of ovo-lacto vegetarians may be valuable if only by adding more variety.

To be sure you get enough calcium in your diet, you need to have enough vitamin D, which promotes the uptake of calcium in your intestine. The best source of vitamin D is definitely sunlight, but there is a fear of overexposure to sunlight, which might lead to skin cancer or possibly malignant melanoma. And there are many places far from the equator where the sun comes in at such an angle in the winter that you get little or no vitamin D from sun exposure. You can get some vitamin D from food, especially from milk and fatty fish like salmon, but the easiest source is a little gel capsule, which is cheap and available in any drugstore.

TIP

If you are concerned that you are not getting enough vitamin D, ask your doctor to perform a blood test for your level.

Being vegan

The word *vegan* describes a person who eats only foods from plants, or in some cases, avoids using any animal products at all, like leather or silk. With respect to diet, you have already seen how plants can provide well-balanced nutrition. Plants are a primary source of carbohydrates in any diet, plant protein is sufficient when the diet is varied, and plant fats are, for the most part, healthy unsaturated fats. There's one nutrient that vegetarians, and especially vegans, cannot get in a plant-based diet, and that is vitamin B12.

Eggs and dairy products do contain vitamin B12, but there are no reliable sources of this essential vitamin from plants. Vitamin B12 has some very important responsibilities, including brain and nervous system function, and a deficiency of this vitamin can lead to severe neurological damage. Vegans must either consume foods fortified with vitamin B12 or take a vitamin supplement.

TIP

Breakfast cereals are commonly fortified with vitamin B12 and provide a convenient source for vegans. Soy and nut milks are often fortified, as are meat substitutes, and vegans must look for this nutrient on nutrition labels. Products targeted to vegetarians and vegans are certain to list this essential fact on the nutrition label.

A vegetarian or vegan diet can be completely consistent with diabetes, especially when nonstarchy vegetables are liberally included. The heart benefits to this eating strategy are clear, and as long as you remember that carbohydrates are found in fruits, grains, legumes (beans), and starchy vegetables, you can manage your health and your diabetes quite nicely.

Thinking About Low-Carb Diets

Low-carbohydrate diets have increased in popularity in recent years. In some respects, this is a response to flawed dietary advice from many health professionals, governments, and public health organizations for the last several decades that recommended a low-fat, high-carbohydrate diet. The possible association of saturated fat with heart disease coupled with a lack of understanding of the importance of cholesterol lipid oxidation and inflammation as a contributing factor, resulted in blanket advice to reduce fat consumption. Little distinction was made between healthy unsaturated fats and saturated fats that increased LDL cholesterol.

In addition, despite recognizing that the Mediterranean diet was very healthy indeed, there was little effort to understand and promote the beneficial high-fat foods — such as extra-virgin olive oil and nuts — that contributed to its positive effects, including through bioactive compounds.

There was a focus on calorie counting, and because fats contain approximately three times as many calories per gram when compared with protein and carbohydrates, fats, it was concluded, made people fat. The advice may not have had such negative consequences were it not for the failure to properly describe the difference between good-quality and poor-quality carbohydrates. As the food industry produced more additives and combined sugars and refined carbohydrates in processed convenience foods, claiming products to be low in fat and therefore healthy, rates of obesity, diabetes, and many chronic diseases soared.

The current risk is that the mistakes of grossly oversimplistic advice to change the macronutrient makeup of our diets in the last half of the 20th century may be repeated in the first part of the 21st. What is not in doubt is that in the shortterm, low-carbohydrate diets can result in weight loss and even improvements in markers of diabetes control. It is also clear that many people are consuming too many highly refined, poor-quality carbohydrate foods. If these foods are replaced with healthy fats, proteins, and better quality carbohydrates described in Chapter 6 of this book, and if a diet is rich in micronutrients and bioactive compounds, then that can certainly lead to a healthier weight, a reduced risk of developing type 2 diabetes, better control of established diabetes, and less chance of the complications of diabetes.

The long-term health controversies surrounding such an approach to weight loss are still unresolved, and a few of the concerns relate to diabetes. Some doctors, for instance, worry that high protein consumption over a long term eventually takes a toll on kidney function, and bone loss is another common concern. In practice, the grand celebration over eating all the foods other diet plans look to minimize often gives way to craving the carbohydrates (and maybe other nutrients) you've been missing. Low-carb diets are usually not sustainable.

The meta-analysis, first mentioned in this chapter's section on the Mediterranean diet, included diets described as low carbohydrate and diets described as high protein. Whereas the extent of carbohydrate restriction didn't always fall to the low-carb standards of these diets, that analysis found neither a low-carbohydrate nor high-protein diet reduced A1C as much as the Mediterranean plan.

WARNING

Extremely low-carbohydrate diets may be fun (for some) and effective as a weight-loss option for healthy individuals over a short term, but adding diabetes to the mix is cause for concern. Considering that other dietary approaches are proven to effectively manage diabetes and associated health concerns, low-carbohydrate diets need more research to justify an endorsement for people with diabetes, and we should always consider the effects of the foods that replace the carbohydrates as well as being mindful that foods are made up of much more than their macronutrients.

Atkins diet

The Atkins diet, surely the best-known low-carbohydrate weight-loss plan, is based on a theory that excess weight is mostly related to excess carbohydrates. And this eating plan may be attractive to people with diabetes because the constant focus on carbohydrates in diabetes management plans may be interpreted to confirm the notion that carbs are inherently bad.

The Atkins diet, or other low-carbohydrate diets, aims to switch your body into burning fat as an alternative to glucose, and as a weight-loss strategy, these diets are effective. The popularity of the Atkins plan skyrocketed in 2003, with nearly 10 percent of Americans gloating over the diet that required consumption of bacon and steak. Sales of carbohydrate foods like rice and pasta plummeted, and food manufacturers began marketing low-carb versions of their standard products. The death of Dr. Robert Atkins from a fall in 2003, followed by autopsy results suggesting heart disease and high blood pressure, marked the beginning of the end to this frenzy.

Similar diets have taken the place of the Atkins diet and encourage low or very low carbohydrate intake. These include the "keto" diet and the "paleo" diet.

Keto diet

In comparison with Atkins, proponents of the ketogenic or keto diet, generally advise replacing carbs with more fats, as opposed to more proteins. A typical profile might be 60 to 75 percent of calories from fat, 15 to 30 percent from protein, and 5 to 10 percent from carbohydrates. While the shift of metabolism away from carbohydrates to gaining energy from fats and ketones may well lower blood glucose levels and insulin as well as induce weight loss, the down side is the lack of sustainability and questions about the long-term effects on health.

If reducing carbohydrates also means a loss of fiber, minerals, and bioactive compounds from plants, and the increase in fats results in adverse effects on cholesterol levels, then it is reasonable to predict that a keto diet may increase the risk of the very chronic diseases that are the complications of diabetes we are trying to avoid.

Paleo diet

The paleo diet originates in the idea that we should base our eating on foods that were available before societies became agricultural. A typical hunter-gatherer in the paleolithic period might have consumed more meat (though animals would have led very different lives than the livestock of today) and less grains, legumes, and dairy products. Of course, our ancient ancestors would have benefitted from the absence of processed foods in their environment. The diet is usually classified as a low-carbohydrate diet with the approximate ratios often quoted as being 50 percent of calories from fat, 30 percent from protein, and 20 percent from carbohydrates.

The effects of a paleo diet may be similar to a keto diet, although the emphasis on avoiding industrially produced foods and the conscious inclusion of nuts and seeds may give it a marginal edge. Any increase in farmed meat, however, is likely to have adverse effects on our health and the health of our planet.

Counting Points: Weight Watchers

Weight Watchers, now rebranded as WW, is a successful weight-loss program that is not, by its own admission, "designed for those with diabetes." However, successful weight loss can have profoundly positive effects on blood glucose control and on risk factors for diabetes complications like heart disease. Weight Watchers promotes a healthy lifestyle, including regular exercise, and offers programs that include regular, in-person meetings as well as an online program.

A basic Weight Watchers philosophy is that foods are not forbidden. Instead, foods are assigned a specific point value, and the participant budgets for a daily points target. The targets are designed to provide a daily calorie deficit, resulting in weight loss. Foods that are low calorie, low fat, and high fiber are assigned a lower point value than high-calorie, high-fat, low-fiber foods. The advantage to the participant is in being able to see the relative advantage to choosing healthier foods, even though less healthy options can be freely chosen as long as the higher points are counted.

Additionally, following the Weight Watchers program requires at least some focus on food portion sizes in order to arrive at the points value for any particular food. Diabetes management also requires an understanding of portion sizes.

So, on the positive side, Weight Watchers has the following benefits:

>> Potentially helps some achieve weight loss

>> Can be a positive and shared social experience

>> Encourages healthier foods and physical activity

>> Teaches that all foods can fit into a healthy diet

>> Requires a focus on portion size and the nutritional quality of food to arrive at a point value

WARNING

On the cautionary side, the points are completely unrelated to the carbohydrate content of food. In practice, that means that tracking Weight Watchers point values is no substitute for tracking carbohydrates in your meals and snacks. Carbohydrate foods are some of the healthiest foods around, and Weight Watchers often assigns a lower point value based upon the calorie, fiber, and fat content. In fact, a recent attempt to encourage healthier choices left some fruit as point-free foods. For effective diabetes management, eating healthy food is important, but so is managing the volume and timing of your carbohydrates, and you can't ignore the carbs in a fruit even if Weight Watchers says so.

Secondly, there is, of course, a financial cost to the Weight Watchers program. Expect an initial sign-up fee and a monthly fee for both the traditional and online programs. Weight Watchers doesn't require the purchase of its branded food products, but should you decide to go for Weight Watchers foods or its *Smart Ones* brand frozen entrees (found in a store near you) be aware that the cost of food is extra.

Lastly, weight loss is an appropriate goal for many people with diabetes — remember that more than 80 percent of people with type 2 diabetes are overweight or obese. Diabetes is a serious condition and is often joined by other related health problems. You should discuss any plan to modify your diet with your doctor, and with your registered dietitian. Severely limiting calories or restricting food choices without considering health conditions and your medications shouldn't be undertaken without consulting your medical team. And remember to appreciate that much dietary advice included in these plans fails to appreciate the importance of bioactive compounds including polyphenols.

Food By Mail

Some weight-loss programs claim to do all the work for you by delivering your meals already made. But, is doing all the work for weight loss the same as doing all the work for controlling blood glucose?

Nutrisystem

Nutrisystem was founded in 1972, and in 1999 began its current business model selling prepackaged foods directly to customers. The current Nutrisystem program offers weight-loss programs tailored to men or women, each with a subcategory for seniors, vegetarians, or people with diabetes. The plans are calorie-restricted for weight loss, and deliver meals and snacks for 28 days each month to the participant's door. Fresh produce, dairy, and some protein foods must be purchased separately. Nutrisystem offers transition and maintenance plans when you're ready to leave the program, or to maintain a target weight. A members' website offers educational information and tracking tools, and some membership levels include telephone counseling.

The Nutrisystem plan is built, according to its promotional information, on the *glycemic index*, and its diabetes plan, called Nutrisystem D, offers access to Certified Diabetes Educators at all membership levels. The women's diabetes plan is 1,250 calories per day, and 2,300 milligrams sodium. Many of the food choices are specifically for the diabetes plan, and the cost at the lowest level for 28 breakfasts, lunches, dinners, and snacks is advertised at $260.00 per month for men (slightly less for women) if you select the automatic shipping option. Remember, the participant must supply some food.

A 2009 study involving 69 obese participants, funded by Nutrisystem, concluded that the Nutrisystem D was significantly more effective for weight loss, A1C reduction, and other health indicators than a program described as "a diabetes support and education program." This group participated in a group session about diabetes management every four weeks, but its diet was not controlled.

REMEMBER

The Nutrisystem D plan is almost certainly suitable for diabetes management, but some qualification may be necessary. One important note to the Nutrisystem-funded study of the Nutrisystem D plan is that participants consumed a certain number of Nutrisystem food servings as well as additional sources of dairy, fruit, and vegetables. It is fair to deduce that some of the daily carbohydrate choices that are part of the Nutrisystem D plan are purchased weekly at a grocery by the participant, prepared by the participant, and portioned by the participant. Including fresh foods is a good thing, but this element of the Nutrisystem D program suggests that you won't escape thinking about, and planning for, carbohydrates in your diet.

Noom

Noom is a subscription program that helps members meet their goals with yearly prescriptions. It also offers a Diabetes Prevention Program. Noom's philosophy is that "all food — including cheese cake — fits in moderation. And, just as important as tracking calorie or sugar intake is the why behind your eating habits — whether it's related to stress, boredom, or family tradition." The company offers lessons that can help you manage your responses to emotional triggers when eating, support coaches, and peer groups along with meal delivery.

Hello Fresh

At the time of writing, Hello Fresh doesn't have a diabetes-specific menu, but it offers fit and wholesome and low-carb meal kits that might be a fit.

BistroMD

BistroMD is a meal-delivery service "designed by a doctor for diabetics, pre-diabetics, and those who are carb-conscious to achieve long-lasting weight loss results." Its menus consist of 1,200 to 1,400 calories on average per day, and you can choose from various programs that offer 25 grams or less of net carbs per meal from high-quality, complex carbs; 30 grams of lean protein on average per meal; 5 grams of fiber on average per meal; and 3 grams of saturated fat on average per meal. It also offers a diabetic-friendly program that limits sodium to 500 milligrams or less per meal to help members with diabetes meet their health goals.

Resisting Fads

The cabbage soup diet of the 1980s is alive and well, apparently outliving cabbage patch dolls of the same period. But, those who own the original dolls may find they still have value — those who tried the diet lost any value almost immediately. In fairness to the cabbage soup diet, it only claims on its website that you can lose ten pounds in seven days. If you're 28 years old and want to drop a few pounds before your ten-year class reunion, it may be that feeling light-headed, weak, and unable to concentrate is worth a week of cabbage. If you have diabetes, however, the cabbage soup diet is maybe not such a great idea.

Americans are on a constant search for an easy way to lose weight, spending more than $2 billion each year on ineffective weight-loss supplements. Fad diets, although not nearly so expensive (cabbage is cheap), somehow seem irresistible to many. And, while you might be perfectly able to see through the claims of diet plans like the Hot Dog Diet or Dr. Siegal's Cookie Diet, the desperation that comes from unsuccessful efforts at weight loss can cloud judgment. The guilt about weight that sometimes goes with diabetes can increase that sense of desperation, too, but having diabetes makes fad diets potentially dangerous.

Promising the quick fix

Medical professionals generally consider weight loss of about 1 to 2 pounds per week fast enough unless close supervision is provided. Diet plans that guarantee rapid weight loss, perhaps by resetting or revving up your metabolism, are either fraudulent or dangerous.

The HCG diet, where HCG stands for *human chorionic gonadotropin,* is an excellent example. The plan focuses your attention on injections of this special hormone recovered from the urine of pregnant women, but the extreme weight loss is actually related to the diet's 500 calories per day food allowance. A diet that includes only 500 calories per day is not safe. The U.S. Food and Drug Administration issued warning letters to companies that market HCG as a natural weight-loss supplement, but startling claims and persuasive testimonials are everywhere still.

The bottom line is that ultra-quick weight loss is unhealthy, is often only a loss of water (the weight is regained immediately), and the method is not sustainable. Just ask those who tried the Apple Cider Vinegar Diet.

Trumpeting miracle weight-loss foods

Sorry, there are no miracle foods or secret combinations of foods that burn fat while you sleep. The constantly resurrecting Grapefruit Diet, or the Wu-Yi Tea Diet are examples — there are others, and there will always be new ones.

Losing weight and losing fat is about using more calories than you ingest, and any of these plans that actually leads to weight loss inevitably does so by coming in with low calories. Unfortunately, these plans also restrict foods that are healthy, and sometimes essential.

A few other keys to recognizing fad diets would include the following:

>> It sounds too good to be true (your mother was right!).

>> It's the food (or diet) they don't want you to know about (if it was healthy, they really would want you to know about it).

>> Claims are based on a single unpublished study, or simple conclusions are drawn from a complex study.

>> A diet special for only some people (the Blood Type Diet).

>> It includes a miracle food only available from one place (at a low price today only, plus shipping and handling).

REMEMBER Having diabetes makes it especially important that you not waste time (or money) or risk your health by looking for shortcuts to better health. The sooner you decide to follow a proven path, the better your future looks.

Chapter **15**

What's on the Menu: Having a Plan for Eating Out

Eating out can be one of life's greatest pleasures. While we advocate preparing meals yourself as much as possible so that you can control the quality and nutrients in your food, there's no need to swear off restaurants and prepared food forever if you have diabetes. That said, it's important to realize that if you don't manage exactly what, how, and when you eat, your health will surely suffer.

This chapter helps you find a balance between diabetes management and eating away from home by employing the same strategies that can keep you on track at home — planning ahead. And, if planning is your key to conquering impulsive eating at home — and it is — imagine how important planning can be when you're enveloped by the sights and sounds and aromas that encourage you to eat with abandon.

Making Decisions First

If you don't plan carefully, eating away from home almost certainly means eating less healthy foods overall. Studies show that people eating away from home are consistently confronted with higher-calorie foods, larger portion sizes, and an atmosphere that encourages overindulgence. Consequently, eating away from home results in a higher intake of calories, fat, saturated fat, and sodium as well as a lower intake of fiber, vitamins A and C, carotenes, calcium, and magnesium. With diabetes wellbeing so closely connected to food, eating away from home, while staying true to your medical nutrition therapy, is definitely a challenge.

Table 15-1 compares a full day's recommendations for carbohydrate, fat, and sodium for a 1,700-calorie eating plan to a few single meals at popular restaurants. Remember, the first line is the recommendation for a whole day.

TABLE 15-1   **Restaurant Meals Compared to Daily Recommendations**

Sample Meal	Calories	Carbohydrate	Fat	Sodium
Daily calories and nutrients for diabetes	1,700	212 grams	56 grams	1,500 milligrams
Honey chipotle chicken	1,700	200 grams	77 grams	4,110 milligrams
Hibachi chicken skewers	1,330	187 grams	41 grams	4,760 milligrams
Angus deluxe, large fries, large diet soda	1,260	124 grams	64 grams	2,025 milligrams
Tostada chicken salad	1,551	102 grams	94 grams	2,480 milligrams

Standing face to face with food, or with images of food like in a menu, is not the time to be making decisions about healthy eating. The thinking part of your brain is no match for biology in the spur of the moment — it needs time to consider all variables and reach a logical conclusion. Giving your thinking brain the time and information to do what it does best is one thing that makes meal planning so powerful.

So, making decisions first, before you're confronted with overwhelming choices, means actually making decisions. It doesn't mean considering in some general way whether you might go for the salad at dinner tonight. Your thinking brain needs information, and it's up to you to collect the facts.

FROM THE AUTHORS

We talk about calories in this chapter not only because your dietician or nutritionist may have advised you to closely count the calories you eat, but also because restaurants are increasingly listing the calories with each meal they serve. Counting calories can be a useful guide to the amount of energy you are taking in, but it is important to also understand that not all calories are the same. Some heart-healthy high-fat foods like extra-virgin olive oil, olives, nuts, and avocados may increase the calorie numbers but may not necessarily increase your risk of putting on weight, and even have a beneficial effect on glucose regulation.

On the other hand, some artificial sweeteners, while sparing the calories, have been shown to lead to a less healthy gut microbiome and increase the risk of putting on weight. Calorie "light" products where fats are reduced may be higher in refined sugars that are lower in calories gram for gram, but are not good for diabetes control. The answer is to use calorie counts as one of several strategies you have learned from reading this book to help you achieve the best diet for your diabetes and your general health.

Remembering your meal plan

If you don't have a personalized meal plan from a registered dietitian or nutritionist as part of your diabetes *medical nutrition therapy*, get one. Food is extremely important to controlling your diabetes, and a personalized meal plan tells you how many grams of carbohydrate to eat at each meal, what your daily calorie goal should be, how to best address blood pressure and cholesterol, how your diabetes medications work most effectively, and includes nutritional guidance for other medical conditions.

The most unique element of your diabetes meal plan is its focus on carbohydrates, because carbohydrates raise blood glucose levels directly. Because diabetes is all about unhealthy high blood glucose levels, it makes perfect sense that managing the foods that raise blood glucose levels is important. The amount and timing of carbohydrate foods you eat works hand in hand with the amount and timing of your medications, including insulin, to keep blood glucose levels as close to normal as possible. When you can keep these levels as close to normal as possible, your risk for serious diabetes complications is reduced, so keeping your blood glucose under control makes perfect sense too. Your thinking brain is pleased when things make perfect sense.

Your meal plan helps this whole process by recommending a specific number of grams of carbohydrate with each meal and by giving general guidance on which carbohydrate foods give you the most nutrition-related bang for your buck. Generally, about 50 percent of your daily calories comes from carbohydrates — 1,000 calories from carbohydrates if your calorie recommendation is 2,000 calories per day. Because carbohydrates store 4 calories of energy per gram, 1,000 calories translate to 250 grams of carbohydrate per day.

Carbohydrates, in diabetes-related nutrition, are discussed in 15-gram portions called a *carbohydrate* (or carb) *choice*. Your 2,000 calories per day eating plan, therefore, recommends about 16 carb choices per day — maybe 5 with each meal, and one 15 gram snack, depending upon your personalized plan. Your meal plan never recommends that you save all, or even most, of your 16 carbohydrate choices for the all-you-can-eat buffet. So, making decisions in advance about what you're going to eat for a meal away from home should include a strong preference for about four to six carb choices, whatever is consistent with your meal plan, for the entire meal — drinks, finger food, appetizers, soup, salad ingredients and dressing, entree and sides, and dessert.

TIP

Food that's sitting around in plain view — bar snacks, appetizers, or bread — is difficult to ignore. Try taking a small serving, then have the food removed from your sight. Most people believe they are not influenced by such temptations, but studies show that having food in reach translates to eating more.

REMEMBER

With the immediate focus on carbohydrates, don't forget your healthy eating recommendations for protein, fat, and sodium. A 2,000-calorie eating plan would call for about 100 grams of protein per day, and about 67 grams of total fat, only about 15 grams of that from saturated fat. And, the daily recommendation for sodium is 1,500 milligrams per day. Going off the tracks for protein, fat, or sodium in one meal away from home may not have the same immediate impact that a surge in blood glucose levels from excess carbohydrates has, but if excess protein, fat, and sodium become routine, the long-term negative impact on heart health is clear.

Checking ahead

You can't always tell what you're eating by looking. Some things you'll know, such as the carbohydrates in a giant baked potato, but other dishes are a mystery. For instance, from the dishes in Table 15-1 is there anything in the name *hibachi chicken skewers* that would tip you off that this entree would be 12 carb choices, 72 percent of your daily carbohydrate budget, and more than three times your recommended daily sodium limitation? The only thing you can be sure about is that it isn't the chicken. It's probably not the skewers, either. So, either a hibachi is a terribly salty and starchy food, or there are added ingredients (soy sauce would be a prime suspect for the sodium) that aren't given away by the dish's name.

Fortunately, you don't have to find out that the hibachi chicken skewers were not a good choice for diabetes after you've already eaten them. There are great resources online and in print that give nutrition information for many specific restaurant menus. And most restaurant websites provide the information, too. As long as you know where you're going to eat, it's usually possible to pull the information for virtually every food item you find at any larger restaurant.

Chapters 9 and 13 offer a great deal of information on meal planning success. Those same principles that are discussed in those chapters can be implemented while dining out. Here are a few tips:

>> **Follow the diabetes-friendly "MyPlate" method.** Fill half of your plate with green leafy or other nonstarchy vegetables, one quarter of your plate with good-quality complex carbs, and one quarter with good-quality lean protein such as fish or chicken.

>> **Think of how those items are prepared.** Grilled, roasted, sautéed, stewed, poached, and baked foods are your best bet along with fresh leafy greens at every meal.

>> **Forgo sauces and heavy dressings when you are eating out.** At home, you can control what goes into those items and may come up with very tasty yet healthy versions such as those included in the recipes in Chapter 18. In the restaurant setting, however, dressings and sauces are hideout spots for tons of sugar and artificial sweeteners, sodium, fat, and other unwanted ingredients.

>> **Create your own seasonings.** Ask for extra fresh herbs when possible, drizzle your foods with extra-virgin olive oil, lemon juice, and vinegars for extra flavor.

Sticking to a plan

Having a plan goes a long, long way in helping you resist impulse eating, but it's up to you to stick to your plan. There may be chef's specials you didn't know about in advance, finger foods in the bar or appetizers somebody wants to share, and one of your companions may rave about the meal that they had last week — "you have to try it."

Sticking with your plan is a matter of your overall commitment to diabetes self-management, and having the confidence that you've made the right choices. But, here's an important point: The fact that you took a few minutes to actually think ahead about what you see as the best choices for you is most of the battle. Whether you made the perfect choices is almost beside the point — it's virtually certain that your advance choices were better than the ones impulsive eating would have led you to make.

TIP

We recommend browsing the menu for sharable items beforehand. That way when a friend or dining companion recommends something, you can offer, "Why don't we share (fill in the blank) instead?" Or just simply say that it sounds great but that you need to follow a specific meal plan and ask everyone to order for themselves. Splurging on a meal that is outside of the diabetes-friendly guidelines a few times a year won't hurt anyone in the long term. Not developing the confidence and determination to say no to the suggestions of others on a regular basis, however, will.

Dining Out

A few generations ago, dining out was a luxury afforded by the few. Nowadays, however, many people in industrialized countries eat out more than not. A lack of skill or interest in the kitchen coupled with a perceived lack of time and easy-to-obtain, affordable dining options have changed the way our world nourishes itself. Because of this, if you want to stay healthy or become healthy, you have to make the restaurants work for you. You also have to, as much as possible, frequent them only occasionally and not as a lunch or dinner solution on a daily basis.

It's easy to see how deciding on an eating plan ahead of time is a great idea — you can ignore the temptations and be confident you've accounted for your health. But, what if your eating-out opportunity comes up suddenly or isn't at a restaurant with nutrition information available? There are visits with friends, parties, banquets, and unexpected schedule changes. How can you get the information you need when you don't have time or access to the menu in advance, and how can you make good decisions if you can't get the information?

Analyzing the menu

If an occasion to eat at a restaurant comes up without time for preplanning, you can still make the healthier choices. The biggest difference is that you're making your choices surrounded by distractions and engulfed in an atmosphere created to trigger your eating instincts. These are powerful influences, but you can make healthy choices if you concentrate on what you know about your diabetes meal plan — manage carbohydrates from all sources, look to reduce dietary fat unless it is a known healthy good-quality fat (such as extra-virgin olive oil, almonds, walnuts, avocado, omega-3s in fish), and reduce sodium. Try to identify options that are less likely to have added preservatives and other unwanted ingredients. This is sometimes difficult to do, but some foods like processed cheeses and meats might be more obvious.

TIP

You can access nutrition information from your table on mobile devices, either from websites or apps. Alternatively, you can request nutrition information from the restaurant — most are able to bring you the information at your table, or while you're waiting. It is perfectly acceptable to ask polite questions about ingredients and even to ask what cooking oil a restaurant uses. If the waiter is offended by such a question, you should probably go to a different restaurant.

In addition, the menu descriptions can give some valuable clues about healthy and not-so-healthy choices that can help you narrow your options down to a few, check the details on those, make a choice, and join the conversation.

Here are some tips for analyzing menu items:

>> Look for clues in the cooking method. Healthier cooking styles include baked, grilled, steamed, poached, and broiled. Not-so-healthy methods are deep fried, flash fried (unless in a good-quality oil like olive oil), scalloped, or creamed.

>> Be careful with breaded or batter-dipped foods, crusts or double crusts, sweet-and-sour dishes, or syrups because of the added carbohydrates.

>> Be cautious about sauces and glazes — most are high in calories and fat, and some are sweetened.

>> Be aware of portion sizes for foods you know are carbohydrates — bread, pasta, rice, and potatoes are often served in liberal portions. One slice of bread, 3 ounces of baked potato, and ⅓ cup of cooked rice or pasta are all 15 grams of carbohydrate.

>> Don't assume that a meal-sized salad is healthy just because it's a salad — read the ingredients and take the dressing on the side (or go for an alternative nonfat dressing like lemon or lime juice, or plain balsamic vinegar).

>> Look at the appetizer menu. Often it's possible to get similar foods in smaller portions.

There's not much you can do differently when it comes to fast foods. Go for broiled or grilled rather than fried (unless in a healthy fat), avoid mayonnaise and special sauces when possible (you can scrape them off), watch the carbohydrates in bread, buns, French fries, and sweetened drinks, and go for thin-crust pizzas to minimize the carbohydrates from thick crusts. When traveling, in lieu of eating at a fast-food restaurant, we recommend seeking out shops or cafes that sell unsweetened Greek yogurt, almonds, fruits, crudités with hummus, salads (remember to swap out extra-virgin olive oil and vinegar for dressings when possible), and other simple foods that can be eaten on the run but are still good for you.

TIP

Nonstarchy vegetables, like lettuce and tomato, can fill you up and add almost no carbohydrates to your meal. Fast-casual Mexican, Middle Eastern, and Asian eateries offer many options along with lean proteins. Sandwich shops and pizza joints always offer a variety of nonstarchy vegetables as well.

REMEMBER

One way to know whether you've made the best choices is to test your blood glucose levels two hours after you eat. Over time, patterns can inform your choices the next time you find yourself choosing from the same menu. If you have access to continuing glucose monitoring, it's even easier to analyze the effect.

Asking the right people

Don't be shy — what's in your food has a direct effect on your health, and just because this information isn't required to be provided by law, doesn't mean it isn't important. Some countries even tell you which farm grows the food so that you can be ensured it's good quality. There is a stigma in the United States around diabetes, unfortunately, and it makes people embarrassed to inquire about menu items and ask for substitutions. But it shouldn't be that way. There are more people who suffer from diabetes than allergies and celiac disease, and restaurants should cater to them. In addition to helping your own health condition, your questions may help influence restaurants to offer diabetes-friendly options, as we believe they should, from the beginning.

If you're taking insulin to match your carbohydrate consumption, it's not just about your long-term health either — having accurate information helps you avoid dangerous low or high blood glucose levels after you eat. So, whether you're at a restaurant, a banquet, a party, or eating at a friend's home, ask questions — somebody has information you can use. There are basically two barriers to quizzing others about what's in your food.

First, you might be uncomfortable being assertive, or you may feel that asking about food is bad manners. You're more likely to feel reluctant about quizzing friends than about asking questions in a restaurant — most everyone is comfortable getting details when they're paying. But, if someone else is buying, or if the food is at a party or a friend's house, there can certainly be a reluctance to ask questions. You may feel you're insulting the person who prepared the dish — trying to determine whether it's good enough for you to eat. Everyone will be more comfortable if you acknowledge that your concerns are health-related and not about whether you think the food is tasty. And, if you say you're trying to determine how much you should eat, as opposed to whether you can eat a certain dish or not, people will understand.

TIP

When going to a friend's home for a meal, call ahead and tell them you are on a special diet. Ask what they are planning to prepare. If it doesn't meet your needs, let them know that you'll bring a dish to share that meets your needs and others can enjoy. Or let them know that you'll bring part of a meal so that you can stay within your guidelines.

Second, you need to know what you're wanting to know. Again, because carbohydrates have a direct and immediate impact on blood glucose levels, carbohydrates are your main concern. That's not to say that calories, unhealthy fat, sodium, and added ingredients aren't important, but it's difficult to focus on too many things unless you've been able to give your thinking brain the time to evaluate all the options. You want your overall lifestyle to manage calories, unhealthy fat, and sodium, too, but an occasional adventure won't have the same effect that overloading on carbohydrates can have. Plus, you can control your calorie intake to some extent based simply on how much you eat.

Your search for carbohydrates is most effective if you can simply know the recipes for the foods you're planning to eat — so ask. Ultimately, it's the hidden carbohydrates you want to find. You know that potatoes, corn, peas, beans, rice, pasta, bread, and fruits contain carbohydrates. Sugars, honey, syrups, flour, cornmeal, fruit juice, milk, yogurt, and other carbs can be unseen in sauces, gravy, stuffing, spreads, dips, or drinks. Bar-b-que sauces, for instance, are almost always high in carbohydrate. If you can't get a peek at the recipe, consider asking questions about the possible hidden carbs.

REMEMBER

If food isn't already prepared, don't be shy about asking for modifications. Your options might be limited at parties or fast-food restaurants, but full-service restaurants are generally more than happy to modify a menu item. You should feel free to request a healthier cooking method, different sauces, added or omitted ingredients, or menu substitutions for the side dishes. Don't forget, restaurants want you back, and most of the changes are really no big deal.

Bringing your own

Bringing your own food may not be a good option in some cases, but for a family get-together or meals with close friends it's a surefire way to make sure you've got food that fits your meal plan perfectly. If you know what's on the menu, you can bring food when the foods available don't work well for diabetes, or perhaps you bring a healthy salad to help dampen your appetite. Bringing your own food can work for office lunches, on trips, or anyplace else your choices are going to be limited.

TIP

Anytime you're going to a potluck or bring-a-dish affair, bring a dish that you know works well with your diabetes eating plan. In addition, Chef Amy likes to bring good-quality extra-virgin olive oil and vinegar as a gift for the host. They are lovely items to receive, and it ensures that you have the type of ingredients you need to dress your food. This way, you know you have options. Bringing a delicious and nutritious dish to a party is always a good idea anyway because it demonstrates that taste and nutrition aren't mutually exclusive.

Taking some home

Refer to Table 15-1 and notice that the nutrition information shows that all of the listed dishes give you your lion's share of daily calories, carbohydrates, and fat — although protein isn't provided in the table, it's the same story. In today's food environment, this is common. Even menu choices labeled as "lighter" or "lunch portions" are likely to give you more than one meal's share of calories, fat, protein, and carbohydrate when you divide up a daily total.

One can make a strong case that the excess food Americans have become accustomed to getting at restaurants carries over into other meals and has contributed to the skyrocketing rates of obesity and type 2 diabetes. Nutrition professionals call this *portion distortion*. As you look over the menu nutrition information from any restaurant, this becomes obvious. And such distorted portion sizes are not only true in the United States and does not just apply to food. A large glass of wine in most U.K. restaurants is 250 milliliters. If you top up with another glass then you will have drunk two thirds of a standard bottle of wine!

So, it's fair to say that with most any meal you eat from the menu at a restaurant, you can't eat the entire meal and at the same time stay somewhat committed to your meal plan. That means that unless you're splitting the meal with someone else, which is often a great idea, you'll have leftovers to take home.

TIP

Now, if you already know in advance that you shouldn't eat the entire meal, there's a secret to making sure that you don't. Because eating behavior is so subconscious, ask for a take-home container as soon as your food is served and stash the excess amount out of sight while you eat. You can be almost certain that you won't take your doggy bag out of its hiding place to add more food to your plate — you can't be certain that you won't nibble away until the entire meal is finished if you leave the food on the plate. You can also ask the kitchen to plate half and wrap up the other half in advance.

Taking food home isn't always practical — maybe you're traveling with no way to refrigerate or reheat the food later. But if you're just going to a movie after dinner, bring along an insulated bag and some ice packs. Cooling your leftovers to 40 degrees Fahrenheit keeps it safe until you make it home. Don't forget that if you separate your leftovers before you ever begin eating, you can send them home with somebody else without sending your germs along, too.

Keeping It Honest

Don't be offended — maybe honest isn't the best choice of words, but keeping it accurate sounds too nitpicky. The point is, it's possible to pile on calories, unhealthy fat, sodium, and carbohydrate a little at a time when you're in a social environment, and calories, unhealthy fat, sodium, and carbohydrates count just the same whether you get them in many small packages or all at once from the hibachi chicken skewers. So, in a real sense it's important to be honest about being accurate, even if that's both offensive and nitpicky.

Drinks and bar snacks

Alcohol is not a carbohydrate, so alcohol doesn't raise blood glucose levels directly; however, alcohol stores more energy per gram than the 4 calories per gram in carbohydrates or protein, and almost as much as the 9 calories per gram stored in fat. So, at 7 calories per gram, 1 ounce of 80-proof liquor adds about 60 calories to your day. Alcoholic beverages are rarely just alcohol, however, and a 12-ounce beer can come in at 150 calories, a glass of wine about the same, and mixed drinks or liqueurs can bring along two or three times as many calories. Beer, wine, and many mixed drinks and liqueurs also contain carbohydrate, and the grams can vary significantly by brand or according to the mixer.

REMEMBER

Often mixers are sodas with artificial sweeteners, promoted as having reduced sugar and calories, but be aware that some artificial sweeteners have been shown to have an adverse effect on blood glucose and are coming under scrutiny for possible links with cancers.

Bar snacks aren't free foods, either. Twenty pretzel sticks is 120 calories and 26 grams of carbohydrate, and 1 ounce of beer nuts can bring along 185 calories, 15 grams of fat, and 6 grams of carbohydrate — 1 ounce of beer nuts is only about 25 or 30 nuts. Many snack mixes get their calories from carbohydrate and fat, complicating blood glucose control if you're eating mindlessly. A 1-ounce nibble of some snack mixes can add 15 to 25 grams of unexpected carbohydrate to your diabetes meal plan.

If you have a tequila sunrise with 1 ounce of the free snack mix before dinner, you're starting out with 325 calories and three carb choices (45 grams carbohydrate) already in your tank. That may be okay if you made the drink and snacks part of your advanced meal planning, but if you're not planning on a drink and bar snacks, be sure to make a specific plan not to have a drink and bar snacks. Leaving more than 300 calories and 45 grams of carbohydrate up to chance is no way to do meal planning unless you're equally prepared to deduct that amount from what you intended to have for dinner.

Just to be clear, you can have a drink and some bar snacks without cashing in the big calories and carbohydrates before your meal. Drinks are easy to research, and you can find one you like that's lower in calories and carbohydrates than the 200 calorie, 25 grams of carbohydrate tequila sunrise. A glass of wine usually has less than 5 grams of carbohydrate, and low-carb beers are popular still. Plus, you can ask the bartender to modify recipes just like you're prepared to ask a chef. Alternatively, feel free to ask for water with a slice of lemon.

WARNING

The snacks are a different story. Most nuts might load in extra calories but are very low in carbohydrate; however, the mixed snacks with crackers, pretzels, and sesame sticks are going to be carbohydrate-rich. If you can't avoid them completely, put a small amount on a napkin or plate to eat slowly, and ask someone to remove the remainder from your field of vision.

Hors d'oeuvres, appetizers, bread, and dessert

These are the foods that seem to find you, even if you're trying to hide from them, especially hors d'oeuvres — with those little party bites it may seem there's a conspiracy at work to put you face-to-face with a tray of bacon-wrapped scallops. Once again, these are foods that seem to just appear, are powerfully tempting, can seem insignificant, but can add up quickly.

Technically, hors d'oeuvres are not necessarily associated with a meal, so they're often circulated at parties or events where an actual meal isn't included. In some ways this can be a good thing. If you keep reasonable track of what you've eaten from passing trays or long tables, you can potentially adjust your foods at a later meal to compensate. In theory there's nothing wrong with, and even some benefits to, eating more than three smaller meals in a day. But, the operable word is smaller. There can be a tendency in some circumstances to try and make a meal of hors d'oeuvres, and that can make keeping track of what you've eaten very difficult. These finger foods can disappear in one bite, and large events can have many different varieties floating around. Plus, hors d'oeuvres aren't necessarily healthy choices, and nutrition information may be hard to find.

TIP

If you're at a party or an event, have an hors d'oeuvre or two, preferably something without carbohydrates, and then have a reasonable dinner later. Don't try and make a dinner from finger foods unless you're confident you have options that are healthy and let you keep reasonably accurate track of what you've eaten.

Appetizers and bread often appear before a meal and are intended to stimulate an appetite or to keep you busy while waiting for the food you ordered to be prepared. Most often the bread is standard, but appetizers are part of an order. Even if you don't order an appetizer, somebody will almost surely want you to share theirs.

REMEMBER

The story with appetizers and bread is the same — if you have planned ahead to include these foods in your advance meal plan, and chosen healthy options, then dig in. Unplanned food sitting in plain sight, however, makes healthy eating more difficult than it has to be. If possible, let the unplanned appetizers and bread be quickly passed and removed from the table.

Dessert is purely optional but can be one of the great pleasures of eating out. However, restaurant desserts can be 500 calories or more and almost by definition include a sizable dose of carbohydrates. Sorbets, sherbets, or fresh fruit are your best options. For most other desserts, splitting them four ways may still leave you with 300 extra calories and 30 to 40 grams of carbohydrate.

Salad bar foolers

Since the appearance of salad bars in restaurants, people have often seen them as the healthy choice. Even though salad greens make a great foundation for a healthy meal, the range of ingredients available to add to your salad can leave you with an unexpected load of calories, unhealthy fat, and refined carbohydrates. It's the small amounts you add that can lead you to consider those ingredients as irrelevant.

A salad bar may have plenty of great lettuce choices, but the best are the lettuces with colored leaves and a peppery taste over iceberg, which contains much lower levels of polyphenols. Add in carrots, tomatoes, beans, peppers, onions, and cucumber to make a great base. You may also find olives, nuts, seeds, avocados, tuna, and even some good-quality cheese on offer. Although these items increase the overall calorie count, they are healthy choices and tend not to translate into fat around our waistline.

It is the croutons — often poor-quality bread fried in unhealthy fat — and the bacon, ham, chicken strips fried in breadcrumbs, processed cheeses, and factory-produced salad dressings that can add both calories and unhealthy ingredients to a salad. Coleslaws and macaroni, pasta, and potato salads often include mayonnaise, which adds unhealthy calories. A simple dressing with extra-virgin olive oil and balsamic vinegar is the best dressing for your final salad choice.

REMEMBER

Keeping an eye on the carbohydrates is especially important because losing track of your carbohydrate food is losing control of your blood glucose. Watch for carbohydrates in fresh or canned fruits, raisins and dried fruit, beans and peas, potatoes, croutons, crackers, rice, pasta, and any mixed or creamy salads that include these items — potato salads and three-bean salads are common.

The point is not to declare salad bars off limits or label them as a bad choice without reservation. The point is to demonstrate that it's not only possible to lose track of what you're eating from the salad bar, it's easy to lose track. If your dinner meal recommendations are in the 700-calorie and 90-grams carbohydrate neighborhood, it's difficult to imagine you can sail past those numbers scooping ingredients with a tablespoon but it is certainly possible.

TIP

Here's the secret. Start your salad with nonstarchy or low-calorie vegetables like lettuce, spinach, alfalfa sprouts, bean sprouts, broccoli, carrots, cauliflower, celery, cucumber, peppers, mushrooms, onions, radishes, tomatoes, and zucchini. Then, if you need to add carbohydrates to your meal, add them from beans, potatoes, corn or peas, whole-grain bread or crackers, and fresh or dried fruit. Find some healthy protein — tuna, egg, or soy — and a little healthy fat from nuts, olives, or a touch of extra-virgin olive oil if available.

Buffets: Wanting it all

If the salad bar is no place for amateurs, access to the dinner buffet should require a year of classes with a final exam. Buffets are tempting because of the variety of food and the price. In fact, it's easy to get swept up into a competition, where the more you eat the better the deal. This kind of fun may work well for active teens, but managing diabetes requires a little discipline, as you know.

The buffet is a challenging assignment not only because of the variety of foods available, but also because planning ahead isn't possible. There is only one inherently positive thing about the all-you-can-eat buffet. The owners are aware of mindless eating cues, and almost always provide small plates — people who eat from smaller plates tend to eat less. From the business owner's perspective, five trips through the buffet with a smaller plate saves money compared to five trips with a larger plate. From your perspective, taking diabetes and weight management into account, the small plate is only a benefit for one trip through — without stacking.

So, how can you responsibly approach eating from a buffet? First, take your seat as far away from the buffet line as possible — out of sight, if feasible. Then, do a reconnaissance mission to look specifically for foods that seem healthiest. Finally, eat responsibly.

In evaluating the foods and making your eating plan, consider the following:

» If there's a salad bar, go for a salad of nonstarchy vegetables with vinegar or lemon or lime juice as a dressing. If you skipped the previous section of this chapter on salad bars, go back and see why you should avoid many of the add-ons provided for your salad.

» If there's a broth-based soup, have a little. A healthy salad and broth-based soup helps reduce your appetite without adding excess calories to your meal, but salad fixings and creamy soups only add calories, fat, and even carbohydrates. (Broth-based soups in restaurants are likely to be very high in sodium, so if you eat out often, this strategy may have a downside over the long term. Broth-based soups can include added carbohydrates, like noodles, as well.)

» Look for meat or fish that has been roasted, poached, or steamed, and is not floating in buttery-looking sauce. A plain fish filet or the carved roast beef may be your best choices — pick one.

» Go for vegetables with the same idea — no sauces, not fried, and be careful about casseroles and mixed dishes.

>> Get your carbohydrates from whole-grain bread, fruit, or grain and potato dishes without added fat from cooking methods or sauces.

>> Be cautious with desserts.

Don't be shy about asking questions of the servers, and even the chefs. Somebody has information you may need to decide on certain dishes, and it's perfectly reasonable that you should have it.

The greatest challenge with eating away from home, however, may be the greater need for planning because the food can be so extreme. Eating away from home is seen as an opportunity to relax from all things stressful, like meal planning. Just when the need for planning is greatest, the temptation to avoid thinking about food is strongest. What will it hurt to splurge just this once? Eating out has become so routine for some people that the splurging may happen three, four, or five times a week, and that makes it a lifestyle. Plus, the food you encounter when eating out is likely to be way beyond the bounds of a normal meal and can have immediate consequences. The carbohydrate content of some entrees and most desserts can send blood glucose levels to dangerous heights, especially for someone with type 1 diabetes who underestimated his insulin requirements.

Having a plan in advance equips you to resist the powerful biological, psychological, and social influences that lead to overconsumption and consumption of the wrong foods. When your advanced plan is consistent with healthy eating for diabetes management, you can not only leave the stress of thinking about food behind while you're eating out, but also can truly enjoy and feel good about what you're eating.

Chapter **16**

Choosing Sensible Beverages and Snacks

O ffering liquid refreshment and nourishment to guests is good manners, sound business practice, and in many cultures, a formal offer of goodwill. In today's ultra-commercial, convenience society, however, drinks and snacks have taken on a much bigger and less nutritious role. You've probably noticed that every commercially available drink or snack also comes with great friends, vitality, perfect weather, peak athletic performance, never-ending fun, a bonfire on the beach at sunset, and maybe even world peace. Your main choice, it appears, is which kind of wonderful life is right for you.

So, you're not completely convinced by billions of advertising dollars that every drink or snack is the one missing piece that can make your life perfect? In that case, maybe it's a good time to take a closer look at how drinks and snacks best fit into your regular life. In this chapter, you explore how to manage drinks and snacks without sabotaging your diabetes management plan. You also find some drinks and snacks that are surprisingly healthy.

Beverages

Beverages can make or break a healthy lifestyle plan. While drinking plenty of water and staying hydrated is crucial, sugary drinks and artificial ingredients can set you up for failure. What you drink should be taken every bit as seriously as what you eat if you want to balance your blood sugar.

Water

In a world full of sugary beverages loaded with preservatives and artificial flavors, plain water can be a hard sell. But the truth is that whether you have diabetes or not, water should be the main liquid you consume to keep your body running optimally.

ASK THE DOCTOR

Some medical conditions can result in different fluid requirements. Always check with your doctor to ensure that you are properly hydrated considering your medical history, activity level, diet, and medications.

For those with diabetes, drinking water can help reduce blood sugar (glucose) levels by diluting the amount of sugar in the bloodstream. Consuming the proper amount of water can also help prevent dehydration that can be caused by high glucose levels. You can use various figures from reliable sources as a starting point to determine your hydration needs. For example, 1.6 liters or 6.5 cups of water per day for women, and 2 liters or 8.5 cups per day for men is a standard measurement to use as a benchmark. Keep in mind that extreme cold and hot temperatures and increased physical activity all require additional hydration.

Some medications and foods can have a dehydrating effect on the body, and it is a good idea to drink even more water while taking them if advised to do so by your health professional. There are also some medical conditions where different fluid intake is recommended. Again, follow the advice of your doctor.

Alcohol

Alcohol in beer, wine, or spirits has been around for millennia. At certain times in history it was safer to drink beer or wine than the contaminated local water supply. The pleasantly intoxicating effects of alcohol, its potentially addictive properties, and its capacity in excess to cause physical, mental, and social harm have been apparent since it was first discovered.

Until recently, public health guidelines in most countries recommended that it was safe to consume alcohol in moderation, described as a number of "units" of alcohol per week. Many people drink above these limits, some drink particular types of alcoholic drinks regularly and in modest amounts, and some abstain completely for religious or other reasons.

A number of studies actually support the notion that, for example, the daily consumption of a small amount of red wine (100 to 200 milliliters of an average strength wine) each day is associated with a reduced risk of heart disease, and can improve brain function in later years. However, in 2023, a review paper that looked at many studies that included more than 4 million individuals, concluded that there was, in general, an increased risk of cancer, some types of heart disease, and early death when consuming even modest amounts of alcohol. This led some public health agencies to conclude that "there is no safe level of alcohol."

But it may not be quite as simple as this. People drink alcohol in different contexts, and the type of drink as well as the pattern of drinking varies in different cultures. Many researchers suggest that studies that look at large numbers of drinkers might not recognize smaller subsets of people whose patterns of drinking might not only be safe, but perhaps provide some of the benefits to health that have been seen in earlier studies. There is clearly a significant difference between risky binge drinking of mixtures of high-alcoholic spirits on an empty stomach on the weekend in comparison with having a small glass of wine most days with a meal.

Evidence suggests that consumption of red wine (and to a lesser extent white wine) provides healthy bioactive polyphenols, which may benefit cardiovascular health. There is also research confirming that consuming red wine with a meal rich in extra-virgin olive oil increases the activity of the polyphenols of the wine and also the extra-virgin olive oil and creates new polyphenols. The association of alcohol consumption with an increased risk of breast cancer in western cultures does not appear to be seen in Mediterranean regions, and studies that include counting moderate consumption of red wine as part of the Mediterranean diet have been linked with lower rates of many cancers including breast cancer. It is possible that healthy bioactive components of extra-virgin olive oil such as lignans or polyphenols from other components of the diet may even mitigate the increased risk of breast and other cancers associated with alcohol in other dietary patterns.

The effects of alcohol are certainly modified when consumed with food, and it may even be that the way we drink, in friendly company and while enjoying a meal, may have a big impact on its effects on health.

TIP

For people with diabetes, there are specific dangers of excess alcohol consumption including a risk of hypoglycemia, so it is especially important if you want to enjoy an alcoholic drink that you drink in moderation, perhaps enjoying a small glass of wine with a meal.

WARNING

However, even moderate alcohol consumption may not be right for some people with diabetes. Diabetes-related problems with sensation called neuropathy can be made worse by even small amounts of alcohol. As a general rule, nondrinkers should not begin drinking for the potential health effects. Anyone with diabetes should honestly discuss their alcohol consumption patterns with their health-care team.

Finding the calories and carbohydrates

Alcohol is not a carbohydrate, and by itself has virtually no impact in raising blood glucose levels. Alcohol, however, does have calories. In fact, alcohol stores 7 calories per gram — significantly more than the 4 calories stored by 1 gram of carbohydrate or protein, and only slightly less than the 9 calories stored by fat. So, the calories in alcohol can mount up, with a 1½–ounce jigger of 80-proof spirits like gin or whiskey packing about 100 calories.

Many alcoholic beverages, like wine and beer, do include carbohydrates, and mixed drinks bring along whatever carbohydrates and calories are in the mixer. Table 16-1 shows common alcohol-containing beverages with the typical serving size, and the calories and carbohydrate grams per serving.

TABLE 16-1 **Nutrition Information for Alcoholic Beverages**

Beverage	Typical Serving	Calories	Carbohydrate
80-proof spirits	1.5 ounces (jigger)	97	0 grams
Light beer	12 ounces	60–100	2–8 grams
Beer	12 ounces	120–150	10–12 grams
Stout beer	12 ounces	up to 300	up to 20 grams
Cabernet red wine	5 ounces	120	4 grams
Riesling white wine	5 ounces	120	6 grams
Sweet dessert wine	3.5 ounces	170	15 grams
Piña colada	4.5 ounces	245	32 grams
Coffee liqueur	3 ounces	275	44 grams
Irish cream	3 ounces	351	22 grams
Margarita	8 ounces	368	16 grams

You can see that a relaxing margarita every night before dinner equals 25 percent of a 1,500-calorie eating plan, making weight management very difficult. Sipping Kahlua on ice grabs not only 18 percent of your calories, but also 25 percent of your daily carb choices.

REMEMBER

For weight management and blood glucose control it's important to evaluate both the calorie and carbohydrate content of alcoholic beverages. When you look carefully, you may be surprised to find that reducing the calories and carbs you're drinking every day results in more effective weight and blood glucose control. All calories and carbohydrates count.

Caution about hypoglycemia

In certain cases, alcohol consumption can contribute to dangerous, even life-threatening, low blood sugar. Anyone who is taking insulin or other diabetes medication, or combination of medications, where low blood glucose is a possible side effect must be extremely careful with alcohol.

Falling blood glucose levels normally stimulate a release of stored glucose from liver cells, but alcohol interferes with this process. Recent research also suggests that alcohol stimulates insulin secretion by changing blood flow patterns in the pancreas. As a consequence, if alcohol is being consumed without food, blood glucose levels in people with diabetes can continue to fall at an uncommon rate. Because the symptoms of hypoglycemia and alcohol intoxication are similar, you (or those with you) may attribute the telltale signs of acute low blood glucose to the alcohol. In circumstances where alcohol consumption goes beyond moderate, hypoglycemia can be extremely serious.

TIP

To avoid the dangers of alcohol-induced hypoglycemia follow this advice:

>> Always drink in moderation.

>> Have your alcoholic beverage with your meal.

>> Always test your blood glucose levels, even in the morning, and especially after excessive consumption.

>> Make sure your companions are aware of the potential for low blood glucose, and always wear medical alert identification.

Coffee and tea

Coffee and tea may be best known for delivering the stimulant caffeine, but evidence is mounting to support significant health benefits for both. On the caffeine point, coffee takes the prize, delivering about two to five times as much per cup.

That's good news for sleepy heads, but most of the health benefits of coffee and tea seem unrelated to the caffeine. And, caffeine is not well tolerated by some people. Coffee, by the way, is more popular than tea in the United States by about 2.5 to 1 in gallons consumed annually, but worldwide, tea is in second place as a beverage, behind only water.

Both coffee and tea appear to reduce the risk of cardiovascular disease, and while the effect is often attributed to the antioxidants contained in both, the actual mechanisms are not clear. Recent research shows a decreased risk for stroke for both coffee and tea drinkers. Coffee drinking has a fairly clear association with reduced risk for dementia and Parkinson's disease. And, studies involving hundreds of thousands of subjects show heavy coffee consumption may reduce the risk for diabetes by more than 30 percent. A review of weight-loss supplements found that only green tea provided a genuine benefit to weight management.

All in all, the health data on coffee and tea looks solid, and both can be recommended as being consistent with effective diabetes management. Like alcohol, however, the pitfalls can be in added ingredients. Sugar and creamers can add calories, fat, and carbohydrates, and specialty coffee or tea drinks can take a significant bite from your daily calorie and carbohydrate budget. A large white chocolate mocha Frappuccino weighs in at 440 calories, 16 grams total fat, with 69 grams carbohydrate if made with whole milk — a green tea latte is 390 calories, 7 grams fat, and 57 grams carbohydrate.

Soft drinks and flavored waters

Soft drinks are sometimes called soda, pop, soda pop, Coke, or something else, in large part depending upon where you live. And, soft drinks have been around for a long, long time. Soft drinks are, of course, carbonated.

Flavored waters, on the other hand, are newcomers to the commercial drink market. They come ready-to-drink in bottles or cans, and some varieties are carbonated like soft drinks. The difference between carbonated flavored water and a soft drink may be only a question of the manufacturer's target market. Flavored water also comes as a dry powdered mix that can be added to water. Many flavored waters advertise certain formulas of vitamins and nutrients, or are labeled with descriptive words hinting at a particular effect — relax, flex, think. View these claims as advertising's subtle attempt to convince you there are no other options for finding these nutrients, and always check the nutrition facts label for calories and carbohydrate.

As you might suspect, the primary issue with soft drinks and flavored waters related to diabetes is whether the drinks are sweetened with sugar. A 12-ounce, sugar-sweetened soft drink has 140 calories and 39 grams of carbohydrate. Soft drinks are commonly packaged in 20-ounce bottles, too, listed as one serving on the nutrition labels with 240 calories and 65 grams carbohydrate. Supersized fountain drinks — 32 ounces or more — can pack 300 calories and 80 grams carbohydrate.

Of course, most soft drinks and flavored waters come in no-calorie varieties, meaning they are either not sweetened, or are sweetened with non-nutritive sweeteners. For diabetes and blood sugar management, unsweetened drinks and water are your best bets.

WARNING

A final thought on soft drinks relates to excessive consumption. The acid in soft drinks can contribute to dental cavities by eating away at the enamel coating of teeth. There is also some evidence that the phosphoric acid content in some soft drinks can contribute to bone loss.

You may think that if you consume drinks that are sweetened with sugar substitutes containing no calories that you have reduced your energy intake by a large number of calories. For example, 12 ounces of Coca-Cola has 140 calories, but Diet Coke has none. In fact, studies have shown that you tend to replace those calories to the extent of 25 percent or more with other foods. Artificial sweeteners used in soft drinks are under scrutiny at the moment with concerns about possible cancer-causing effects. We recommend avoiding them.

Sports and energy drinks

The advertising behind sports drinks is slightly different than for soft drinks. Sports drinks actually do provide benefits in carbohydrate replacement and in electrolyte replacement. But the need to quickly replace carbohydrates and electrolytes comes as a result of intense exercise. If you're not a marathoner, or participating in some other high-intensity exercise for an hour or longer, chances are you don't need a sports drink.

Sports drinks contain varying amounts of carbohydrate from sugar, and the electrolytes potassium and sodium. If you're eating a balanced diet, you're already getting enough carbohydrates and potassium — and sodium, almost certainly more than you need. Sports drinks have a high glycemic index value, to rapidly raise blood glucose and make that energy available. Again, this is essentially the opposite of what you want from your carbohydrates.

Sports drinks may have some use among athletes with type 1 diabetes in combating hypoglycemia during and after intense workouts, but that's a specific use that is uncommon to the great majority of people with diabetes. Unless you can realistically see yourself in head-to-head competition with the athletes starring in sports drink commercials, sports drinks aren't really for you.

Today's advertising for energy drinks definitely targets youth, and annual sales in the United States topped $7.8 billion in 2022 and is anticipated to have the value of $15.7 billion by 2027. Adults with diabetes may be tempted to try these products because their energy levels can be chronically low as a consequence of diabetes. So, energy drinks deserve a closer look.

The secret to the energy in energy drinks is caffeine — lots of caffeine. Many energy drinks also contain carbohydrate in the form of sugar, although most offer sugar-free versions, too. The list of special ingredients can feature a range of B vitamins, ginseng, taurine, guarana, and glucuronolactone. The consensus among experts, however, is that energy drinks have no effect other than the effect of caffeine and sugar. The additional, often featured, ingredients are lacking sound evidence for any benefit whatsoever. It's also important to read the nutritional labels to make sure that the sugar and sodium quantities are low or non-existent.

Ultimately the question becomes one of purpose and cost. It's fair to say that people with diabetes don't need additional carbohydrate. Many of these drinks also include unwanted sodium, which makes people thirsty and continue to drink more of them. Regular consumption of these drinks may push someone with pre-diabetes into the diabetes zone. Some research suggests that caffeine has a negative effect on blood glucose and insulin balance in people with type 2 diabetes that is not well controlled. And, whereas caffeine does raise blood pressure, the effect seems to be temporary. Nevertheless, consuming caffeine when you already have high blood pressure should be discussed with your physician, and caffeine in the amounts contained in many energy drinks is unnecessary. Lastly, the cost of energy drinks, at $2.50 to $3.50 per container, is an expensive way to get caffeine, which inevitably also comes with ingredients you don't need.

Snacks

Healthful snacking is an important part of any healthy eating plan, and in some ways especially important for managing body weight and blood glucose when you have diabetes. But, when people think of snacks, they often think of the high-calorie, high-carbohydrate, and high-fat kind like chips, cookies, or candy bars on racks in your local convenience market. Healthy snacks can help reduce between-meal hunger, give a boost of energy, and even reduce mealtime calorie intake, all without piling on extra calories, unhealthy fats, or excess carbohydrates.

Nuts and seeds

Portion control is always important and so are added ingredients like salt, but all in all nuts and seeds fit the bill for diabetes snacking pretty well.

TIP

In the practical sense, nuts and seeds contain enough protein, fiber, and fat to help you feel full. You can easily guess that managing hunger can go a long way toward reducing impulsive eating. Nuts and seeds are relatively low in carbohydrate, too, so they work well for most people with diabetes by not raising blood glucose levels. In fact, if you've been advised to have a snack during the day or in the evening to avoid periods of low blood glucose, nuts or seeds are not your best choice. Later in this chapter you find a list of healthy snacks that do offer enough carbohydrate to stabilize lower blood glucose levels between meals.

The real story with nuts and seeds is fat — healthy mono- and polyunsaturated fats, to be specific. One ounce of nuts contains 13 to 22 grams of these heart-healthy fats. Walnuts, Brazil nuts, pumpkin seeds, and sunflower seeds contain more polyunsaturated fats. Almonds, cashews, pecans, hazelnuts, macadamia nuts, peanuts, and sesame seeds contain more monounsaturated fats. Although the fat in nuts is predominantly these healthy fats, any fat is calorie dense. A 1-ounce serving of nuts packs 150 to 200 calories. Packaged nuts and seeds often include added salt or sugar, neither of which are helpful for the main purpose of snacking, so check the nutrition label on packaged foods.

Several studies have looked at nuts and seeds as a desirable element of diabetes management. Research found the consumption of nuts and seeds to be a favorable replacement for carbohydrate snacks when a group with type 2 diabetes showed improvements in A1C and bad LDL cholesterol after three months. A study involving 13,000 subjects by Louisiana State University found consumers of tree nuts (the study excluded peanuts, which are a legume) had smaller waist measurements, lower weight, lower blood pressure, lower fasting blood glucose, higher levels of HDL ("good") cholesterol, and lower levels of proteins linked to inflammation and heart disease. In fairness, regular nut eating was also linked with higher consumption of whole grains and fruits, and lower consumption of alcohol and sugar. Still, the association between nuts, seeds, lower weight, and better cardiovascular health is strong.

Yogurt

Yogurt, especially the Greek-style plain variety that is produced around the world now, is high in protein and vitamin B12, which is mostly found in animal products, making it a great protein choice for those who don't eat meat. The original Greek variety is made from a combination of goat's and sheep's milk, and those types of milks offer additional nutrient profiles. Even cow-based milk contains a healthful dose of calcium, vitamins B2 and B12, potassium, and magnesium. Yogurt with live active cultures (probiotics) is known to help maintain the natural balance of organisms, known as *microflora,* in the intestines.

TIP

Yogurt also may contain an ingredient called *inulin,* which looks similar to insulin without the letter "s." Inulin helps to regulate blood sugar levels and we recommend it for a snack anytime. Eaten at bedtime, it can help to keep you full and your glucose balanced during your hours of fasting.

WARNING

While natural, plain, or authentic Greek-style yogurts are healthful options, it is a good idea to always check the ingredients because some contain added sugars, artificial flavors, and stabilizers. It is best to enjoy plain varieties and add raw honey and fresh fruit or extra-virgin olive oil as flavor enhancers.

ASK THE DOCTOR

Unlike most other foods, yogurt contains all three macronutrients (carbohydrates, fat, and protein) in a healthy form. Consuming the three macronutrients at each meal or snack is extremely important for those with diabetes. It is an easy no-brainer when you need good fuel fast. If you combine the yogurt with fresh fruit you can enjoy the benefits of even more powerful antioxidants, fiber, and energy-boosting carbohydrates.

Fruit

A piece of whole, fresh fruit is a great snack at any time of day. Even though fruit contains natural sugars, it also contains vitamins and minerals.

FROM THE AUTHORS

It is a good idea to eat a few almonds, walnuts, or a bit of plain, Greek-style yogurt along with the fruit so that it doesn't spike your blood sugar.

Veggies and dips

Mouthwatering Mediterranean-style dips such as tzatziki, hummus, baba ghanouj, pesto, and tahini are all examples of foods that those with diabetes can feel good about eating, especially if the dips are made from scratch. If you're purchasing the dips, be sure to read the labels to ensure that only a few, fresh, quality ingredients are used in making them. One quarter cup of one of these dips with a small plateful of crudités — raw broccoli, cauliflower, tomatoes, carrots, celery, and more — make a filling and nutritious way to fill up between meals.

Dark chocolate

Does any food product have a greater connection to emotions than chocolate? There's a chocolate associated with virtually every holiday, especially the Valentine's Day celebration of romance. And most people — at least those raised in the United States — hold an affection for chocolate that goes back to childhood. But mentioning chocolate in a discussion about weight management and diabetes has a hint of the proverbial good news/bad news conclusion. Well, not so fast. There's still some room for love.

If you're interested in improving your health, you'll want to skip both sugary candies and chocolates and opt for dark chocolate instead. Polyphenol antioxidant-rich dark chocolate, which should be eaten in extreme moderation for its fat content, is known to balance blood sugar levels in people with diabetes when eaten in small quantities, which means no more than 30 to 60 grams of dark chocolate (70 percent cocoa content or higher) per day. Enjoy it with plain almonds for a snack in-between meals or alone after a meal in lieu of dessert.

The specific health benefits identified in studies, often when comparing chocolate eaters to non-eaters, include the following:

>> There's a reduced of risk of stroke in women who ate more than 45 grams (about 1½ ounces) of chocolate per week.

>> In an Italian study, chocolate eaters show improved insulin sensitivity.

>> Improved muscle cell function by production of new mitochondria, the cell structure where glucose is converted to ATP, was seen in profoundly ill subjects with major muscle cell damage. The subjects were fed cocoa fortified with additional epicatechin (an antioxidant flavanol occurring naturally in cacao).

>> Chocolate acts to lower blood pressure and increase good HDL cholesterol.

>> Studies have shown that chocolate improves blood flow.

Is there a catch? Well, the beneficial cardiovascular effects are associated with plant phenols (cocoa phenols), and the darker the chocolate, the higher the levels of these antioxidants. Most experts, therefore, recommend eating chocolate that's at least 70 percent cacao, and, of course, consuming this dark chocolate in moderation — perhaps 1 ounce per day.

Low-Carb Healthy Snacks

So far you've gotten relatively good news about nuts, seeds, and chocolate — eat in moderation, watch the fat, and know your carbohydrates. You may now be asking if there are low-calorie and low-carb snacks. And, what about snacks that are more in the carbohydrate family — grains, fruit, starchy vegetables, or dairy?

There are options here, too, and in some cases carbohydrate snacks are a specific part of your meal plan. In other cases, where insulin or pills that can cause low blood glucose are part of your treatment plan, these snacks may come in handy when blood glucose needs a slight boost between meals or before bedtime. For the most part, these snacks aren't suitable for treating serious low blood glucose levels, where a quick response is preferred.

REMEMBER

Raw vegetables always offer the best deal on volume when trading for carbohydrates, calories, or fat. Cucumbers are particularly refreshing, but bell peppers, zucchini, green beans, carrots, or other choices may suit your tastes even better.

15-gram snacks

Snacks that offer 15 grams of carbohydrate — one carb choice — elevate blood glucose levels 30 to 45 milligrams per deciliter if necessary to head off mild hypoglycemia. For those wearing an insulin pump, carbohydrate snacks when blood glucose levels are normal can be offset with a bolus dose of insulin (a carbohydrate snack may not be worth an injection when low-carb snacks are just as satisfying). A few lower calorie, 15-carbohydrate-gram snacks include the following:

- 1 cup berries or cubed melon

- 6 ounces Greek-style yogurt

- ½ grapefruit or mango

- ¼ cup mixed unsalted nuts

- 1 cup of carrots and chopped bell peppers with ¼ cup guacamole

- ⅓ cup unsweetened granola

- Approximately 20 grapes

30-gram snacks

In general, 30-carbohydrate-gram snacks may be worked into your meal plan in a balance with fewer carb choices at meals. Having one of these two-carb-choice snacks should require an insulin bolus for those with type 1 diabetes, because these snacks may raise blood glucose by 60 mg/dl or more. These snacks are not intended for treating hypoglycemia.

With type 2 diabetes these snacks can be matched to your medication to help spread carbohydrate consumption more evenly throughout the day. A few 30-carbohydrate-gram snacks include the following:

- ¼ cup dried fruit

- ½ cup beans on a 6-inch tortilla

1 large apple or banana

A palmful or ½ cup mixed unsalted nuts

1 avocado with a poached egg

Alternative Sweeteners

The term *alternative sweetener* refers to sweeteners that are alternative to sucrose, which is typical table sugar and primarily produced from sugarcane and beets. Sucrose in different forms is the sugar most people know — table sugar, brown sugar, confectioner's sugar, and so on. But there are many alternatives to sucrose, some confined primarily to commercial food production uses, that can generally be divided into alternatives with equal calories to sucrose or alternatives that are no-calorie (often called non-nutritive). Other common terms attached to some products are *artificial sweetener* and *sugar substitute*.

FROM THE AUTHORS

We believe that artificial sweeteners should be avoided. It's best to derive sweet flavors from natural foods, and for people with diabetes, even those need to be managed carefully. It has been found that the brain doesn't know the difference between a natural or an artificial sweetener. If you consume beverages that are sweetened artificially, you will continue to crave sugary products, even though you have been consuming "sugar-free" products.

No-calorie or zero-calorie sweeteners are manufactured compounds or natural extracts that taste many times sweeter than sucrose, and so they can be added to foods or drinks in extremely small amounts for equal sweetness. The big three in the United States are saccharin (in the pink packets), aspartame (in the blue packets), and more recently sucralose (in the yellow packets). These sweeteners are everywhere, from diet soft drinks to no-sugar-added ice cream, to the table at restaurants and coffee shops, and into your home-baked desserts. No-calorie sweeteners allow people with diabetes to enjoy sweetened food without calories and without carbohydrates from sugar (calories and carbohydrates can come from other sources, like flour in baked goods).

TIP

Some alternative sweeteners provide no caloric or carbohydrate advantage to your eating plan. Raw honey, molasses, dates, fruit juices, maple syrup, and agave nectar are popular alternatives. We recommend using these sparingly when needed.

WARNING

Some artificial sweeteners have now been shown to be possibly associated with an increased risk of cancer, and the World Health Organization has classified aspartame as a possible carcinogen.

5

Putting It All Together: Meals to Manage Your Diabetes

Take a running start on what you need to plan a week's worth of meals.

Enjoy 25 recipes for complete meals to make planning breakfast, lunch, and dinner a cinch.

Savor chef-driven recipes and all the nutritional information you need to take charge of your food and your health.

Learn to love your time in the kitchen and at the table.

Chapter **17**

Reviewing a Seven-Day Menu

One of the most glorious aspects of eating is that several times per day we have the ability to nourish ourselves with flavors, aromas, textures, and tastes that appeal to us individually. Eating, like dressing, are two highly individual and personalized forms of expression and meeting our basic needs. While we much prefer to provide recipes and guidelines to allow people to plan their own meals for themselves, we often get requests to come up with specific meal plans.

The most common comment nutrition professionals hear from people with diabetes has got to be, "just tell me what to eat." And, if this was a line in a Broadway play, the note in the margin would cue the actor to speak this line with extreme exasperation. But, planning healthy meals for diabetes isn't that miserable an experience. If you're exasperated trying to get started with healthier eating habits, it may be something else that's holding you back. Maybe you see this as the first step into a life of restriction and deprivation — no more tasty food, and never again feeling the satisfaction that comes with a good meal.

That would be a misconception, however. To prove the point, this chapter provides a whole week's menu — three meals a day for seven days. The intent is not to tell you what to eat — you'll get pretty tired going through the same food every day, week after week. The idea is to provide a wide range of options that demonstrate how you can plan your meals and to show how diabetes-friendly meals can be marvelous.

The daily menus all take into account the need to have macronutrient requirements met at each meal, and they incorporate diversity and bioactive compounds that are most beneficial to people with diabetes. We purposely included low glycemic index (GI) carb choices that are satisfying and tasty to eat.

You can find the recipes for each of the breakfast, lunch, and dinners listed here in Chapter 18. Your personal meal plan may also include a carbohydrate snack at some point, so a list of various snack choices is provided at the end of the chapter. More snack item suggestions can be found in Chapter 16. It is our hope that the recipes and suggestions in this book inspire you to create your own delicious diabetes-friendly meals, but, in the meantime this chapter offers a good start.

REMEMBER

Keep in mind that differently sized people, with different metabolisms and different activity levels, require different amounts of food. There is no one-size-fits all recipe size when it comes to properly feeding your body and balancing your blood sugar. Be sure to work with a registered dietitian or certified nutrition specialist to ensure that you are eating the proper amounts of foods.

A WORD ABOUT HYDRATION

People with diabetes have an increased risk of dehydration as high blood glucose levels lead to decreased hydration in the body. It's a good idea to keep yourself well hydrated and enjoy water — perhaps enhanced with a lemon slice, mint leaves, or cucumber slices — at each meal and whenever you have a snack. Aim for a daily intake of approximately 2 liters per day. If you drink one 8-ounce glass of water upon waking, one before and during each meal, and one with a snack or before bed, you can ensure that you are well hydrated. Keep in mind that alcohol and some medications deplete hydrating, so if you consume those, be sure to drink additional amounts of water unless you have been advised to limit your fluid intake by your doctor. There are some rare medical conditions where fluid is restricted.

Day 1

The menu for this day includes all the recommended servings of rainbow-colored vegetables and a wide variety of foods from the various food groups. It also incorporates almonds, leafy green vegetables, fish, beans, extra-virgin olive oil, yogurt, and other foods that are specifically beneficial to people with diabetes. Keep in mind that you can switch the meals up and eat them at a time that best fits your schedule. You may want to have the lunch recipe for dinner and vice versa. You may want to add in an extra green leafy salad at dinner.

TIP

If you are in a crunch for time, you can simplify each of these recipes. The fruit salad for breakfast can be a simple piece of fruit with almonds, and the salmon at dinner can be dressed even more simply and roasted in the oven at the same time as your favorite green vegetables. It's not important that you stick to these exact recipes, but that you follow the general principles.

Breakfast

Recipe: Fresh Fruit Salad with Homemade Vanilla and Flaxseed Granola

Black coffee or espresso; herbal, black, or green tea

Lunch

Recipe: Homemade Hummus and Whole Wheat Pita with Fresh Vegetables

Salad with green leafy vegetables, extra-virgin olive oil, lemon juice, or vinegar

Snack

Handful of almonds

Dinner

Recipe: Citrus Marinated Salmon with Fiery Potatoes and Kale

Snack

½ cup unsweetened Greek yogurt with ¼ cup fresh berries or vegetable crudités

Day 2

The menu for your second day offers a cornucopia of fruit and vegetables enhanced with anti-inflammatory spices and intoxicating aromas. You can switch the order of lunch and dinner if you prefer, and instead of kefir at breakfast, you can enjoy unsweetened yogurt with the same pineapple and kiwi. Remember to make extra stir-fry and baba ghanouj to enjoy for lunch another day.

Breakfast

Recipe: Cardamom-Scented Kefir, Pineapple, and Kiwi Smoothie

Black coffee or espresso; herbal, black, or green tea

Lunch

Recipe: Baba Ghanouj with Crudités and Roasted Chickpeas

1 hardboiled egg

Snack

1 serving of 85 percent dark chocolate

5 walnuts

Dinner

Recipe: Asparagus, Red Pepper, and Tempeh Stir-Fry with Soba Noodles and Sesame Seeds

Snack

1 pear

5 almonds

Day 3

Your menu today is especially suited to cool weather days because it involves lots of warmed foods, but we guarantee it is nutritious and delicious any time of year. This menu includes nuts, seeds, lots of fresh fruit and vegetables, beans, and a succulent simmered chicken dish for dinner.

TIP

We recommend making extra of the soup and the chicken. Store leftovers in the refrigerator or freezer and you will have them on hand when you don't have time to cook. Today's menu is so mouthwatering, you might just forget it's good for you.

Breakfast

Recipe: Warm Raspberry and Cocoa Quinoa with Almond Milk and Sesame Seeds

Black coffee or espresso; herbal, black, or green tea

Lunch

Recipe: Broccoli and Pecorino Cheese Soup with Stuffed Baby Portobello Mushrooms

Snack

1 serving unsweetened Greek yogurt with a handful of blueberries

Dinner

Recipe: Chicken Simmered in Tomatoes, Olives, and Capers with Sauteed Dandelion Greens and Salad

Snack

¼ cup hummus or other bean puree with celery and carrot sticks

Day 4

Breakfast on Day 4 can be made in advance and stored in the refrigerator for breakfast on the go. The pinwheels for lunch and the Turkish stew can also be made in advance so that there's no need to cook after a long day of work. Today's menu is full of all the superfoods and flavor you need to keep eating healthy with gusto!

TIP

If you need to cut down on more carbs, you can swap out the brown basmati rice at dinner and serve with a leafy green salad on the side as well.

Breakfast

Recipe: Blueberry-Almond Yogurt Bowls with Honey, Cinnamon, and Chia Seeds

Black coffee or espresso; herbal, black, or green tea

Lunch

Recipe: Cucumber and Smoked Salmon Pinwheels with Mixed Green Salad

Snack

1 cup assorted raw vegetables (crudités) with 1 serving cottage cheese or hummus (preferably homemade)

Dinner

Recipe: Turkish-Style Eggplant and Chickpea Stew with Brown Basmati Rice Pilaf

Green salad

Snack

1 small banana with 1 tablespoon peanut butter

Day 5

The menu on Day 5 transports your taste buds to North Africa and the Middle East with traditional, nutritious, and flavorful fruits, vegetables, grains, and pulses. Both satisfying and delicious, these items prove that good taste and good health don't need to be mutually exclusive. If you are in a hurry, or don't feel like eating a savory Egyptian breakfast complete with beans and eggs in the morning, you can easily swap the recipe out for another breakfast recipe. The fuul medammes recipe can also be enjoyed at lunch or dinner another day. Leftover grilled or rotisserie chicken can be used in the salad for lunch, and the Moroccan soup can be made in a completely vegetarian or vegan manner as well. If you do make the soup, be sure to make it in larger quantities so that you can freeze some to enjoy at another time. The recipe is also a crowd-pleaser, so it's great for entertaining.

TIP

If you need to cut down on more carbs, omit the whole wheat pita from the breakfast and serve it with celery sticks or broccoli flowerets instead. You can also omit the rice from the soup.

Breakfast

Recipe: Egyptian Fuul Medammes with Extra-Virgin Olive Oil, Tomato, and Eggs (or hummus) and 1 serving whole wheat pita

Black coffee or espresso; herbal, black, or green tea

Lunch

Recipe: Lebanese Fattoush Salad with Citrus-Infused Chicken

Snack

Carrot and celery sticks with tzatziki (cucumber yogurt sauce)

Dinner

Recipe: Moroccan Rice, Lamb, Vegetable, and Lentil Soup

Snack

3 unsweetened dried figs

5 unsalted almonds

Day 6

Today's recipes also incorporate flavors from around the globe, but you can make them in a more simple fashion, if desired. For breakfast, for example, you can enjoy a hardboiled egg with a bit of Greek yogurt and vegetables instead of in the Middle Eastern fashion as noted here. For lunch, the quinoa and sweet potatoes can be made in advance to be assembled quickly. The fish dinner is both elegant and tasty. Even though it can be made in minutes, it's worthy of a special occasion.

Breakfast

Recipe: Middle Eastern–Style Breakfast Platter (labneh, vegetables, za'atar, eggs)

Black coffee or espresso; herbal, black, or green tea

Lunch

Recipe: Roasted Sweet Potato, Avocado, and Quinoa Bowls with Honey-Lime Dressing and Cashews

Snack

1 small apple with 1 teaspoon peanut butter

Dinner

Recipe: Fresh Herb and Parmigiano Crusted Fish with Apple, Beet, and Carrot Salad with Citrus Vinaigrette

Snack

½ cup unsweetened Greek yogurt with ¼ cup chopped fresh strawberries

Day 7

You can end your week in style with Poached Egg and Avocado Toast with Warm Cherry Tomatoes and Sea Salt. This recipe does double duty as a fast weeknight dinner or a quick lunch at home. The farro minestrone can also be made with barley or rice instead of farro, if desired. We recommend making it in large portions and freezing it for later. The dinner is a perfect weekend delight that can be prepared in minutes. If you want to make the cannellini bean puree in advance, it will be even easier to prepare at the last minute. We recommend making extra cannellini bean puree to enjoy as a snack with crudités when needed.

TIP

If you need to cut down on even more carbs, serve the breakfast without the toast or swap out the toast for grilled zucchini or Portobello mushrooms. You can also leave the farro or other grains out of the soup and prepare it with a bit of leftover chicken or meat instead.

Breakfast

Recipe: Poached Egg and Avocado Toast with Warm Cherry Tomatoes and Sea Salt

Black coffee or espresso; herbal, black, or green tea

Lunch

Recipe: Hearty Farro and Five-Vegetable Minestrone

Snack

¼ cup olives (rinsed if in brine and drizzled with extra-virgin olive oil and spices of your choice)

Dinner

Recipe: Sizzling Rosemary Shrimp over Cannellini Bean Puree and Sautéed Greens with Mixed Peppers

Snack

1 cup raw broccoli and/or cauliflower with 2 tablespoons Greek yogurt or hummus

Snacks

It's likely your personalized meal plan includes a carbohydrate snack or two, and it's important to choose snacks that don't impact your blood glucose dramatically yet fill you up. Nothing on this list of snacks is appropriate for treating low blood glucose, where you do want to raise blood sugar quickly.

Each of these snacks provides 15 grams of carbohydrate, but one carb choice, small amounts of nuts or any nonstarchy vegetable, can provide a snack with virtually no impact on blood glucose levels provided the calories, and fat in the case of nuts, fit into your meal plan.

The following snacks provide one carbohydrate choice, 15 grams of carbohydrate, to your daily eating plan:

- ½ cup sugar-free pudding
- 3 graham cracker halves with 1½ teaspoon peanut butter
- Raisin bread with 1 teaspoon margarine
- 1 small granola bar
- ½ cup no-added-sugar ice cream
- 3 ginger snaps
- 5 vanilla wafers

REMEMBER

Having diabetes doesn't mean you avoid carbohydrates — it's hard to say that too often. Having diabetes means you choose your carbohydrates wisely, and you spread them throughout the day. Carbohydrate foods like fruit, whole grains, starchy vegetables, beans and legumes, and milk or yogurt, are nutritious and delicious. Getting your carbohydrates from sugar and refined grains, which often come with little redeeming nutritional value, is not a successful strategy for managing diabetes effectively. Ultimately, it's you who makes the choices about how you're going to eat, and what effect your eating has on your long-term health.

Chapter **18**

Creating Delicious and Nutritious Meals

MEAL RECIPES IN THIS CHAPTER

Bountiful Breakfasts

Poached Egg and Avocado Toast with Warm Cherry Tomatoes and Sea Salt

Blueberry-Almond Yogurt Bowls with Honey, Cinnamon, and Chia Seeds

Fresh Fruit Salad with Homemade Vanilla and Flaxseed Granola

Warm Raspberry and Cocoa Quinoa with Almond Milk and Sesame Seeds

Middle Eastern–Style Breakfast Platter

Egyptian Fuul Medammes with Extra-Virgin Olive Oil, Tomato, and Eggs

Cardamom-Scented Kefir, Pineapple, and Kiwi Smoothie

Looking Forward to Lunch

Homemade Hummus and Whole Wheat Pita with Fresh Vegetables

Moroccan Rice, Lamb, Vegetable, and Lentil Soup

(continued)

Food is one of life's greatest pleasures, and a diabetes diagnosis doesn't need to change that. Food is not only a source of sustenance, but also a source of cultural expression, affection, charity, therapy, and medicine. In modern western culture, food is often thought of as the enemy — something that needs to be avoided. But the truth is, enjoying the right foods in the right amounts is a powerful way to take control of your health and happiness.

Those with diabetes need to pay even more attention to what they're eating. Cooking and preparing food at home is a great way to ensure that you're getting the nutrients and types of food you need at a fraction of the cost as restaurant, fast-food, and take-out meals. Cooking itself can also be incredibly therapeutic. It is our hope that these recipes inspire you to enjoy yourself in the kitchen.

It's important that people with diabetes consume nutrient-dense food and quality macronutrients (carbohydrates, fat, and protein) in each meal. For this reason, the

(*continued*)

- Roasted Sweet Potato, Avocado, and Quinoa Bowls with Honey-Lime Dressing and Cashews
- Lebanese Fattoush Salad with Citrus-Infused Chicken
- Asian Noodle and Seven-Vegetable Salad with Sweet and Tangy Ginger Sauce
- Broccoli and Pecorino Cheese Soup with Stuffed Baby Portobello Mushrooms
- Hearty Farro and Five-Vegetable Minestrone
- Cucumber and Smoked Salmon Pinwheels with Mixed Green Salad
- Baba Ghanouj with Crudités and Roasted Chickpeas

Delicious Dinners

- Citrus-Marinated Salmon with Fiery Potatoes and Kale
- Red Lentil Croquettes over Baby Spinach with Tzatziki Sauce
- Chicken Simmered in Tomatoes, Olives, and Capers with Sautéed Dandelion Greens and Salad
- Turkish-Style Eggplant and Chickpea Stew with Brown Basmati Rice Pilaf
- Fresh Herb and Parmigiano Crusted Fish with Apple, Beet, and Carrot Salad with Citrus Vinaigrette
- Pasta with Pistachio Pesto, Fresh Tuna, and Yellow Tomato Sauce
- Sizzling Rosemary Shrimp over Cannellini Bean Puree and Sauteed Greens with Mixed Peppers
- Assorted Seafood Tartines with Microgreen, Red Cabbage, Carrot, and Corn Slaw
- Asparagus, Red Pepper, and Tempeh Stir-Fry with Soba Noodles and Sesame Seeds

Must-Have Base Recipes

- Dried Beans
- Lentils
- Homemade Stock
- Fresh Bread Crumbs
- Fresh Tomato Sauce

recipes in this chapter were designed to be complete meals. Instead of having to pair foods together to create a complete meal, these recipes enable you to cook a full meal all in one recipe. In addition, each recipe is folded into the sample week's menu in Chapter 17. With all you've learned about healthy eating and meal planning, you can find thousands more recipes that fit the bill. It may take a little time and effort, but the payoff is worth the effort.

Good cooking is an investment in time, but it is also an investment in your health, in your happiness, and in your future wellbeing. The meals you choose to eat today not only help you feel better now, they also prevent long-term illness as well. Just as working out, learning a new skill, or any other new habit takes time, so can cooking. If you make it a priority, however, and commit to enjoying yourself in the process, you will be amazed at the results.

Bountiful Breakfasts

A nutritious and blood glucose–balancing meal that also tastes great gets your day off to a good start. Breakfast recipes are among the most challenging to prepare because people have very distinct ideas of what constitutes the first meal of the day. Some enjoy sweet breakfasts, others savory, and some people eat breakfast on the run. For this reason, the meals in this chapter are varied — some can also be eaten for lunch or as a snack.

For those with diabetes, eating a balanced meal within the first few hours of waking can really help keep blood glucose levels in check throughout the day. No matter which style of breakfast you prefer, if your first meal of the day consists of diabetes-friendly foods with additional health benefits for diabetes, it will be good for you.

TIP

If you're short on time in the morning, prepare your breakfast the night before. Even a piece of fruit or some plain Greek yogurt and a handful of plain, unsalted almonds on the run are much better than skipping a morning meal.

Poached Egg and Avocado Toast with Warm Cherry Tomatoes and Sea Salt

PREP TIME: 5 MINUTES	COOK TIME: 12 MINUTES	YIELD: 4 SERVINGS

INGREDIENTS

4 slices good-quality whole wheat, barley, or oat bread

4 teaspoons Amy Riolo Selections or other good-quality extra-virgin olive oil

2 ripe avocadoes, halved and pitted

4 eggs

½ cup cherry tomatoes, halved

⅛ teaspoon unrefined sea salt or fleur de sel, plus extra for water

DIRECTIONS

1 Toast the bread in a toaster or under the broiler to desired doneness.

2 Drizzle ½ teaspoon of olive oil over each piece of bread.

3 Scoop the avocado out of the shell and place the flesh from ½ of each avocado on each of the pieces of bread.

4 To poach eggs, bring a pot of water to a gentle boil, then salt the water.

5 With a spoon, begin stirring the boiling water in a large, circular motion.

6 When the water is swirling like a tornado, add the eggs. If it's your first time, try one at a time until you get the hang of it. Cook for 2½ to 3 minutes.

7 Using a slotted spoon, remove the eggs and place on top of the toast.

8 Heat a small skillet over medium-high heat and add the remaining 2 teaspoons of olive oil.

9 Add the cherry tomato halves and stir to coat. Cook for 2 to 3 minutes until warm and the tomatoes release their juices or are cooked until your preferred texture.

10 Scatter the tomato pieces and salt over the top of the toast and serve.

PER SERVING: Calories 315 (From Fat 191); Fat 21g (Saturated 4g); Cholesterol 212mg; Sodium 248mg; Carbohydrate 24g (Dietary Fiber 7g); Protein 11g.

TIP: This simple toast can do triple duty as lunch or dinner paired with a green leafy salad.

NOTE: Avocados are full of vitamins, nutrients, and heart-healthy fats, while also being cholesterol-free. It is believed that adding avocado to the diet may help those with diabetes to lose weight and increase insulin sensitivity while lowering cholesterol.

VARY IT! Use hardboiled egg slices or crumbles or Greek yogurt to make this dish even easier. If avocados aren't ripe or are too pricy, substitute sautéed fresh spinach, collards, or kale.

Blueberry–Almond Yogurt Bowls with Honey, Cinnamon, and Chia Seeds

PREP TIME: 5 MINUTES	COOK TIME: 0 MINUTES	YIELD: 2 SERVINGS

INGREDIENTS

1 cup organic blueberries

½ cup plain, unsalted, whole almonds

1 cup plain (unsweetened) Greek yogurt

2 tablespoons chia seeds

2 teaspoons raw honey

1 teaspoon ground pure (ceylon) cinnamon

DIRECTIONS

1 Divide the blueberries and almonds evenly between two bowls.

2 Pour ½ cup of the yogurt over the top of each bowl.

3 Scatter 1 tablespoon chia seeds and 1 teaspoon of honey on top of the yogurt.

4 Sprinkle ½ teaspoon cinnamon over the top and serve.

PER SERVING: *Calories 412 (From Fat 219); Fat 24g (Saturated 3g); Cholesterol 13mg; Sodium 38mg; Carbohydrate 33g (Dietary Fiber 11g); Protein 21g.*

TIP: Make this recipe when fresh berries are in season, otherwise swap out the same quantity for fresh apples or pears or frozen berries if preferred.

NOTE: Blueberries are a great way to get more fiber, vitamin C, and healthy cancer-preventing compounds into your diet. The live cultures along with lactic acid, zinc, and other minerals and enzymes in yogurt as well as probiotics make yogurt a great choice for improving skin condition as well.

VARY IT! You can put the same ingredients and a handful of ice in the blender and blend until smooth for delicious smoothies that also make great postworkout snacks.

Fresh Fruit Salad with Homemade Vanilla and Flaxseed Granola

PREP TIME: 5 MINUTES PLUS 5 HOURS TO OVERNIGHT FOR MARINATING	COOK TIME: 0 MINUTES	YIELD: 4 SERVINGS

INGREDIENTS

1 cup cantaloupe, cubed

½ cup blueberries

½ cup sliced kiwi

1 cup whole rolled oats

¼ cup chopped almonds

2 teaspoons flaxseeds

1 tablespoon pure vanilla extract

¼ cup creamy almond butter

DIRECTIONS

1 In a large bowl, combine the cantaloupe, blueberries, and kiwi.

2 Preheat the oven to 300 degrees Fahrenheit and line a baking sheet with parchment paper.

3 In a medium bowl, combine the oats, almonds, flaxseeds, vanilla, and almond butter.

4 Stir until combined. Scoop the granola onto the baking sheet and press the mixture into a 1-inch-thick oval. This will encourage clumping.

5 Bake for 8 minutes. Use a fork or spatula to flip, turn, and gently break the granola apart.

6 Bake for 15 minutes more, or until golden brown. Use the parchment paper to lift the granola out of the pan and onto a cooling rack and allow to cool completely, approximately 15 minutes.

7 Transfer fruit to individual bowls and top with equal portions of granola.

PER SERVING: *Calories 261 (From Fat 133); Fat 15g (Saturated 1g); Cholesterol 0mg; Sodium 80mg; Carbohydrate 28g (Dietary Fiber 5g); Protein 7g.*

TIP: Make extra granola to store in an airtight container in the refrigerator and to use when needed on yogurt.

NOTE: Substitute all-natural sugar-free granola if you don't have time to make your own, or simply top fruit with chopped almonds and flaxseeds.

VARY IT! Swap out the fruits called for in this recipe with those that are inexpensive and in season. You can also use your favorite frozen fruits.

Warm Raspberry and Cocoa Quinoa with Almond Milk and Sesame Seeds

PREP TIME: 10 MINUTES	COOK TIME: 15 MINUTES	YIELD: 2 SERVINGS

INGREDIENTS

½ cup dry quinoa, rinsed

2 teaspoons plain, powdered cocoa (unsweetened), Fair Trade Certified, if possible

1 teaspoon pure vanilla

½ cup unsweetened almond milk

2 teaspoons pure raw honey, if desired

1 cup fresh raspberries or blueberries

2 tablespoons raw sesame seeds

DIRECTIONS

1 Bring 1 cup of water to a boil in a medium saucepan over high heat.

2 Add the quinoa, cocoa, and vanilla, stir, reduce heat to low, and cover. Allow to simmer until all liquid is absorbed, 10 to 15 minutes. Remove from the heat and allow to cool completely.

3 Stir in the almond milk and honey to sweeten, if desired.

4 Place the quinoa in two bowls and top with raspberries and sesame seeds.

5 Serve warm.

PER SERVING: *Calories 262 (From Fat 73); Fat 8g (Saturated 1g); Cholesterol 0mg; Sodium 4mg; Carbohydrate 42g (Dietary Fiber 7g); Protein 9g.*

TIP: Quinoa is considered a complete protein, so it is a great alternative to meat, fish, and dairy for lunch. Prepare it in advance to toss it into salads, or eat with a few berries, nuts, and a drizzle of cinnamon and honey with almond milk for breakfast.

NOTE: Warm quinoa puts a surprising spin on breakfast and the addition of cocoa adds rich, chocolaty taste and antioxidants.

VARY IT! You could swap out other whole grains, such as rice, barley, millet, or oats in this warm breakfast. Because quinoa has more protein though, it's best to add a handful of chopped almonds if you're swapping out a grain that has less protein.

Middle Eastern–Style Breakfast Platter

PREP TIME: 5 MINUTES	COOK TIME: 0 MINUTES	YIELD: 2 SERVINGS

INGREDIENTS

2 Persian cucumbers or 1 English cucumber, sliced

2 Roma tomatoes, sliced

1 handful fresh mint or parsley, or a combination of both, cleaned

½ cup labneh cheese or Greek yogurt

2 hardboiled eggs

2 tablespoons Amy Riolo Selections or other good-quality extra-virgin olive oil

2 teaspoons Za'atar spice mix, or unrefined sea salt

DIRECTIONS

1 On two separate plates or a large platter, arrange cucumber slices and tomatoes in a decorative pattern on half of the plate.

2 Add fresh mint and/or parsley to the center of the plate.

3 Dollop the labneh or Greek yogurt on one quadrant of the plate.

4 Slice the hardboiled eggs into quarters and place next to the labneh.

5 Drizzle the egg and labneh with olive oil and sprinkle with Za'atar or sea salt.

PER SERVING: *Calories 277 (From Fat 184); Fat 20g (Saturated 4g); Cholesterol 218mg; Sodium 287mg; Carbohydrate 10g (Dietary Fiber 3g); Protein 14g.*

TIP: This quick and nutritious Middle Eastern power plate can be a great portable lunch or dinner as well.

NOTE: Za'atar is a wild thyme spice mix that hails from the Middle East. It usually contains sumac, sea salt, coriander, and sesame seeds. If you can't find it, substitute your favorite spice or unrefined sea salt.

VARY IT! Use a combination of your own favorite vegetables and cook the egg in a different way if you choose.

Egyptian Fuul Medammes with Extra-Virgin Olive Oil, Tomato, and Eggs

PREP TIME: 2 MINUTES	COOK TIME: 5 MINUTES	YIELD: 4 SERVINGS

INGREDIENTS

5 teaspoons Amy Riolo Selections or other good-quality extra-virgin olive oil

1 (15-ounce) can cooked fava beans with juice

½ teaspoon cumin

½ teaspoon dried ground coriander

⅛ teaspoon unrefined sea salt

Freshly ground black pepper, to taste

4 hardboiled eggs, quartered

4 Roma tomatoes, diced

4 pieces whole wheat pita bread for serving, if desired

DIRECTIONS

1 In a medium frying pan, add 1 teaspoon of olive oil and warm over medium–low heat. Add the beans and juice from the can, cumin, coriander, salt, and pepper. Stir well to combine. Cook until most of the liquid has absorbed, about 5 minutes.

2 Reduce the heat to low and mash slightly with a fork or potato masher, cooking just until the mixture is slightly looser than refried beans, about 1 minute. Serve immediately.

3 Spoon evenly onto four plates. Place egg quarters around the edges. Make a hole in the center and drizzle the remaining 1 teaspoon of olive oil into each.

4 Garnish with tomatoes on top and serve with pita bread.

PER SERVING: *Calories 213 (From Fat 101); Fat 11g (Saturated 2g); Cholesterol 211mg; Sodium 682mg; Carbohydrate 16g (Dietary Fiber 5g); Protein 13g.*

TIP: Fuul medammes is a time-honored Middle Eastern street food. These are a blank culinary canvas for lots of toppings — just like baked potatoes or nachos are in the United States. Restaurants and food carts selling *fuul* will give you your choice of diced fresh vegetables (tomato, cucumber, onion), olive oil and lemon, tahini sauce, and other options for enjoying them in addition to this version.

NOTE: Protein- and fiber-dense fava beans are believed to be the world's oldest agricultural crop — they're said to have been one of the pharaoh's favorites. This traditional Egyptian dish is still a popular breakfast and snack food. This can also be a fast lunch or dinner dish.

VARY It: Swap out chickpeas or cannellini beans in this recipe if needed. The name would then need to be changed to match whichever bean you use, but it would still make a delicious and nutritious dish.

Cardamom-Scented Kefir, Pineapple, and Kiwi Smoothie

PREP TIME: 5 MINUTES	COOK TIME: 0 MINUTES	YIELD: 2 SERVINGS

INGREDIENTS

1 cup kefir

1 teaspoon ground cardamom

½ cup fresh pineapple chunks

2 kiwis

1 cup ice

DIRECTIONS

1 Place all ingredients into a blender and blend on high power until smooth and creamy.

2 Pour into two glasses and serve cold.

PER SERVING: *Calories 116 (From Fat 14); Fat 2g (Saturated 1g); Cholesterol 5mg; Sodium 131mg; Carbohydrate 22g (Dietary Fiber 3g); Protein 5g.*

TIP: Yogurt could be used in place of kefir in this recipe if desired.

NOTE: Pineapple is a good source of vitamins A, B, C, manganese, and fiber, as well as a compound called bromelain, which offers many health benefits. Be sure to use fresh pineapple or frozen pineapple instead of sugar- and sodium-laden canned versions. Cardamom is correlated with supporting glucose metabolism.

VARY IT! Any fresh fruit — bananas, pomegranate seeds, berries, apples, oranges, or a combination — can be made in this recipe. Be sure to choose those like cherries, grapefruit, and apples that have a lower glycemic index for best results.

Looking Forward to Lunch

According to many of the world's most known healing culinary traditions, such as those found in Ayurveda, the Mediterranean diet, and traditional Chinese medicine, it is believed that the largest and most important meal of the day should be eaten at lunch (or when the sun is hottest).

While many of our modern workday lunches don't exactly follow the patterns of the sun, it's still a safe bet to say that this is the time of day when our body most needs nourishment and can handle fuller meals. Just because we may work in an office or a factory, which makes lunch time less of a ritual, doesn't mean we shouldn't take the time to pause and nourish ourselves with the foods that are best for us.

TIP

The recipes in this chapter run the gamut from different cultural traditions to nutritious foods on the go. Some of them can and should be made in advance and can be quickly packed for lunch the night before. Keep in mind that left-over portions from the dinner recipes can also be great for lunch the next day.

Homemade Hummus and Whole Wheat Pita with Fresh Vegetables

PREP TIME: 10 MINUTES	COOK TIME: 0 MINUTES	YIELD: 4 SERVINGS

INGREDIENTS

1 cup cooked or no salt added canned chickpeas (see recipe at the end of this chapter)

1 garlic clove, minced

⅓ cup tahini sauce (sesame puree)

3 teaspoons Amy Riolo Selections or other good-quality extra-virgin olive oil

½ teaspoon unrefined sea salt

2 ice cubes

Dash of paprika, for garnish

2 cups broccoli flowerets, for serving

2 cups cauliflower flowerets, for serving

1 English cucumber, sliced, for serving

1 cup cherry tomatoes, for serving

4 pieces whole wheat (4-inch) pita bread, cut into triangles

DIRECTIONS

1 Peel chickpeas and place them in a food processor, reserving a few for garnish.

2 Add the garlic, tahini sauce, 2 tablespoons of olive oil, and salt, to a food processor. Puree until smooth.

3 Add the ice cubes and continue to puree.

4 If the hummus isn't creamy enough, add water, tablespoon by tablespoon, to get an extra-creamy consistency. (You should need less than ¼ cup in total.)

5 Scrape down the sides of the food processor and puree for 1 to 2 additional minutes. Taste and adjust seasonings if necessary.

6 Spoon into a small round dish. Using the back of a spoon, make dents in the top and fill the dents with the remaining tablespoon of olive oil.

7 Sprinkle paprika and arrange the remaining chickpeas on the top. Serve with broccoli, cauliflower, cucumbers, tomatoes, and pita bread.

PER SERVING: *Calories 329 (From Fat 139); Fat 15g (Saturated 2g); Cholesterol 0mg; Sodium 426mg; Carbohydrate 0g (Dietary Fiber 9g); Protein 13g.*

TIP: If not serving immediately, store hummus in a container with a lid in the refrigerator.

NOTE: In the Eastern Mediterranean countries, hummus can be served with slices of meat or chicken on top. If you have leftover meat, this is a great way to make another meal out of it.

VARY IT! You can make a delicious, nutritious, and creamy puree out of all kinds of beans and lentils. Just don't call it hummus! The word means "chickpea" in Arabic.

Moroccan Rice, Lamb, Vegetable, and Lentil Soup

PREP TIME: 15 MINUTES	COOK TIME: 50 MINUTES	YIELD: 4 SERVINGS

INGREDIENTS

1 medium yellow onion, diced

1 pound lamb leg meat, cut into ½-inch pieces

½ cup brown lentils, sorted, rinsed, and drained

½ cup tomato puree

4 cups homemade vegetable or chicken stock (see recipe at the end of this chapter) or water

1 teaspoon ground coriander

½ teaspoon ground cumin

½ teaspoon ground ginger

½ teaspoon unrefined sea salt

¼ teaspoon freshly ground black pepper

¼ cup medium grain rice

4 stalks celery, finely chopped

4 carrots, peeled and diced

¼ cup fresh cilantro, roughly chopped

¼ cup fresh parsley, finely chopped

DIRECTIONS

1 Place onions, lamb, lentils, tomato puree, stock, coriander, cumin, ginger, salt, and pepper in a large saucepan or stockpot.

2 Bring to a boil over high heat, stir, and reduce heat to low. Simmer for 20 minutes.

3 Add rice, celery, carrots, cilantro, and parsley and bring to a boil over high heat.

4 Once boiling, reduce heat to low, cover, and simmer for another 30 minutes or until all vegetables and lamb are tender.

PER SERVING: *Calories 419 (From Fat 88); Fat 10g (Saturated 3g); Cholesterol 67mg; Sodium 825mg; Carbohydrate 49g (Dietary Fiber 11g); Protein 33g.*

TIP: This soup tastes even better when reheated the next day, so it's great to prepare in advance. You can also make extra portions and freeze for another occasion.

NOTE: To make a vegan variation, replace lamb with chickpeas and use vegetable stock instead of chicken.

VARY IT! You can omit the rice or use vermicelli, quinoa, or barley in its in place.

Roasted Sweet Potato, Avocado, and Quinoa Bowls with Honey–Lime Dressing and Cashews

PREP TIME: 20 MINUTES	COOK TIME: 15 MINUTES	YIELD: 2 SERVINGS

INGREDIENTS

1 sweet potato

½ cup quinoa

1 pound fresh baby spinach (or kale, dandelion greens, arugula)

1 avocado, sliced

¼ cup unsalted cashews (or almonds)

4 tablespoons Amy Riolo Selections or other good-quality extra-virgin olive oil

Juice and zest of 2 limes

1 teaspoon raw honey

⅛ teaspoon unrefined sea salt

¼ teaspoon freshly ground black pepper

DIRECTIONS

1 To cook the sweet potato, prick it with a fork and either microwave it per instructions or roast it in the oven at 425 degrees Fahrenheit for 30 minutes or until tender.

2 Bring a cup of water to boil over high heat. Add quinoa, stir, and reduce heat to medium–low. Cook until tender (approximately 10 minutes), and then drain and allow to cool.

3 Place spinach at the bottom of two bowls or carryout containers.

4 Chop sweet potato into large chunks and place on top of the spinach.

5 Scatter cooled quinoa over each. Scatter the avocado slices and cashews over the top.

6 In a medium bowl, whisk together the olive oil, lime juice, honey, salt, and pepper until creamy and emulsified.

7 When it is time to serve the salad, drizzle the vinaigrette over the top and garnish each with lime zest.

PER SERVING: *Calories 727 (From Fat 436); Fat 48g (Saturated 7g); Cholesterol 0mg; Sodium 328mg; Carbohydrate 65g (Dietary Fiber 15g); Protein 18g.*

TIP: If you have prepared quinoa in advance, this salad is a cinch to prepare. Store vinaigrette separately until serving.

NOTE: Any combination of greens, grains, and legumes can be used in this salad.

VARY IT! Leftover proteins can be added to this salad as well.

Lebanese Fattoush Salad with Citrus-Infused Chicken

PREP TIME: 10 MINUTES	COOK TIME: 15 MINUTES	YIELD: 4 SERVINGS

INGREDIENTS

1 pound boneless chicken breast, sliced into thin strips (or leftover rotisserie or roasted chicken)

4 tablespoons Amy Riolo Selections or other good-quality extra-virgin olive oil

2 tablespoons pomegranate molasses

Juice of 2 lemons (about ½ cup)

2 teaspoons white wine vinegar

1 teaspoon dried mint

¼ teaspoon kosher salt

¼ teaspoon freshly ground pepper

1 cucumber, diced

4 Roma tomatoes, finely chopped

1 medium red onion, thinly sliced

1 green pepper, seeded and diced

2 teaspoons sumac

1 piece whole wheat (6-inch) pita bread or gluten-free bread, cut into 12 pieces

DIRECTIONS

1 Preheat the oven to 425 degrees Fahrenheit and place the chicken strips on a baking sheet.

2 Add the olive oil, pomegranate molasses, lemon juice, white wine vinegar, mint, salt, and pepper to a medium bowl. Whisk vigorously to form a smooth dressing.

3 Pour half of the dressing over the chicken strips and toss to combine.

4 Roast the chicken strips in the oven until cooked through (registering 165 degrees Fahrenheit on a meat thermometer), approximately 15 minutes.

5 In another large bowl, combine the cucumber, tomatoes, red onion, and green pepper.

6 Sprinkle the pita pieces with sumac, and place under the broiler and toast for 2 to 4 minutes, or until golden on both sides. Remove from the oven and set aside to cool.

7 Add the pita chips and chicken to the vegetables and toss to combine. Pour the dressing over salad and toss again to combine. Serve immediately.

PER SERVING: *Calories 245 (From Fat 132); Fat 15g (Saturated 2g); Cholesterol 11mg; Sodium 232mg; Carbohydrate 25g (Dietary Fiber 3g); Protein 7 g.*

TIP: Fattoush is often served alongside other popular Lebanese dishes without meat as well.

NOTE: Sumac is a traditional spice that gives a tangy flavor and ruby red color to the dish.

VARY IT! Any leftover beef, lamb, or fish could also work in this recipe.

Asian Noodle and Seven-Vegetable Salad with Sweet and Tangy Ginger Sauce

PREP TIME: 20 MINUTES	COOK TIME: 10 MINUTES	YIELD: 4 SERVINGS

INGREDIENTS

8 ounces brown rice dry noodles

4 cups mix of red cabbage, carrots, and radish, shredded

1 red bell pepper, finely sliced

2 cups broccoli and cauliflower flowerets

1 cup frozen edamame, thawed

½ bunch cilantro, chopped

Dressing:

¼ inch fresh ginger root or ½ teaspoon dried ground ginger

2 cloves garlic

¼ cup almond butter

¼ cup fresh orange juice (about 1 large orange)

¼ cup fresh lime juice (about 2 limes)

1 tablespoon low-sodium tamari sauce

2 tablespoons raw honey or agave

2 tablespoons toasted sesame oil

1 teaspoon chili paste, or to taste

Garnish:

¼–½ cup roasted, crushed peanuts

DIRECTIONS

1 Prepare rice noodles according to package directions. When tender, drain and rinse.

2 While noodles are cooking, place cabbage, carrots, radish, bell pepper, broccoli and cauliflower, edamame, and cilantro in a large bowl.

3 Toss noodles into vegetables with tongs.

4 Combine all dressing ingredients in a blender and blend until smooth. Taste and adjust if necessary.

5 Pour dressing over vegetables and noodles. Toss to coat. Serve with peanuts on top, if desired.

PER SERVING: *Calories 553 (From Fat 205); Fat 23g (Saturated 3g); Cholesterol 0mg; Sodium 406mg; Carbohydrate 79g (Dietary Fiber 8g); Protein 14g.*

TIP: Prepare the dressing and vegetables one day in advance and store separately for a quick meal.

NOTE: This salad makes a great meal on the go.

VARY IT! You can substitute rice noodles for rice, wild rice, or other grains, if desired.

Broccoli and Pecorino Cheese Soup with Stuffed Baby Portobello Mushrooms

PREP TIME: 10 MINUTES	COOK TIME: 20 MINUTES	YIELD: 4 SERVINGS

INGREDIENTS

4 tablespoons Amy Riolo Selections or other good-quality extra-virgin olive oil

1½ pounds fresh broccoli, cut into flowerets and small pieces

1 large onion, chopped

1 carrot, peeled, trimmed, and chopped

½ teaspoon unrefined sea salt

¼ teaspoon freshly ground black pepper

3 tablespoons all-purpose flour

4 cups Homemade Chicken or Vegetable Stock (see recipe at the end of this chapter)

¼ cup plain Greek-style yogurt

For the mushrooms:

4 Portobello mushrooms, rinsed and rubbed dry

4 tablespoons Amy Riolo Selections or other good-quality extra-virgin olive oil

½ cup fresh bread crumbs (see recipe at the end of this chapter)

¼ cup Pecorino or Parmigiano-Reggiano cheese, grated

DIRECTIONS

1 Heat olive oil in a heavy-bottomed Dutch oven or saucepan over medium-high heat.

2 Add broccoli, onion, carrot, salt, and pepper. Sauté stirring occasionally until onion is translucent, approximately 5 minutes.

3 Add the flour, stir, and cook for another minute, until the flour takes on a golden hue. Add stock, increase heat to high, and bring to a boil.

4 Reduce heat to medium-low and simmer, uncovered, until broccoli is tender, approximately 15 minutes.

5 With an immersion blender (or in a blender with the center spout removed and the hole covered with a clean kitchen towel), puree the soup.

6 Return to the saucepan and stir in the yogurt.

7 Serve warm with mushrooms.

To make the mushrooms:

1 Preheat the broiler to 500 degrees Fahrenheit.

2 Trim stems off mushrooms and chop the tender parts into fine pieces, reserving the tough bottom parts for use in stock or stew. Place mushroom pieces in a large bowl.

(continued)

(continued)

¼ cup mozzarella cheese, shredded

1 tablespoon fresh basil, chopped

Unrefined sea salt, to taste

Freshly ground black pepper, to taste

2 cups fresh baby arugula or other greens

1 lemon, juiced and zested

¼ cup freshly chopped parsley

3 Pour 2 tablespoons of olive oil into the bowl with chopped mushroom stems, and add the bread crumbs, Pecorino, mozzarella, and basil. Stir to combine and season with salt and pepper.

4 If the undersides of the mushroom caps contain large brown gills, lightly scrape them away with the back of spoon and discard. Distribute the filling evenly among mushroom caps until full, and place on a baking sheet.

5 Place the mushroom caps under the broiler (use the second rack to top so that they don't burn), and bake for 3 to 5 minutes or until the mushrooms are golden and cooked through and the cheese has melted.

6 Remove the mushroom caps from the oven, and place on a platter filled with arugula leaves. Drizzle the remaining olive oil over the top, along with the juice of the lemon. Use the lemon zest to garnish the dish, and top with parsley.

PER SERVING: *Calories 534 (From Fat 302); Fat 32g (Saturated 6g); Cholesterol 18mg; Sodium 548mg; Carbohydrate 45g (Dietary Fiber 8g); Protein 21g.*

TIP: You can stuff the mushrooms one day in advance and bake them before serving. The soup can be made one day ahead.

NOTE: Leftover soup makes great pasta sauce. Leftover mushrooms can be chopped and added to whole-grain and pasta dishes.

VARY IT! Substitute cauliflower for broccoli in soup if desired. Mushrooms, while a plant-based food, offer nutrients similar to those found in meat. If you don't have time to stuff the mushrooms, you could sauté them in olive oil and stir into the soup instead.

Hearty Farro and Five-Vegetable Minestrone

PREP TIME: 15 MINUTES	COOK TIME: 50 MINUTES	YIELD: 8 SERVINGS

INGREDIENTS

2 tablespoons Amy Riolo Selections or other good-quality extra-virgin olive oil

1 stalk celery, diced

1 carrot, diced

1 large yellow onion, diced

2 cloves garlic, peeled and finely diced

¼ cup dried porcini mushrooms, soaked in water for 20 minutes, drained, and rinsed

2 cups Fresh Tomato Sauce (see recipe at the end of this chapter) or boxed or canned no salt added diced tomatoes

2 cups chopped savoy cabbage

¼ cup brown lentils, rinsed and sorted

½ teaspoon unrefined sea salt

¼ teaspoon freshly ground black pepper

4 cups Homemade Chicken Stock or Vegetable Stock (see recipe at the end of this chapter), reduced-sodium stock, or water

1 cup farro, barley, or whole wheat pasta

DIRECTIONS

1 Add olive oil to a large, heavy-bottomed saucepan or Dutch oven over medium heat. Add celery, carrot, onion, and garlic.

2 Sauté until golden, approximately 5 minutes. Stir in the mushrooms and sauté for another 2 to 3 minutes. Add tomatoes, cabbage, lentils, salt, and pepper. Stir and simmer for 5 minutes.

3 Add stock or water. Bring to a boil over high heat and then reduce heat to medium-low and simmer, covered, for 40 minutes.

4 Add farro, and cook until pasta is done and lentils are tender, approximately 10 minutes. Serve hot.

PER SERVING: *Calories 196 (From Fat 44); Fat 5g (Saturated 1g); Cholesterol 0mg; Sodium 180mg; Carbohydrate 32g (Dietary Fiber 8g); Protein 9g.*

TIP: This soup gets better as it sits, making it the perfect cook-ahead dish.

NOTE: You can also freeze it in individual containers to reheat later. This soup can be served by itself with bruschetta and salad or precede a hearty winter roast.

VARY IT! This recipe is just a base. In Italy, cooks literally use what is on hand. The only guideline is that this soup contains a mixture of legumes, vegetables, and grains.

Cucumber and Smoked Salmon Pinwheels with Mixed Green Salad

PREP TIME: 20 MINUTES   COOK TIME: 0 MINUTES   YIELD: 4 SERVINGS

INGREDIENTS

4–6 ounces plain Greek yogurt

1 tablespoon chopped fresh dill

2 tablespoons Amy Riolo Selections or other good-quality extra-virgin olive oil

Juice and zest of 1 lemon

2 burrito-style spinach wraps (or any burrito-sized wrap)

2–3 cups spinach

2 Persian cucumbers or 1 English cucumber, sliced thin lengthwise into strips

4–6 ounces smoked salmon

DIRECTIONS

1 In a small bowl combine the yogurt, dill, olive oil, and lemon juice and zest. Mix until well-incorporated and creamy.

2 Lay out both wraps and evenly spread the yogurt mixture onto each one. Be sure to spread the mixture out to the edge on one side, as you'll use this side to "seal" the pinwheel.

3 Evenly distribute the spinach between the two tortillas, followed by the cucumber strips. Top with the smoked salmon.

4 Tightly roll up each wrap, tucking in the ends as you go.

5 With a serrated knife, cut the edges off of each wrap, and then cut each one into ½-inch rounds. You should get about 14 to 16 pinwheels, 7 to 8 per wrap.

PER SERVING: *Calories 250 (From Fat 105); Fat 12g (Saturated 3g); Cholesterol 12mg; Sodium 472mg; Carbohydrate 24g (Dietary Fiber 2g); Protein 13g.*

TIP: This is a fun recipe to get the kids involved with.

NOTE: Pinwheels are a fun lunch and entertaining option for a buffet.

VARY IT! You can omit the burrito wrappers and use lettuce leaves instead for a gluten-free option.

Baba Ghanouj with Crudités and Roasted Chickpeas

PREP TIME: 15 MINUTES	COOK TIME: 20 MINUTES	YIELD: 4 SERVINGS

INGREDIENTS

2 medium eggplants

2 tablespoons tahini sauce (sesame puree)

4 tablespoons Amy Riolo Selections or other good-quality extra-virgin olive oil

Juice of 1 lemon

1 garlic clove, minced

Unrefined sea salt, to taste

Freshly ground black pepper, to taste

2 cups broccoli florets, for serving

2 cups carrot sticks, for serving

1 English cucumber, sliced, for serving

For the chickpeas:

1½ cups cooked chickpeas (see recipe at the end of this chapter)

Amy Riolo Selections or other good-quality extra-virgin olive oil, for drizzling

½ teaspoon unrefined sea salt

1 teaspoon paprika

DIRECTIONS

1 Preheat the broiler to 500 degrees Fahrenheit. Cover a baking sheet with aluminum foil.

2 Place the eggplants on the baking sheet and prick the eggplant in various places (as you would a baked potato). Place the baking sheet in the oven on the highest rack, closest to the broiler, but without touching it. Broil for a few minutes on each side, watching carefully, until the eggplants are completely charred (like roasted red peppers) in several places. This could take anywhere from 5 to 15 minutes, depending on how close the eggplants are to the broiler. Be sure to watch them carefully and use potholders and large tongs to turn them. The eggplants are done when they're so soft that they shrivel and collapse when held up by tongs. When done, remove from the oven and set the eggplants in a colander over a bowl.

3 As soon as they're cool enough to touch, cut off the tops and remove the skins. Allow the eggplants to drain until all the liquid comes out of them.

4 Take the eggplant pulp out of the colander and transfer it to a large bowl. Mash the pulp with the back of a fork or by squeezing it in your hands until it becomes a mashed consistency.

5 Add the tahini sauce, olive oil, lemon juice, and garlic; stir vigorously to combine. Taste and season with salt and pepper, if needed. Cover and store in the refrigerator until needed.

(continued)

(continued)

To make the chickpeas:

1 Preheat the oven to 425 degrees Fahrenheit. Spread the chickpeas on a kitchen towel and pat them dry. Remove any loose skins.

2 Transfer the chickpeas to the baking sheet and toss them with a drizzle of olive oil and salt.

3 Roast the chickpeas for 20 to 30 minutes, or until golden brown and crisp. Remove from the oven and, while the chickpeas are still warm, toss with salt and paprika.

4 Store the roasted chickpeas in a loosely-covered container at room temperature.

To serve:

1 Spoon the baba ghanouj onto a large platter, make a well in the center, and drizzle with olive oil to taste.

2 Scatter the roasted chickpeas on top. Serve with broccoli, carrots, and peppers, or other crudités.

PER SERVING: *Calories 275 (From Fat 84); Fat 9g (Saturated 1g); Cholesterol 0mg; Sodium 441mg; Carbohydrate 43g (Dietary Fiber 15g); Protein 10g.*

TIP: If you're grilling, you can roast the eggplants on the grill in advance.

NOTE: Both the baba ghanouj and the roasted chickpeas can be made one day in advance.

VARY IT! Baba ghanouj is a classic recipe, so Chef Amy doesn't recommend changing it too much. However, if you want an eggplant dip without the tahini sauce, you could add Greek yogurt and pomegranate seeds for a delicious variation.

Delicious Dinners

Adding more vegetables to your diet, even going vegetarian now and then, is the key to healthy eating. In many cultures in the world where people enjoy the best health, meals are planned around fresh produce, not protein. The breakfast, lunch, and dinner meals in this chapter are full of rainbow-colored fruits and vegetables to help you get the 9 to 12 servings of produce your body needs daily with ease. Vegetables help fill you up, they are packed with healthy nutrients and bioactive compounds like polyphenols, they give you important fiber, they add a boost of color to your plate, and most have a very low glycemic index, especially when combined with ingredients like extra-virgin olive oil.

Some of these recipes are vegetarian, but you could add bits of meat, chicken, fish, or eggs to them if desired. And remember, when it comes to nonstarchy veggies, you can usually add more to your meal without increasing your blood glucose level or your weight. When in doubt, an extra side salad of green leafy vegetables is a great way to get more nutritional bang out of your meals.

TIP

If you live alone, portion these meals out to enjoy them for lunch or dinner the following day. If you have a family, you may want to double or triple the meal quantities so that you can enjoy the leftovers at other times. Keep in mind that the lunch recipes also work well for dinner.

Citrus–Marinated Salmon with Fiery Potatoes and Kale

PREP TIME: 15 MINUTES	COOK TIME: 45 MINUTES PLUS 1 HOUR MARINADE	YIELD: 4 SERVINGS

INGREDIENTS

6 tablespoons Amy Riolo Selections or other good-quality extra-virgin olive oil

¼ cup orange juice

½ teaspoon unrefined sea salt, plus extra

Freshly ground black pepper

4 (4-ounce) salmon fillets, skin on

4 medium Yukon gold potatoes, chopped into bite-size pieces

4 cloves garlic, finely chopped

Crushed red chili pepper

Unrefined sea salt, to taste

Freshly ground black pepper, to taste

½ pound fresh kale, rinsed with stems and tough ribs discarded, then roughly chopped

1 sweet onion, thinly sliced

1 cup plain Greek yogurt

2 oranges, 1 zested, 1 thinly sliced

DIRECTIONS

1 In a small bowl, whisk 2 tablespoons of olive oil, orange juice, salt, and pepper together until emulsified.

2 Place the salmon fillets in a glass baking dish and pour marinade over the top. Allow to marinate for 1 hour.

3 In the meantime prepare the potatoes. Preheat the oven to 400 degrees Fahrenheit.

4 Place the potatoes on a baking sheet and toss with 2 table-spoons of olive oil, garlic, crushed red chili pepper, salt, and pepper. Bake for 15 to 20 minutes, or until golden and soft.

5 In a large bowl, toss the kale with the remaining 2 tablespoons of olive oil and salt and pepper to taste. When the potatoes have roasted, remove from the oven and scatter the kale on top. Return to the oven and roast for another 10 minutes, or until kale is crisp. Serve hot.

6 Scatter the onion slices around the salmon and cover the baking dish with aluminum foil. Bake until the fish flakes easily with a fork and is opaque in color, 20 to 30 minutes.

7 While the fish is baking, combine the Greek yogurt with the orange zest. Remove the fish from the oven and place on a serving plate. Dollop with about ¼ cup of yogurt mixture and garnish with orange slices.

8 Serve potatoes and kale on the side.

PER SERVING: Calories 559 (From Fat 214); Fat 24g (Saturated 5g); Cholesterol 69mg; Sodium 198mg; Carbohydrate 51g (Dietary Fiber 6g); Protein 36 g.

Red Lentil Croquettes over Baby Spinach with Tzatziki Sauce

PREP TIME: 15 MINUTES	COOK TIME: 30 MINUTES	YIELD: 4 SERVINGS (2 CROQUETTES EACH)

INGREDIENTS

1½ cups plain organic full-fat yogurt

1 English cucumber, peeled and diced

¼ teaspoon unrefined sea salt, plus more to taste

2 tablespoons fresh dill or mint, chopped

1 clove garlic, minced

1 small yellow onion, grated and drained

For the lentil croquettes:

1 cup dried red lentils, rinsed

2 cups vegetable or chicken stock (see recipe at the end of this chapter) or water

1 tablespoon tomato paste

5 garlic cloves, finely chopped

¼ teaspoon unrefined sea salt

Freshly ground black pepper, to taste

4 tablespoons Amy Riolo Selections or other good-quality extra-virgin olive oil

16 ounces fresh spinach, cleaned and dried

DIRECTIONS

To make the tzatziki sauce:

1 Place the yogurt in a medium bowl.

2 Place the cucumbers in a colander and sprinkle with salt. Let stand for 20 minutes. Rinse off the salt and add the cucumbers to the yogurt.

3 Stir in the dill. Add the garlic and onion, and season with salt to taste.

4 Serve immediately to prevent the salad from becoming runny. If storing, place in an airtight container in the refrigerator and drain off excess liquid before serving.

To make the lentil croquettes:

1 Place the lentils, stock, tomato paste, garlic cloves, salt, pepper, and 1 tablespoon of olive oil in a medium saucepan.

2 Bring to a boil over high heat, reduce heat to medium, and simmer, stirring occasionally, for 5 minutes, or until lentils are cooked and the mixture resembles a puree.

3 Remove from heat and allow to cool.

4 Heat 1 tablespoon of olive oil in large, wide skillet and add the spinach. Stir to coat and cook over medium heat for 2 to 3 minutes, or until the spinach is wilted. Season with salt and pepper to taste.

(continued)

(continued)

5 Arrange the spinach on a serving platter. Drain any liquid from the skillet and set aside.

6 When the lentil mixture is cool enough to handle, use a ¼-cup measure or an ice cream scoop to form balls of the mixture.

7 Using two spoons or your fingers, shape the mixture into oval (football) shapes.

8 Once cool enough to handle, dry the skillet that was used to cook the spinach with paper towels.

9 Heat the remaining 2 tablespoons of olive oil in the skillet over medium-high heat. Using two spoons, lower the lentil croquettes into the hot oil. Allow to cook 2 to 3 minutes per side, turning until each side is golden.

10 Arrange the lentil croquettes in an attractive pattern on top of the spinach. Serve with the tzatziki sauce.

PER SERVING: *Calories 433 (From Fat 170); Fat 19g (Saturated 4g); Cholesterol 12mg; Sodium 418mg; Carbohydrate 49g (Dietary Fiber 9g); Protein 22 g.*

TIP: Make extra tzatziki sauce to enjoy with crudités or whole wheat pita bread as a snack.

NOTE: When made into larger patties, the lentil croquettes make great natural veggie burgers. You can serve them in buns, in a lettuce wrap, or in large Portobello mushroom caps.

VARY IT! If you want to alter the recipe, use brown lentils, cannellini beans, or chickpeas instead of lentils. Note that these ingredients take longer to cook than red lentils (see the recipes at the end of this chapter), but if you have them already on hand, they are a simple variation.

Chicken Simmered in Tomatoes, Olives, and Capers with Sautéed Dandelion Greens and Salad

PREP TIME: 15 MINUTES	COOK TIME: 45 MINUTES	YIELD: 4 SERVINGS

INGREDIENTS

6 tablespoons Amy Riolo Selections or other good-quality extra-virgin olive oil

3 pounds chicken thighs and legs with skin and bones

1 medium onion, diced

2 cups fresh diced tomatoes

½ teaspoon freshly ground black pepper, plus more to taste

¼ cup capers, rinsed well to remove salt, and drained

1 cup homemade chicken stock (see recipe at the end of this chapter) or water

1 cup Kalamata or your favorite olives, pitted and rinsed

2 bunches fresh dandelion greens, roughly chopped

4 cups mixed field greens

Juice of 1 lemon

DIRECTIONS

1 In a large skillet, warm 2 tablespoons of olive oil over medium-high heat.

2 Add the chicken pieces and sauté until golden brown in color, about 3 minutes per side. Remove from the pan and set aside.

3 To the same skillet, add the onions, tomatoes, pepper, and capers. Stir and sauté until the onions are tender, about 10 minutes.

4 Return the chicken to the skillet and add just enough stock to cover. Add the olives. Stir and lower the heat to medium-low. Cover and simmer until the chicken is cooked through and registers 165 degrees Fahrenheit on a meat thermometer, about 45 minutes.

5 While the chicken is simmering, prepare the dandelion greens. In a large, wide skillet, heat 2 tablespoons of olive oil over medium heat. Add the dandelion greens and stir to coat. Season with salt and pepper to taste and cook for 3 to 4 minutes, stirring occasionally, until wilted.

6 Spoon the dandelion greens onto a large serving platter.

7 Make the salad by placing the mixed greens in a large bowl. Drizzle the remaining 2 tablespoons of olive oil, lemon juice, and a pinch of pepper over the top. Using tongs, toss to combine.

8 When the chicken has finished cooking, arrange on top of the greens and serve.

PER SERVING: *Calories 509 (From Fat 346); Fat 38g (Saturated 8g); Cholesterol 83mg; Sodium 708mg; Carbohydrate 21g (Dietary Fiber 7g); Protein 23g.*

Turkish-Style Eggplant and Chickpea Stew with Brown Basmati Rice Pilaf

PREP TIME: 10 MINUTES	COOK TIME: 50 MINUTES	YIELD: 4 SERVINGS

INGREDIENTS

4 tablespoons Amy Riolo Selections or other good-quality extra-virgin olive oil

2 medium yellow onions, 1 diced and 1 sliced

3 garlic cloves, minced

1 pound eggplant, cubed

2 cups cooked chickpeas (see recipe at the end of this chapter)

1 teaspoon ground cumin

1 teaspoon ground cinnamon

1 teaspoon ground coriander

1 (28-ounce) can reduced-sodium diced or chopped tomatoes

½ teaspoon unrefined sea salt

¼ teaspoon freshly ground black pepper

1 cup brown basmati rice, soaked in water for 20 minutes or more

¼ cup freshly chopped cilantro

1 pound fresh collard greens, or kale, washed, dried, and chopped

2 red bell peppers, diced

1 small red chili pepper or ¼ teaspoon chili paste

DIRECTIONS

1 Heat 2 teaspoons of olive oil in a large saucepan over medium heat.

2 Add the onions and garlic and cook until the onions are soft.

3 Stir in the eggplant, chickpeas, cumin, cinnamon, coriander, tomatoes, salt, and pepper.

4 Increase the heat to high and bring to a boil. Reduce the heat to low and cover.

5 Cook the stew for 45 minutes, or until the eggplant is very tender.

6 In the meantime, drain the basmati rice and stir in the cilantro. Add 1 tablespoon of olive oil to a medium saucepan with a fitted lid and heat over medium heat.

7 Add the basmati rice and stir well to coat. Add ¼ teaspoon salt, stir, and cover with 1½ cups water. Bring to a boil over high heat. Reduce heat to low, stir, and place a paper towel over the top of the saucepan. Place the lid on top of the paper towel, being sure to cover the saucepan tightly (this ensures the rice doesn't become mushy). Simmer on low for 10 minutes, or until the liquid is evaporated.

8 Heat the remaining 1 tablespoon of olive oil in a large, wide skillet over medium-high heat.

9 Add the collards, bell peppers, chili pepper or chili paste, and a pinch of salt. Sauté until the greens and pepper are tender, 8 to 10 minutes.

10 When rice is done, add the collard green mixture and toss to coat. Serve pilaf and stew together, warm.

PER SERVING: *Calories 614 (From Fat 167); Fat 19g (Saturated 3g); Cholesterol 0mg; Sodium 330mg; Carbohydrate 100g (Dietary Fiber 19g); Protein 19g.*

Fresh Herb and Parmigiano Crusted Fish with Apple, Beet, and Carrot Salad with Citrus Vinaigrette

PREP TIME: 15 MINUTES	COOK TIME: 10 MINUTES	YIELD: 4 SNGS

INGREDIENTS

½ cup whole cornmeal or polenta

1 tablespoon Parmigiano-Reggiano cheese

¼ cup mixed fresh herbs (fresh parsley and basil work well), finely chopped

Juice of 2 lemons

4 (4-ounce) tilapia or other tender white fish fillets

4 tablespoons Amy Riolo Selections or other good-quality extra-virgin olive oil

¼ cup orange juice

Freshly ground black pepper, to taste

2 large red beets, peeled and quartered

2 carrots, peeled and quartered

2 apples, peeled, cored, and quartered

DIRECTIONS

1 Combine cornmeal, Parmigiano, and herbs on a large shallow dish.

2 Place lemon juice in a wide, shallow bowl.

3 Dip the tilapia fillets in the lemon juice to coat. Dredge them in the cornmeal mixture and turn to coat on all sides. Place on a platter and set aside.

4 In a small bowl, whisk 2 tablespoons of olive oil, orange juice, and pepper together until emulsified and set aside.

5 Heat the remaining 2 tablespoons of olive oil in a large, wide skillet over medium-high heat. Add the tilapia fillets and cook for 4 to 5 minutes per side and cooked through. (Fish is finished cooking when it flakes easily with a fork and is opaque in color.)

6 While the fish is sautéing, place the beet, carrots, and apple in a food processor with the shredder attachment (or use a box grater) and pulse until shredded. The end result should look like tiny coleslaw-like pieces of vegetables.

7 Toss the vegetables with the reserved dressing.

8 To serve, place tilapia on plates with the salad mixture spooned over the top, or on the side, if desired.

PER SERVING: Calories 436 (From Fat 150); Fat 17g (Saturated 3g); Cholesterol 58mg; Sodium 337mg; Carbohydrate 47g (Dietary Fiber 6g); Protein 27g.

Pasta with Pistachio Pesto, Fresh Tuna, and Yellow Tomato Sauce

PREP TIME: 15 MINUTES	COOK TIME: 10 MINUTES	YIELD: 4 SERVINGS

INGREDIENTS

3 tablespoons Amy Riolo Selections or other good-quality extra-virgin olive oil

1 cup yellow grape tomatoes

1 teaspoon capers

1 clove garlic

1 handful fresh parsley, rinsed and dried

¼ cup plain pistachios, shelled

4 fresh (3-ounce) tuna fillets, cut into 1-inch chunks

1 handful fresh basil, rinsed, dried, and finely chopped (reserve a few leaves for garnish)

½ cup dry white wine

½ teaspoon unrefined sea salt, to taste

¼ teaspoon freshly ground black peppers, to taste

½ pound whole wheat pasta (paccheri, ziti, or penne work best)

DIRECTIONS

1 Place 2 tablespoons of olive oil, ½ cup grape tomatoes, capers, garlic, parsley, and pistachios in a food processor and process until smooth. Set aside.

2 Heat 1 tablespoon of olive oil in a large, wide skillet over medium-high heat. Add the tuna chunks and turn to brown on all sides. Add the remaining tomatoes and basil, and stir to combine.

3 Add the wine to the pan, increase the heat, and cook until most of wine is absorbed, about 5 minutes.

4 Season with salt and pepper, and stir mixture to combine. When tuna is cooked through and flaky, remove from heat and cover with a lid.

5 Prepare the pasta according to package directions until al dente, reserving ¼ cup of the pasta water.

6 Drain the pasta, and immediately stir in the reserved pesto from Step 1.

7 Toss the pesto-coated pasta into tomato and tuna sauce, tossing well to coat. Serve hot, garnished with additional basil, if desired.

PER SERVING: *Calories 682 (From Fat 177); Fat 20g (Saturated 3g); Cholesterol 38mg; Sodium 324mg; Carbohydrate 90g (Dietary Fiber 1g); Protein 39g.*

TIP: You can omit the pesto sauce and serve the pasta with the tuna and tomato sauce if you'd prefer.

VARY IT! You could skip right to Step 2 and prepare the tuna (or your favorite fish) in the same way. Instead of pasta you could serve it with another grain or greens and a salad, if desired.

Sizzling Rosemary Shrimp over Cannellini Bean Puree and Sautéed Greens with Mixed Peppers

PREP TIME: 10 MINUTES	COOK TIME: 10 MINUTES	YIELD: 4 SERVINGS

INGREDIENTS

2 cups cooked cannellini beans (see recipe at the end of this chapter)

4 tablespoons Amy Riolo Selections or other good-quality extra-virgin olive oil

Juice and zest of 2 lemons

½ teaspoon unrefined sea salt

½ teaspoon freshly ground black pepper

4 cloves garlic, minced

1½ pounds jumbo shrimp, peeled and deveined

2 teaspoons freshly chopped rosemary

Dash of crushed red chili flakes

3 bell peppers (red, green, orange, or yellow), cut into 1-inch pieces

4 cups baby kale or spinach

DIRECTIONS

1 Combine the cannellini beans, 1 tablespoon of olive oil, ½ of the lemon juice and zest, ¼ teaspoon salt, and ¼ teaspoon pepper in a food processor. Process until smooth, about 3 minutes. Add an ice cube or a bit of water, if needed.

2 Heat 2 tablespoons of olive oil in a large skillet over medium-high heat. Add ½ of the garlic and stir. Add the shrimp, rosemary, chili flakes, and the remaining salt and pepper.

3 Cook, uncovered, for about 2 minutes per side, or until shrimp turn pink.

4 Heat the remaining tablespoon of olive oil in a large, wide skillet over medium-high heat. Add bell peppers and stir to coat. Cook for 3 to 4 minutes, or until they start to soften. Stir in the kale or spinach and stir to combine. Cook until the greens are wilted. Stir in the remaining lemon juice and season with salt or pepper, as needed.

5 Spoon the cannellini puree onto a serving platter evenly, and flatten with the back of a spoon.

6 Spoon the greens and pepper mixture over the top. Place shrimp on the top of the plate and serve.

PER SERVING: *Calories 471 (From Fat 158); Fat 18g (Saturated 3g); Cholesterol 259mg; Sodium 520mg; Carbohydrate 34g (Dietary Fiber 10g); Protein 45g.*

TIP: Make extra cannellini bean puree to serve as a dip or in a wrap on another day.

NOTE: Shrimp cooked this way also make great, last-minute toppings for salads or protein plates.

VARY IT! Use fish or scallops in place of the shrimp and/or use chickpeas or lentils instead of cannellini beans.

Assorted Seafood Tartines with Microgreen, Red Cabbage, Carrot, and Corn Slaw

PREP TIME: 15 MINUTES	COOK TIME: 5 MINUTES	YIELD: 4 SERVINGS

INGREDIENTS

5 tablespoons Amy Riolo Selections or other good-quality extra-virgin olive oil

1 teaspoon honey mustard or Dijon mustard

Juice of 1 orange

2 tablespoons Amy Riolo Selections white balsamic (or your favorite) vinegar

2 cups microgreens, or your favorite green leafy vegetable, shredded

2 cups shredded red cabbage

1 cup shredded carrots

½ cup corn kernels

½ pound shrimp, peeled and deveined

Juice and zest of 1 lemon

4 (½-inch) slices country wheat French bread (boule, harvest)

4 teaspoons Boursin cheese, room temperature

8 ounces smoked salmon (or leftover flaked fresh fish)

¾ pound English or Persian cucumbers, thinly sliced

DIRECTIONS

1 In a small bowl, whisk together 3 tablespoons of olive oil, mustard, orange juice, and balsamic vinegar until emulsified.

2 Place microgreens, cabbage, carrots, and corn into a large bowl. Drizzle dressing over the top and toss to coat. Set aside.

3 Heat 1 tablespoon of olive oil in a large skillet over medium-high heat.

4 When olive oil begins to release its aroma, add shrimp and lemon zest.

5 Cook for 2 to 3 minutes per side, or until shrimp are bright pink and cooked through. Squeeze lemon juice over the shrimp.

6 Place bread slices on a work surface and slather 1 teaspoon Boursin on each slice.

7 Place smoked salmon on top.

8 Place a thin layer of cucumber slices on top of each bread slice, reserving extra if necessary.

9 Place shrimp on top of the cucumbers and drizzle with the remaining tablespoon of olive oil.

10 Serve one tartine on each plate with ¼ of the slaw.

PER SERVING: *Calories 393 (From Fat 177); Fat 20g (Saturated 4g); Cholesterol 105mg; Sodium 712mg; Carbohydrate 28g (Dietary Fiber 4g); Protein 27g.*

Asparagus, Red Pepper, and Tempeh Stir-Fry with Soba Noodles and Sesame Seeds

PREP TIME: 15 MINUTES	COOK TIME: 15 MINUTES	YIELD: 4 SERVINGS

INGREDIENTS

2 tablespoons sesame oil

1 bunch fresh asparagus, trimmed, and cut into 3-inch pieces

2 red peppers, sliced thinly

2 (8-ounce) packages tempeh, cut into 2-inch cubes

3 cloves garlic, minced

1½ tablespoons low-sodium tamari

¼ cup raw honey

¼ cup raw sesame seeds

1 (9.5-ounce) package soba noodles

DIRECTIONS

1 Heat oil in a large, wide skillet or wok over medium-high heat.

2 Add the asparagus, peppers, and tempeh, and brown on all sides.

3 Combine garlic, tamari, honey, ½ cup water, and sesame seeds in a small bowl.

4 Pour over the vegetables and allow them to simmer 5 to 7 minutes, stirring occasionally, until everything is tender.

5 Prepare soba noodles according to package directions. Drain and toss into the vegetable mixture. Turn with tongs to coat. Serve warm.

PER SERVING: *Calories 621 (From Fat 218); Fat 24g (Saturated 4g); Cholesterol 0mg; Sodium 731mg; Carbohydrate 79g (Dietary Fiber 4g); Protein 34g.*

TIP: Tempeh and tofu are similar because they are both made from soy, except tempeh is fermented and provides more protein per serving; contains iron, potassium, and a prebiotic fiber; and is less processed.

NOTE: If you don't have tamari on hand, you can substitute 1 tablespoon of soy sauce for flavor, but keep the quantity down because it is saltier.

VARY IT! You can use pieces of chicken instead of tempeh in this recipe, if preferred. Soba noodles can be swapped out for black rice or another grain as well.

Must-Have Base Recipes

Most commercially prepared bread crumbs, canned beans and stocks, prepared tomato sauce, and salad dressings are full of preservatives, hidden ingredients, sugar or artificial sweeteners, and unnecessary amounts of sodium. Replacing store-bought ingredients with these homemade staple ingredients will improve the overall taste of your dishes and save you time and money, while cutting excess sodium, calories, and preservatives from your meals.

Whenever Chef Amy prepares these base recipes, she makes them in large quantities and stores them. In fact, every recipe in this chapter can be prepared and then frozen for later use. With your own tomato sauce, stocks, beans, lentils, and fresh bread crumbs in your freezer, you'll always be prepared to whip up healthful, inexpensive soups, pastas, salads, and purees in no time! Use extra-virgin olive oil and your favorite vinegars or citrus juice on salads instead of prepared dressings.

TIP

If for some reason you absolutely have to use packaged and processed pantry items instead of these, be sure to read the labels to get the lowest amounts of unwanted ingredients possible. Otherwise, try swapping those ingredients out for healthier options. It is better to use plain water with herbs and/or spices than have to buy a packaged stock that is full of sodium and ingredients you can't pronounce.

Dried Beans

PREP TIME: 1 HOUR | COOK TIME: 30 MINUTES | YIELD: 8 SERVINGS

INGREDIENTS

1 cup dried beans (any variety)

¼ teaspoon unrefined sea salt

DIRECTIONS

1 Place the beans in a stockpot and cover with cold water; leave to soak overnight. (If short on time, place the beans in a stockpot, cover with boiling water, and leave to soak for 1 hour.)

2 Drain the beans and place in a saucepan. Add the salt, cover with water, and bring to a boil over high heat.

3 Reduce the heat to medium-low, cover, and let cook until the beans are tender, about 25 to 50 minutes.

4 Drain and cool. If not using right away, store in an airtight container in the refrigerator for up to 1 week.

PER SERVING: Calories 40 (From Fat 0); Fat 0g (Saturated 0g); Cholesterol 0mg; Sodium 4mg; Carbohydrate 10g (Dietary Fiber 6g); Protein 4g.

Lentils

INGREDIENTS

1 cup dried lentils (any variety)

¼ teaspoon unrefined sea salt

¼ teaspoon freshly ground black pepper

1 bay leaf

DIRECTIONS

1 Rinse the lentils in a colander.

2 Place the lentils in a saucepan and add enough water to cover them twice (you should have twice as much water as lentils). Add the salt, pepper, and bay leaf. Bring to a boil over high heat. Reduce the heat to low and simmer, uncovered, until the lentils are tender, about 5 to 30 minutes depending on the variety.

3 Store cooked lentils in an airtight container in the refrigerator for up to 1 week.

PER SERVING: Calories 113 (From Fat 3); Fat 0g (Saturated 0g); Cholesterol 0mg; Sodium 3mg; Carbohydrate 19g (Dietary Fiber 10g); Protein 8g.

Homemade Vegetable Stock

PREP TIME: 5 MINUTES	COOK TIME: 30 MINUTES	YIELD: 8 SERVINGS

INGREDIENTS

1 medium onion, halved (not peeled)

1 medium carrot, trimmed and halved

1 medium stalk celery, trimmed and halved (can include leaves, if desired)

4 ounces cherry tomatoes

4 sprigs fresh basil, with stems

1 small bunch fresh flat-leaf parsley, with stems

½ teaspoon unrefined sea salt

DIRECTIONS

1 In a large stockpot, place the onion, carrot, celery, tomatoes, basil, and parsley. Cover with 16 cups water. Bring to a boil over high heat. Reduce the heat to medium–low. Add the salt and simmer, uncovered, for 30 minutes.

2 Drain the stock, reserving the liquid. Discard the rest. If you're not using it right away, allow to cool and then store in the refrigerator or freezer.

PER SERVING: *Calories 11 (From Fat 0); Fat 0g (Saturated 0g); Cholesterol 0mg; Sodium 145mg; Carbohydrate 2g (Dietary Fiber 0g); Protein 1g.*

Homemade Seafood Stock

INGREDIENTS

1 medium onion, halved (not peeled)

1 medium carrot, trimmed and halved

1 medium stalk celery, halved

Shells from 2 pounds shrimp

½ teaspoon unrefined sea salt

1 dried bay leaf

1 tablespoon whole black peppercorns

DIRECTIONS

1 In a large stockpot, place the onion, carrot, celery, and shrimp shells. Cover with 16 cups water. Bring to a boil over high heat. Reduce the heat to medium-low.

2 Skim off the residue that forms on top of the stock and discard. Add the salt, bay leaf, and peppercorns. Simmer, uncovered, for about 30 minutes.

3 Drain the stock, reserving the liquid. Discard the rest. If you're not using it right away, allow to cool and then store in the refrigerator or freezer.

PER SERVING: *Calories 39 (From Fat 7); Fat 1g (Saturated 0g); Cholesterol 0mg; Sodium 145mg; Carbohydrate 1g (Dietary Fiber 0g); Protein 5g.*

Homemade Chicken Stock

INGREDIENTS

1 medium onion, halved (not peeled)

1 medium carrot, trimmed and halved

1 medium stalk celery, halved

1¼ pounds chicken bones or carcass from cooked chicken

1 teaspoon whole black peppercorns

1 dried bay leaf

½ teaspoon unrefined sea salt

DIRECTIONS

1 In a large stock pot, place the onion, carrot, celery, chicken bones, peppercorns, and bay leaf. Cover with 16 cups water. Bring to a boil over high heat. Reduce the heat to medium-low.

2 Skim off the residue that forms on top of the stock and discard. Add the salt and simmer, uncovered, for 40 minutes.

3 Drain the stock, reserving the liquid. Discard the rest. If you're not using it right away, allow to cool and then store in the refrigerator or freezer.

PER SERVING: *Calories 39 (From Fat 11); Fat 1g (Saturated 0g); Cholesterol 0mg; Sodium 145mg; Carbohydrate 1g (Dietary Fiber 0g); Protein 5g.*

Fresh Bread Crumbs

INGREDIENTS

1 (8-ounce) loaf dense, day-old country-style bread

DIRECTIONS

1 Cut the bread into 1-inch cubes and, working in batches, place them in a food processor, being careful not to fill it more than halfway. Pulse on and off until the crumbs are as fine as possible.

2 If not using immediately, freeze bread crumbs in a plastic freezer bag for up to 1 month.

PER SERVING: *Calories 41 (From Fat 2); Fat 0g (Saturated 0g); Cholesterol 0mg; Sodium 92mg; Carbohydrate 8g (Dietary Fiber 0g); Protein 2g.*

Fresh Tomato Sauce

INGREDIENTS

2 tablespoons Amy Riolo Selections or other good-quality extra-virgin olive oil

2 large garlic cloves, peeled and minced

1½ pounds strained (seeded and skinned tomatoes) boxed or jarred tomatoes, such as Pomi brand, or 2½ pounds fresh, ripe tomatoes (if in season) (see Tip for instructions)

Unrefined sea salt, to taste

Freshly ground black pepper, to taste

4–5 leaves of fresh basil, oregano, or parsley

Parmigiano-Reggiano or Pecorino Romano cheese, freshly grated, for garnish

DIRECTIONS

1 Heat olive oil in a medium saucepan over medium heat. Add garlic, and reduce heat to low.

2 When garlic begins to release its aroma (before it turns color), add tomatoes.

3 Stir and allow mixture to come to a boil to create caramelization on the side of the pan.

4 Add salt, pepper, and fresh herbs; stir and cover. Reduce heat to low, and simmer for 10 to 20 minutes, or until it has thickened slightly. Taste and adjust seasonings. Serve with grated cheese.

PER SERVING: *Calories 74 (From Fat 44); Fat 5g (Saturated 1g); Cholesterol 0mg; Sodium 10mg; Carbohydrate 7g (Dietary Fiber 2g); Protein 2g.*

TIP: If you are using fresh tomatoes, place them in boiling water until their skins peel (just a few minutes), strain, and allow them to cool to the touch. Peel, remove the seeds, and cut into chunks. Use in place of boxed or jarred tomatoes in Step 2 above.

Most Italians make large batches of this sauce so that they can have one recipe on hand at all times in the refrigerator and a spare or two in the freezer. This sauce keeps in the refrigerator for up to 1 week or in the freezer for a few months.

NOTE: If you are serving this sauce with pasta as a first course, the second course should not contain tomatoes. Simple grilled or pan-fried chicken, veal, beef, or seafood are natural accompaniments. This simple sauce is the base for Italian tomato soups. In addition to pasta, you can use it to top pizza, eggplant parmigiana, and keep a little extra on hand to dip meatballs and croquettes into.

VARY IT! If using fresh tomatoes, try experimenting with different varieties including heirlooms. You may be surprised how much the recipe changes with each new type. Stir leftover beans and vegetables into this sauce and toss with pasta for a quick weekday meal.

6

The Part of Tens

IN THIS PART . . .

Discover ten diabetes "power foods," including dairy, nuts, beans, and even dark chocolate.

Check out ten diabetes-friendly ways to save while shopping.

Find out how swapping out one of your favorite foods for another can keep you on track and lower your calorie intake.

Discover little changes that are simple and easy and can become new habits that eventually happen without thinking.

IN THIS CHAPTER

» **Getting extra benefits from extra-virgin olive oil**

» **Fueling up with omega-3 fatty acids**

» **Keeping leafy greens on the plate**

» **Enjoying dark chocolate**

» **Settling the score about soy**

Chapter **19**

Ten Diabetes "Power Foods"

E verybody understands that some foods are better than others. If you made your list of best foods, however, chances are that subjective measures — taste, texture, and your emotional attachment to particular foods — would be your main focus. That's how most people think of food. However, nutritional value isn't subjective, and certain foods help people with diabetes more than others. Why not plan your daily meals around them to get the maximum benefits from the food you consume?

The ten foods we highlight in this chapter can provide amazing benefits to your health; however, they are just a small sampling of the powerful, delicious, and healing foods that can help you look and feel your best. Berries, seafood, spices such as ginger and cinnamon, seeds, and countless varieties of vegetables and fruits can also be very beneficial and are highlighted throughout the book.

Extra-Virgin Olive Oil

Extra-virgin olive oil is our single favorite ingredient. In fact, Simon published an entire book called *The Olive Oil Diet* (Robinson), and Amy dedicates a significant amount of each of her books to the topic and markets her own brand of high-quality privately labeled extra-virgin olive oil. We even met giving a lecture about the health benefits of extra-virgin olive oil for those with diabetes years ago in New York.

Because olives and olive oil are a common denominator in the countries surrounding the Mediterranean, they are often the ingredients that are analyzed in Mediterranean diet–based research. Antioxidants such as vitamin E, carotenoids, and phenols such as hydroxytyrosol and oleuropein (known for their anti-inflammatory and antibacterial effects) are found in olive oil.

ASK THE DOCTOR

Antioxidants are important in the prevention of aging. *Oxidation* refers to the complex manner in which cells age. Cells in those following olive oil–rich diets have been proven to be stronger and more resistant to oxidation, and therefore age more slowly. Extra-virgin olive oil (olive oil that has not been refined or industrially treated) is particularly rich in antioxidants, which protects against damage from free radicals and against the formation of cancer.

Consuming high-quality extra-virgin olive oil on a regular basis can help prevent heart disease, lower cholesterol, improve rheumatoid arthritis, and reduce the risk of developing Alzheimer's disease, diabetes, and various types of cancer. Further, various studies have shown that olive oil or an olive oil–rich diet can protect against malignant tumors; reduces the risk of breast, colon, and bowel cancer and the incidence of melanoma; prevents the formation of blood clots; lowers the levels of total blood cholesterol (believed to be responsible for the low incidence of heart problems in countries where olive oil is the main cooking fat); boosts the immune system against the negative effects of toxins, microorganisms, parasites, and other foreign substances; can improve calcium absorption in the body and prevent osteoporosis; may prevent memory loss in healthy elderly people; and may lead to less risk of developing rheumatoid arthritis.

TIP

Best of all, adding extra-virgin olive oil to carbohydrates has the remarkable effect of slowing their absorption as well as increasing insulin sensitivity. It also leaves your appetite more satiated sooner and your gut microbes happier. This combination results in a reduced glycemic load of a meal.

Beans

Beans and legumes are the most underappreciated superfood in Western cultures. Beans are good for your heart by providing both soluble and insoluble fiber, as well as folate, magnesium, and potassium. That makes beans a cholesterol-reducing, blood-pressure-lowering, and gas-producing powerhouse. But, beans also improve blood glucose control, having a low glycemic index due to the fiber and protein content.

Speaking of protein, beans are an invaluable source for vegetarians and the best dollar value on protein for anyone. One-half cup of beans has as much protein as an ounce of meat. Ultimately, these complex legumes are starchy vegetables, so don't forget that your daily ½-cup serving is a 15-gram carbohydrate portion after you deduct half of the fiber from total carbohydrate. Black beans, cannellini, kidney, chickpeas, and lentils are all great options.

TIP

If you are new to legumes, begin slowly so that your body can adapt and synthesize the enzymes you need. If beans give you gas, try taking some Beano.

Salmon and Tuna

Salmon and tuna are fatty fish that are readily available fresh, frozen, or canned. Both are excellent sources of complete protein, some of the best sources of dietary vitamin D, excellent sources of niacin (vitamin B3), and good sources of selenium, vitamin B6, and omega-3 fatty acids. Wild salmon offers some nutritional benefits over farmed salmon, like less saturated fat, but salmon is a power food either way.

TIP

Be sure to check with your supermarket or fishmonger for the most sustainable types of fish possible. In the United States, an app produced by the Monterey Bay Aquarium (www.seafoodwatch.org) is continuously monitored and updated so that you can look up any type of fish and immediately find out whether it is a sustainable choice.

Omega-3 fatty acids may be specifically important in reducing the chronic state of inflammation that's associated with insulin resistance. Research from the University of California at San Diego Medical School identified how omega-3 fatty acids can activate a receptor associated with immune responses, and commonly associated with fat tissue, to reduce inflammation and insulin resistance in obese mice.

Salmon and tuna are great grilled, broiled, on salads, or packed into patties. The bones in canned salmon add to its calcium content, and both salmon and tuna can be an essential source of vitamin B12 and protein for pescatarians.

Nuts

Nuts come in an amazing variety of tastes — walnuts, almonds, pecans, cashews, Brazil nuts, hazelnuts, macadamia nuts, and even peanuts (which are actually legumes). Nuts are a good source of B vitamins, vitamin E, fiber, iron, protein, magnesium, and zinc, and are a great source of mono- and polyunsaturated fats. Nuts are also low in carbohydrate, making them a great snack food for people with diabetes who aren't snacking to raise blood glucose levels.

Peanuts, almonds, and walnuts are all associated in studies with improved insulin sensitivity, and improvements in A1C among people with diabetes. Nuts have been shown to improve cholesterol levels as well, and without weight gain; walnuts even provide valuable omega-3 fatty acids.

TIP

Watch for added salt or sugar in packaged nuts, but otherwise nuts make great snacks, a tasty addition to salads or yogurt, an interesting crusting for fish, and, of course, the marvelous nut butters. Try an ounce of your favorite nut, or a tablespoon of nut butter, the next time you're tempted to reach for a snack.

Oranges and Lemons

Oranges are a great source of the cholesterol-reducing soluble fiber called *pectin*, as well as folate and potassium. Oranges also contain the antioxidant *hesperidin*, which can help prevent damage to cells. And face it, sometimes it's great to have something really sweet, and it's hard to top an orange when it comes to sweet. A medium-sized orange is one 15-gram carbohydrate choice, making one orange or ½ cup of orange juice an effective treatment for moderate hypoglycemia.

TIP

If you want the full bang for your nutrition buck, however, go for the orange instead of the juice. You get more fiber and a better dose of antioxidants. Try eating them as a snack in-between meals with a handful of unsalted, unroasted almonds or tossing orange segments into a salad of spinach and avocado in lieu of tomatoes for a change. Freshly squeezed orange and lemon juice with good-quality extra-virgin olive oil should be your antioxidant-rich dressing of choice for salads and for drizzling over foods that need extra flavor.

Lemons are a great source of vitamin C, and like vinegars, their acidity decreases the glycemic load when combined with carbohydrates in a meal. Adding a squeeze of lemon juice to water is a wonderful way of staying hydrated while balancing the body's PH levels. It's also a wonderful detoxifier and has antimicrobial properties.

Kale (and Other Leafy Greens)

Kale is a fabulous representative of a star group of nonstarchy vegetables, belonging to the same species of plants as cabbage, broccoli, cauliflower, collards, Swiss chard, kohlrabi, and Brussels sprouts. Try to incorporate at least one serving of each of these nutritional power houses with each meal.

From a nutrition standpoint, kale is rich in vitamin A, vitamin B6, vitamin C, vitamin K, folate, calcium, magnesium, fiber, and powerful flavonoids and antioxidants. Kale also contains substances known as bile acid sequestrants, which reduce cholesterol levels and limit the absorption of dietary fat. Kale is great steamed, added to salad, or even sprayed lightly with oil and baked until a crispy chip.

WARNING

Kale contains oxalates, which can interfere with calcium absorption, and can be an issue for people prone to kidney stones.

Kale may be the superstar, but leafy greens are an important part of a healthy diet. Even iceberg lettuce, nearly absent in nutritional value, can help fill you up, and Popeye's affinity for spinach was on target. Chef Amy also snatches up fresh dandelion greens whenever they are available. Similar to kale in flavor and high in fiber, dandelion greens provide 535 percent of the recommended daily value of vitamin K, which may be the most important source of any other plant-based food to strengthen bones, and may also play a role in fighting Alzheimer's disease by limiting neuron damage in the brain.

Dark Chocolate

British researchers looked at the chocolate eating habits of more than 100,000 people from seven previous studies and divided them into groups ranging from never to more than once a day. The analysis produced consistent results, that those who ate the most chocolate had a 37 percent reduced risk of heart disease, a reduced risk of stroke, and a reduced risk of diabetes when compared to subjects who ate the least chocolate.

For the most part this analysis adds to evidence that chocolate, especially dark (more than 60 percent cocoa) chocolate, has benefits related to cardiometabolic health. These benefits are likely related to polyphenols present in cocoa and the beneficial effects on blood pressure, insulin resistance, and blood lipids of these compounds.

So, can chocolate fit into your diabetes management practices? Of course! In an effective diabetes management lifestyle, mindfulness and moderation are keys to good health. But, don't forget that mindfulness and moderation should be keys for everyone else too — this isn't punishment, it's being responsible. A square or two of dark chocolate is a great addition to your day and can help to keep cravings for less beneficial sweet treats at bay. For ethical reasons, we recommend purchasing from bean-to-bar purveyors or Fair Trade Certified chocolate whenever possible.

Soybeans

The soybean is a remarkable little fellow. It's relatively close to one-third each of protein, fat, and carbohydrate. Also, it's the only source of plant protein that is *complete*, which means it provides all the amino acids humans can't make internally, and soy protein is highly digestible, too. The fat content of soybeans is 88 percent healthy monounsaturated or polyunsaturated fatty acids, and the soybean even includes omega-3 fatty acids. And whole soybeans, as opposed to soy processed into tofu, have 16 grams carbohydrate per cup, but also 8 grams of fiber. The combination of protein, fat, and fiber gives soybeans a very low glycemic index value, meaning its impact on blood glucose levels is very gradual.

Soy has been shown to reduce total cholesterol, reduce bad LDL cholesterol, lower blood pressure, and improve *endothelial function*, a measure of the flexibility of arteries.

Soy also contains *isoflavones*, sometimes called phytoestrogens, and certain isoflavones mimic estrogen. Because some breast cancers are fueled by estrogen, information about the safety of soy, with respect to breast cancer, has been swirling around for years, and the issue is not completely clear. Part of the confusion relates to soy supplements, which concentrate isoflavones to much higher levels than you get from soy foods. Information over the years has gone back and forth about whether soy increases or decreases the risk, and about soy in the diet of cancer patients and survivors.

In Asian populations, soy seems to be protective against breast cancer, but it's not possible to isolate soy from other potential foods or lifestyle factors. But, studies in the United States have shown there is no association between soy consumptions and the risk for breast cancer, and studies of breast cancer survivors have shown that soy reduces the rate of recurrence, especially among cancers that are not *estrogen receptor positive*. The American Cancer Society's guidelines conclude that current research finds no harmful effects to breast cancer survivors from eating soy.

You can increase your soy consumption by adding edamame (green soybeans) to your stir-fry dishes or to salad. Tofu and tempeh make great meat substitutes and are now marketed as substitute chicken or beef strips to use in stir-fry or stroganoff, or to enliven your cooking imagination. Tempeh contains the whole soy-bean, and its fiber; tofu does not.

REMEMBER

Not all soy is created equal. If you live in the United States or another area where the majority of soy cultivated is genetically modified, search out organic and non-genetically modified options. Also, soy sauce often tends to be a highly salty processed food. Choose low-sodium, organic versions such as tamari, and use sparingly when adding to recipes.

Full-Fat Greek-Style Plain Yogurt

Yogurt, especially the Greek-style plain variety that is produced around the world now, is high in protein and Vitamin B12, which is mostly found in animal products, making it a great protein choice for those who don't eat meat. The original Greek variety is made from a combination of goat and sheep milk, and those types of milks offer additional nutrient profiles. Even cow-based milk contains a healthful dose of calcium, Vitamin B2, B12, potassium, and magnesium. Yogurt with live active cultures (probiotics) is known to help maintain the natural balance of organisms, known as microflora, in the intestines. Gut health, which we discuss in Chapter 7, is essential for wellbeing in all people, but especially for those with diabetes.

TIP

Eaten at bedtime, Greek yogurt can help keep you full and your glucose balanced during your hours of fasting. Unlike most other foods, yogurt contains all three macronutrients (protein, carbohydrates, and fat) in a healthy form. Consuming the three macronutrients at each meal or snack is extremely important for those with diabetes. It is an easy no-brainer when you need good fuel fast.

Whole Grains: Oats and Barley

We may have cheated a bit by giving you a "two for one" with this last entry, but as far as healthful foods are concerned, we figure, "the more the merrier." Oats and barley are both whole grains, so they are a great start toward healthy right off the bat.

Oats

Oats are most noted for bringing a specific soluble fiber called *beta-glucans* to the rescue. Beta-glucans, technically in a class of carbohydrates called gums, are especially effective at lowering bad LDL cholesterol levels and reducing the risk for the buildup of plaque in arteries known as atherosclerosis. The effectiveness of the soluble fiber in oats in impacting cholesterol levels has earned authorization from the U.S. Food and Drug Administration to make a heart-healthy claim on the packaging.

Studies have also shown that oats help moderate after-meal blood glucose response and improve insulin sensitivity. Oats also contribute to satiety — fullness — helping to reduce appetite. Oatmeal, of course, has long been a breakfast standard, and it's hard to argue with a strategy that starts your day with this power food.

Barley

A carbohydrate can't improve diabetes, can it? Barley can! A study of people with type 2 diabetes who consumed a healthy diet that included 18 grams of soluble fiber each day from barley showed a reduction in A1C of 30 percent, from an average of 8.4 percent down to 5.9 percent.

That's an incredible result, and you can get barley by using it to make warm breakfast bowls, soups, stews, salads, or as a vegetable pilaf. Barley flour can be used to make wholesome bread as it was used prior to wheat in the ancient Mediterranean region. Remember, ⅓ cup cooked is a 15-gram carbohydrate choice.

Chapter **20**

Ten Inexpensive Diabetes-Friendly Foods

Much about managing diabetes can be costly, but food doesn't need to be one of them. There is a huge misconception that eating healthfully has to cost a lot of money, but that isn't true. A diet that's right for diabetes is a diet that's right for virtually anyone, and there are enough foods that fit the bill for blood glucose control and heart health that your budget can remain flexible, and your choices are still many.

The short version of diabetes nutrition is to eat lean protein, mostly unsaturated fats, whole grains, fruits, dairy, beans, green leafy vegetables, nuts in moderation, sweets in moderation, lots of rainbow-colored fresh vegetables, and all the while keeping sodium low. And preparing foods from scratch is the key to keeping meals affordable.

Following are a few tips to remember when shopping with an eye on the budget:

» Buy fresh, local produce.

» Buy dry goods in bulk (beans, lentils, whole grains).

>> Organic stores usually have an in-store brand that offers organic dairy and dry goods at reasonable prices.

>> Stock up on sale items — put your pantry and freezer to work! When your favorite items are on sale, be sure to stock up on them. Fresh fish and vegetables can be frozen and dry goods kept in the pantry.

See Chapter 12 for more details on shopping. Here are some great items to buy while shopping on a budget.

Beans

Beans are incredibly nutritious and among the most versatile foods you can find. And, at under $1 for four servings of dried beans, it's hard to beat the price. Beans are a carbohydrate-containing food, so you need to count the carbohydrates in your eating plan — ½ cup cooked beans is one carb choice, or 15 grams total carbohydrate, but beans also are rich in fiber, both soluble and insoluble, and work to reduce cholesterol levels. Beans are an important source of protein as well, and ¼ cup dry black beans packs only 70 calories.

Cannellini beans, chickpeas, black, kidney beans and others have similar caloric profiles with various features and benefits for our health. Best of all, beans and legumes can be applied to a wide variety of recipes and techniques. Some people may be put off cooking beans by the need to soak them before cooking, but with good meal planning, and considering freezing batches of prepared beans for later use, the need for some preparation should not deter you from enjoying these nutritional power foods. Chapter 18 offers tips on how to prepare them.

Lentils

Lentils are a legume, and therefore contain carbohydrate — a ½-cup serving of cooked lentils is 15 grams carbohydrate, one carb choice. About 30 percent of the calories from lentils, however, is from protein, making lentils one of the highest protein-containing foods among plants. Lentils also offer soluble and insoluble fiber, folate, magnesium, vitamins B1 and B3, and healthy minerals like iron. Notably, lentils have a very low glycemic index value, which means their impact on blood glucose levels is slow and steady, giving insulin time to act. This makes lentils an excellent carbohydrate for diabetes. Dry lentils cost less than $0.10 per ounce, about a nickel per serving, and have an advantage over dry beans because they don't need presoaking before cooking.

Apples

An apple a day may not keep the doctor away, but apples can play a prominent role in healthy eating for diabetes. Apples, as a fruit, are a carbohydrate food, and a medium apple, about the size of a baseball, counts as one carb choice. Apples also contain both soluble and insoluble fiber and help to control cholesterol levels, and an apple gives you only about 80 calories.

There is an incredible assortment of apple varieties, and they are grown in temperate climates all over the world. Whatever your tastes, there's an apple for you, and you should easily find crisp apples ready to take home for less than $0.50 each. In addition to making a great snack when paired with a few nuts, apples can be chopped and added to salads, yogurt, and baked for dessert, too!

Be sure to wash apple skin with a vegetable spray before eating and buy local and/ or organic apples in the United States if possible. Apples are of course a great source of vitamin C and of antioxidant polyphenols such as procyanidins, catechins, and phloridzin.

Yogurt

Yogurt is fermented milk and includes carbohydrate, healthful fat, and quality protein as macronutrients. For diabetes management, plain, full-fat yogurt is the better choice. Yogurt can be eaten plain, served with fruit, or substituted in dishes for sour cream or mayonnaise. It's an excellent source of protein and calcium, and the fermentation process may improve your absorption of calcium and B vitamins in yogurt as compared to milk.

Greek yogurt, which is strained, contains more protein than other commercially available yogurt. At the time of this writing, you can purchase plain yogurt in larger containers (not single servings) for about $0.60 per 6-ounce serving. Some yogurt also contains inulin, which helps balance blood sugar levels as well as a healthy dose of probiotics. It makes an excellent snack or light meal on the go. We recommend that people with diabetes eat it a few hours before going to bed to make sure sugar levels don't spike or lower too drastically during the evening.

WARNING

Unfortunately, many commercially available yogurts contain added sugars and other ingredients such as stabilizers to give the product a longer shelf life. Yogurt does not need to contain these additives, so we recommend looking closely at the ingredient list or even considering making your own.

Potatoes

The potato sometimes gets a bum rap in the diabetes realm because of its high carbohydrate content and its high glycemic index. About 3 ounces of white potato is 15 grams of carbohydrate. But, this starchy root vegetable is a bargain staple food, and brings its own nutritional contributions to the table, too. Potatoes are high in vitamin C, contain more potassium than any other fruit or vegetable, and are a good source of vitamin B6, which helps your body make its own amino acids.

Whole potatoes are always on sale, and a 12-ounce baking potato should go for something like $0.40 — remember, a 12-ounce potato is four carb choices. By weight, potatoes are the least-expensive vegetable.

TIP

Try topping a 3-ounce baked potato with extra-virgin olive oil, unrefined sea salt, and a tablespoon or two of plain Greek yogurt for a much more nutritious version of the restaurant classic. The addition of yogurt that contains fat decreases the glycemic rise of the carbohydrate in potato by slowing absorption and stimulating insulin secretion.

Bananas

Bananas are popular around the globe, and while you won't find many bananas produced in the United States, bananas don't have any problem finding their way here — Americans eat more than 20 pounds per person per year. Bananas cost less than $0.40 apiece, and they are a rich source of fiber, vitamins C and B6, and especially potassium, which is effective in controlling blood pressure. Bananas are a carbohydrate food, and about half of a medium banana makes one 15-carbohydrate-gram carb choice. Be sure to pair the banana with a bit of plain yogurt or some plain almonds or walnuts for a nutritious snack.

Carrots

Carrots are a colorful and healthy, nonstarchy vegetable, and like many nonstarchy vegetables, their color gives away some of the nutritional benefits — carotenes, and especially beta-carotene, the precursor to vitamin A. Their high levels of beta-carotene are what give carrots such an unblemished reputation for eye health. Carrots also contain other active compounds, antioxidants, and other carotenoids. At the current cost of $0.05 per ounce, $0.50 for a 6-ounce carrot, these roots are a nutritional bargain for certain. Carrots are great raw, and add beautiful color to salads, make a great scoop for healthy dips, or can be steamed or roasted as a side dish for any entree.

Eggs

Eggs are a marvelous source of dietary protein. In fact, the amount and balance of amino acids in eggs sets the standard for how the protein in other foods is measured — eggs are a complete source of high-quality protein, containing all of the essential amino acids. But, that's not all eggs have to offer. You also get vitamin A, vitamin D, vitamin B12, the antioxidant lutein, and choline, a nutrient essential for regulating your nervous system and cardiovascular system.

Eggs have spent time out of favor due to a relatively high content of dietary cholesterol, but recent research has shown that moderate consumption of eggs does not negatively impact blood cholesterol levels. At about $0.37 per egg currently, you get quite a deal for the highest quality protein available. Choose free-range eggs and organic if possible.

Beets

Beets are an interesting addition to a list of diabetes-friendly foods because sugar beets are the source of about 30 percent of the world's sugar, which is the disaccharide sucrose. Sugar beets provided a source of sugar that was easier to acquire in days before high-speed transportation than the sugar from cane, which grows only in tropical zones. While commercial sugar beets contain as much as 20 percent sucrose, *table beets* (also known as beetroot, garden beet, or red beet) aren't nearly as sweet. A 3-ounce table beet contains only 8 grams of carbohydrate, and is about 35 calories, even though table beets and sugar beets are the same species.

For about $0.50 per 4-ounce serving, beets are an amazing find. Fresh beets can be eaten raw by peeling and grating them and adding them to salads. The ABC salad — shredded Apples, Beets, and Carrots — is a great alternative to slaw. Roast beets in the oven as you would potatoes to add to bowls and salads as well.

Peanut Butter

At a cost of about $0.40 per ounce, your favorite childhood food can still be your favorite adult food. Peanut butter has been shown to improve blood glucose control, prevent blood glucose spikes, and lower cholesterol levels in people with type 2 diabetes. The effect on blood glucose may be related to arginine, which causes the body to release more insulin. Peanut butter is best known for its protein and healthy fat, but peanut butter also brings fiber, folate, potassium, vitamin E, thiamine, and magnesium to your table. Although not considered a carbohydrate, peanut butter does contain about 7 grams per 2-tablespoon serving.

Peanut butter contains a relatively balanced mixture of healthy polyunsaturated and monounsaturated fats, which help lower bad LDL cholesterol and blood triglycerides, and help raise good HDL cholesterol. Peanut butter also helps increase satiety (fullness), and has been incorporated into successful weight-loss strategies for this reason. Peanut butter makes an excellent snack for people with diabetes because a small amount is filling, and there is virtually no effect on blood glucose. Peanut butter — still the one.

Chapter **21**

Ten Healthful Food Swaps for Losing Weight

An elevated body mass index (BMI), where the ratio of body weight to height falls into the *overweight, obese,* or even higher category on that scale, is common among people with type 2 diabetes, and it isn't just a coincidence. Excess weight is a distinct risk factor for developing type 2 diabetes, and excess weight makes blood glucose more difficult to control after diabetes is diagnosed. Excess weight is also an independent risk factor for high blood pressure and heart disease, so the combination of excess weight and diabetes, which is also an independent risk factor for heart disease, is serious business. Excess weight results from an accumulation of excess calories stored as body fat.

Fortunately, losing only a modest amount of weight — as little as 7 to 10 percent of your current weight — can have a profound effect on insulin resistance. That's in part because visceral fat appears to be the first fat to disappear as the pounds come off. Modest weight loss can have a huge effect on the course of diabetes.

A list of ten food swaps should not be considered a weight-loss program in any sense. This simple list represents an important concept — little changes make big results. And importantly, little changes that are simple and easy can become new habits that eventually happen without thinking. These swaps are focused on changes that will have a benefit on glucose control, insulin sensitivity, and weight management. They also have anti-inflammatory benefits. It is important to choose quality of carbohydrates, fats, and proteins over quantity, and swap processed ingredients for natural ones. Finally, these swaps are very likely to be more sustainable for the planet on which we live.

Swap Bottled Dressings for Extra-Virgin Olive Oil and Vinegar or Lemon Juice

Industrially prepared bottled salad dressings are often loaded with sodium, sugar, preservatives, and added preservatives — all things no one needs an excess of in their diet. If you are a person who normally tops your salads this way, swapping your topping with a good-quality extra-virgin olive oil and vinegar or fresh lemon or lime juice is a powerful way to increase the antioxidant benefits of the vegetables you're eating as well as getting the additional benefits of consuming the extra-virgin olive oil and juice or vinegar of your choice, both of which reduce the glycemic load of your meal.

Everybody knows that a fresh green salad is a healthy choice, and for diabetes management, nonstarchy vegetables like those commonly included in green salads are especially desirable because of their low carbohydrate content. So, after you've prepared your healthy tossed green salad, how are you going to top the lettuce, spinach, cucumber, tomato, carrots, and peppers? Maybe with three or four tablespoons of honey mustard salad dressing for 220 calories and 16 grams of fat, or blue cheese for 240 calories, Ranch or Thousand Island for 260, or French dressing for 280 calories and 26 grams of fat?

Or, maybe think about swapping any kind of salad dressing for fresh lime juice, with no fat and calories you can count on one hand. Fresh lime juice gives you a burst of flavor and complements the garden vegetables of your salad without compromising your healthy intentions. Salad dressing is one of those condiments people tend to ignore because it's added in what seems to be such small amounts. But, the calories from fat mount quickly, and you can do a lot of damage with a tablespoon.

Make Your Own Fresh Tomato Sauce

Jarred commercially prepared tomato and other sauces are one of the main reasons why eating pasta is considered unhealthful outside of Italy. These prepared sauces contain copious amounts of sodium, sugar (or another chemical sweetener), preservatives, and often unhealthful oils and saturated fats. Packaged in flashy labels that pay homage to a delicious Italian lifestyle that they have nothing in common with, they should be avoided at all costs. If you usually purchase prepared sauces, try reading the nutrition label the next time you pick up a jar. You might be surprised to see ingredients such as soybean oil, beef fat, dehydrated milk, chemicals, and much more lurking in a sauce that is labeled as "fresh tomato basil."

If you make your own fresh sauce, however, which only takes 5 to 10 minutes, you can use good-quality ingredients such as extra-virgin olive oil, garlic, tomatoes, freshly cracked black pepper, a pinch of salt, and fresh herbs. Fresh basil, a key element in tomato sauce, has been shown to help balance blood sugar levels. Chef Amy Riolo offers a recipe in Chapter 18 that can be cooked up anytime. If you don't have time to cook, you can swap out the jarred sauce for raw tomatoes, garlic, basil, and extra-virgin olive oil and still get all the wonderful antioxidants and anti-inflammatory goodness coupled with authentic flavor — without the fat, sodium, and chemicals.

Skip Sour Cream and Go Greek Instead

Sour cream is a popular topping for many foods. When many people see a baked potato, certain Tex-Mex dishes, and soups, omitting the sour cream seems non-negotiable. But, for those with diabetes, or anyone interested in optimal health, there's a much better solution.

Standard toppings for baked potatoes are butter and sour cream, but you can save calories and fat by trying full-fat plain Greek yogurt on your potato instead. And, Greek yogurt has the same thick and creamy consistency of sour cream. Greek yogurt, because it's thicker and creamier than regular yogurt, can replace sour cream or margarine just about anywhere.

TIP

If you eat dairy, plain, full-fat Greek yogurt should be a staple in your diet. In addition to offering a significant amount of protein, it's also one of the rare single ingredients that is considered a "complete food" because it contains protein, carbohydrates, and fat. That means if you need a quick snack or something to eat before sleeping when your body will be deprived of food for hours, ¾ cup of plain Greek yogurt is a good choice. It also contains probiotics — important for gut health and digestion — and inulin, a compound that helps the body maintain even blood sugar levels naturally.

Some Greek yogurts may be made from sheep's or goat's milk. These may be even healthier because the saturated fats from sheep's and goat's milk are different from those in cow's milk (being shorter chain fatty acids) and are less associated with a rise in harmful cholesterol. Having said that, the evidence that consumption of dairy products increases the risk of heart disease or stroke is not convincing, and certainly fermented dairy products like cheese and yogurt seem to have a protective effect when it comes to type 2 diabetes.

Flavor Your Foods with Aromatics

A diabetes-friendly diet doesn't need to be free of flavor. Modern restaurants, food chains, the packaged food industry, and Western cultures often rely upon three things to add flavor to recipes: unhealthful fats, salt, and sugar. Obviously, if you're trying to eat healthfully, those ingredients need to be reserved for very special instances. Nutritious daily meals should be composed of whole, nutritious ingredients. When compared to the rich fare that many people are used to, "plain" ingredients might seem to lack flavor.

The key to unlocking flavor in natural foods while amping up their nutrition quotient lies in what chefs refer to as *aromatics*. Cooking with fresh garlic, onions, leeks, shallots, and a wide range of fresh herbs and spices provides not only mouthwatering tastes to your food, but each one of them also unlocks specific compounds that give you more nutritional bang for your buck. Culinarily speaking, even the humble onion, when sautéed for various amounts of time, can completely enhance and transform a dish while enabling the body to remove more of the waste from our cells, aiding in digestion, and feeding your microbiome. Even a simple dish of rice and lentils turns into a masterpiece when garnished with a healthful portion of perfectly caramelized onions.

TIP

Garlic is nature's antibiotic and has wonderful anti-inflammatory properties. Depending upon how garlic is cooked (or not) can also alter the flavor of our food. Try roasting garlic and using it as a delicious spread instead of mayo.

Garlic roasted in the oven for 30 minutes, or zapped in a terra cotta roaster for only about 2 minutes in the microwave, loses much of its strong, pungent bite and takes on a mild, buttery sweetness. And, roasted garlic can be smashed into a rich paste and used on anything where you would otherwise get your buttery sweetness from butter or margarine — bread, potatoes, vegetables, pasta, or wherever.

One tablespoon of roasted garlic is only 12 calories, with no fat, saturated fat, or sodium. Compared to a tablespoon of margarine, roasted garlic saves you 58 calories, 8 grams of total fat, and 100 milligrams of sodium. And, eating garlic does have some beneficial effects on heart health, specifically lowering blood pressure and helping to prevent atherosclerosis.

ENJOYING HERBS TO THE FULLEST

FROM THE AUTHORS

One of Amy's favorite North African and Eastern Mediterranean customs is to make salads with herbs. In countries like Egypt, Lebanon, and Turkey, for example, the base of the "local salad" is often finely chopped fresh parsley or cilantro instead of plain lettuce. Those two herbs offer many more antioxidants than iceberg and some other types of lettuce. Years ago, Amy developed a mashed potato recipe using good-quality extra-virgin olive oil, lemon zest, and baby dill with freshly cracked black pepper in lieu of adding butter, salt, and cream. At first, even Amy had her doubts because she loves traditional mashed potatoes, but when she tried the recipe, she was pleasantly surprised. She actually liked it more than the classic recipe, and so do her readers and clients.

TIP

We highly recommend falling in love with fresh herbs. Use them in large amounts and as much as you can to supercharge your diet and your dishes. Many Western cookbooks and recipes call for 1 tablespoon or teaspoon of freshly chopped herbs, yet cooks in the Mediterranean, central Asia, and Africa use much more. Discover which herbs you like the most. Fresh cilantro, dill, parsley, basil, tarragon, rosemary, sage, thyme, and oregano were traditional medicines in ancient times. Each one offers a myriad of benefits, which we cover in Chapter 8, and should be used liberally in a variety of ways to add flavor and health benefits to your recipes.

Use Raw Vegetables for Dipping

Snack chips and dips are everywhere, from the office break room to parties to the free sample displays at your grocery. But chips are fried and relatively high in fat. A 1-ounce serving of potato chips, corn chips, or cheese snacks — 10 to 15 chips — packs about 150 calories and 10 grams of fat. Add dip — nacho, queso, onion, ranch, or bean — and you add 50 to 70 more calories per 2-tablespoon serving.

Substituting raw vegetables, however, cuts the calories and fat significantly while providing you with nutrients that can actually alter your DNA. You save calories, fat, and sodium while gaining antioxidant and anti-inflammatory properties and plenty of healthful fiber that fills you up and helps you lose weight.

And, if you adopt salsa as your dipping favorite, you lose 80 percent of the calories and all the fat from the dip, too. Make your own salsa by dicing fresh tomatoes, onions, cilantro, garlic, and peppers, and you can impress your friends with your kitchen skills — and your nutrition knowledge.

Spice It Up

Fat adds flavor to food, and one reason you like higher-fat foods is for the flavor. But, you can add incredible flavor with no calories and no fat by adding spices. When we speak of spices, many people assume we are talking about adding heat to recipes, which certainly is a good anti-inflammatory and flavorful option. But pepperoncino, chili peppers, cayenne, and so on, aren't the only way to kick up the flavor quotient in a meal.

Selecting spices gives you the power to add sweet or savory flavors to your meals and draw upon their nutritious properties to feel better. Adding pure (ceylon) cinnamon to recipes, for example, adds a pleasant sweet note, but also promotes balanced blood sugar levels and anti-inflammatory properties. Turmeric, ginger, and a bit of freshly ground black pepper also pack a powerful punch in terms of combatting inflammation and transforming "plain foods" into culinary champions.

TIP

You can make your own anti-inflammatory sweet spice mix by combining ½ cup pure ceylon cinnamon, ¼ cup turmeric, ¼ cup ground ginger, and 1 teaspoon of freshly cracked black pepper in a jar with a tight-fitting lid. Shake it up and use it to coat chicken, salmon, or other fish. Try adding a teaspoon to the onions your sautéing for a soup or stew. The result is a whole new layer of flavor and depth that you can feel good about (literally).

Reach for a Healthier Chocolate Fix

Chocolate is a food processed from the fermented seeds of cacao trees, coming to Western societies from the Mayan and Aztec cultures. But while the ancient Mesoamericans brewed bitter drinks of chocolate, the addition of sugar and milk to make the chocolate you know today has also added significant calories, carbohydrates, and fat. Chocolate is a non-negotiable dietary must-have for many people, however, and fortunately it brings some clear health benefits along with its addictive stimulation of your brain's serotonin levels.

TIP

Choose 80 percent or higher dark chocolate when shopping and indulge in a few small squares when you need a chocolate fix, and enjoy them with a few raw almonds to prevent your blood sugar from spiking.

Dark chocolate is a rich source of polyphenols and when it comes to taste, "bitter is better," with the higher concentration of cacao providing a real boost in these antioxidant and anti-inflammatory compounds. Research has shown that gradually increasing the strength of chocolate from a "milk" chocolate with low levels of cacao and high levels of sugar to an 80 or 90 percent cacao chocolate adjusts your taste preferences so that soon you will only want the most healthy chocolate and are satisfied by smaller quantities.

Choose Fresh or Frozen over Canned and Jarred

In general, canned and jarred products can be hiding places for the exact ingredients we need to cut if we want to enjoy our best lives. Do your best to choose fresh food when possible. Even frozen food, which often gets a bad rap, can actually be an excellent choice. Stocking a freezer with frozen vegetables and lean proteins such as fish and chicken means that you've always got nutritious ingredients on hand and can create a quick meal in minutes, which prevents the urge and need to eat less healthful convenience foods.

Canned tuna is a great source of high-quality protein and healthy omega-3 fatty acids. But, you can get your tuna packed in water or packed in oil. You guessed it — having tuna packed in water saves you 69 calories, 6 grams of fat, and 14 milligrams of sodium compared to the same 3-ounce serving of tuna packed in oil. In addition, the oil that canned foods are often packaged in is not good-quality extra-virgin olive oil, but soybean or other less expensive oil that is high in unhealthful fats. Buy your products fresh or in water, rinse them, and top with your own extra-virgin olive oil, citrus juices, herbs, and spices, if desired.

Canned and boxed broths and stocks are often another source of hidden enemies to our health. If you purchase prepared stock, be sure to read the nutrition labels. Even what is called "low sodium" can often contain more than half the recommended daily allowance of sodium not to mention other additives. Luckily stock is easy to make and we include the recipe in Chapter 18. If you're in a pinch for time, substitute stock for water with bay leaf and your favorite spices or herbs instead of purchased stock in your recipes.

Opt For Nutrient-Dense Foods over Processed and Packaged Foods

WARNING

When you're watching your weight, packaged foods labeled as "low fat" and "healthy" can be extremely tempting because teams of people have created them (and marketing and packaging campaigns) to make them look that way. Even if these foods have a nutritional facts label that seems innocent, they will never be as good for your health as natural foods, which are rich in vitamins and minerals.

Chapters 15 and 16 offer a great deal of information on choosing the best snacks and which foods are best to eat in general so that you are equipped with solutions before problems occur. Armed with nutritious snacks and meal options, you won't need to rely on packaged foods.

Eat Fresh Fish or Legumes over Red Meat

Not all proteins are created equal. If you're trying to lose weight, select the foods that offer you the most protein and the least fat naturally. Fish, chicken breast, goat meat, lentils, plain Greek yogurt, tofu, venison, egg whites, edamame, turkey breast, shrimp, beans and chickpeas, and quinoa are great options.

Eating for planetary health is increasingly important, and plant-based proteins are a great choice if you want to reduce the carbon footprint of your diet. They also contain fiber, vitamins, and minerals as well as bioactive compounds like polyphenols. If you choose fish, it is good to choose more sustainable species. Red meat protein sources are less environmentally friendly than plant sources.

Appendix A
Diabetes Exchange Lists

Diabetes exchange lists were the best way for patients to learn about healthy eating for diabetes before carbohydrate counting became the standard. It's true that carb counting offers more accuracy and flexibility for managing the foods that directly affect blood glucose levels, especially in matching insulin doses to carbohydrate consumption, and in many circles diabetes exchanges have gone by the wayside as a teaching tool.

But these exchange lists still have some life. Some people with diabetes find exchange lists easier to deal with than carb counting, and exchange lists don't address only carbohydrates, but other food groups as well. In that regard, exchange lists can illustrate healthy eating concepts beyond carbohydrate management better than carb counting. And exchanges encourage people with diabetes to select their carbohydrate choices from a variety of carbohydrate-containing foods, rather than from just one group.

A meal plan incorporating exchanges may suggest, for example, that your breakfasts include one starch, one fruit, and one dairy exchange rather than simply three carb choices. While your carbohydrate intake would be the same either way, exchanges would discourage you from choosing three pieces of toast as your three breakfast carb choices.

Exchanges are also helpful in following a weight management plan, which addresses more than simply carbohydrates. If your registered dietitian has recommended a 1,500-calorie-per-day eating plan, you can find your best choices and the appropriate portions for protein and fat in your daily diet from the meat and meat substitutes list and from the fats list.

TIP

Throughout the exchange lists, foods marked with an asterisk (*) indicate choices that may be high in sodium. People with diabetes should restrict sodium intake to 1,500 milligrams per day.

FROM THE AUTHORS

We include a wide variety of foods in the following exchange lists to illustrate the idea of carbohydrate exchanges. We include foods on these lists that we do not recommend you consume regularly because they are highly processed or contain artificial sweeteners. We list them simply for the sake of completion.

Carbohydrate Exchanges

Exchange lists are an effective way to make sure you get the correct portions of any particular food, especially the carbohydrate foods listed in Tables A-1, A-2, A-3, and A-4. Exchange lists may also help you add a variety of carbohydrate foods to your diet simply by listing many available food types that are all equal to 15 grams of carbohydrate in the portions specified.

Starches

One exchange of a starchy food contains about 15 grams of carbohydrate, up to 3 grams of protein, up to 1 gram of fat, and 80 calories. Beans, peas, and lentils are an exception with respect to protein — each portion includes 7 grams of protein and is considered a very lean meat substitute exchange. Starches in the amounts listed in Table A-1 equal one carbohydrate exchange. Choose whole-grain and low-fat starches when possible.

TABLE A-1 ### Starches

Type	Food	Portion Size
Bread		
	Bagel large (4 ounces)	¼ bagel (1 ounce)
	Bread	1 slice (1 ounce)
	Bread (reduced calorie)	2 slices (1½ ounces)
	Challah	1 slice (1 ounce)
	Dosa, plain	1 piece
	English muffin	½ muffin
	Hamburger or hot dog bun	½ bun (1 ounce)

TABLE A-1 *(continued)*

Type	Food	Portion Size
	Matzah	¾ ounce
	Naan	¼ of 8-x-2-inch piece
	Pita	½ pita
	Pumpernickel bread	1 slice (1 ounce)
	Rye bread	1 slice (1 ounce)
	Pancake (4-x-¼-inch thick)	1 pancake
	Potato pancake	½ pancake
	Roti (6 inches)	½ piece
	Tortilla (6-inches, corn or flour)	1 tortilla
Cereals and grains		
	Barley, cooked	⅓ cup
	Bulgur wheat, cooked	½ cup
	Bran, oats, shredded wheat, frosted cereals	½ cup
	Cereal, puffed, unfrosted	1½ cups
	Cereal, unsweetened, ready to eat	¾ cup
	Couscous	⅓ cup
	Granola, low-fat or regular	¼ cup (+ 1 fat exchange)
	Grits, cooked	½ cup
	Kasha (cooked)	½ cup
	Mumra (puffed rice)	1½ cups
	Pasta, cooked	⅓ cup
	Poha	1 cup
	Quinoa, cooked	⅓ cup
	Rice, cooked, brown or white	⅓ cup
	Tabbouleh, prepared	½ cup
	Wheat germ, dry	3 tablespoons

(continued)

TABLE A-1 *(continued)*

Type	Food	Portion Size
Starchy vegetables		
	Corn	½ cup
	Corn on the cob, large	½ cob (5 ounces)
	Mixed vegetables with peas, corn, or pasta	1 cup
	Parsnips	½ cup
	Potato, baked with skin	3 ounces
	Potato, mashed	½ cup
	Pumpkin, canned	1 cup
	Spaghetti or pasta sauce	½ cup
	Squash, acorn or butternut	1 cup
	Succotash	½ cup
	Yam or sweet potato, plain	½ cup
Crackers and snacks		
	Animal crackers	8
	Graham crackers (2½-inch squares)	3
	Matzah	¾ ounce
	Melba toast (2-x-4-inches)	4
	Oyster crackers*	20
	Popcorn, low-fat microwave* or no-fat air popped	3 cups
	Pretzels*	¾ ounce
	Rice cakes (4 inches across)	2
	Saltine crackers*	6
	Snack chips, baked*	15–20 pieces (¾ ounce)
Beans, peas, lentils (count as 1 carbohydrate and 1 ounce lean meat)		
	Baked beans	⅓ cup
	Black, garbanzo, kidney, lima, navy, pinto, white (cooked)	½ cup
	Lentils, cooked	½ cup
	Black eyed, split, green peas (cooked)	½ cup
	Refried beans, canned, fat-free	½ cup

Fruits

One fruit exchange equals 15 grams of carbohydrate and 60 calories. Watch the serving sizes for dried fruit, and choose whole fruits over juices most of the time. Table A-2 lists a variety of fruits as well as the appropriate portion size equal to 15 grams of carbohydrate.

TABLE A-2 **Fruits**

Type	Food	Portion Size
Fresh		
	Apple, small 2-inches across	1 (4 ounces)
	Apricots	4 (5½ ounces)
	Bael	½ cup
	Banana, extra small	1 (4 ounces)
	Blackberries, blueberries	¾ cup
	Cantaloupe, honey dew, papaya, cubed	1 cup (11 ounces)
	Carambola (starfruit)	1½ cups
	Cherries	12 (3 ounces)
	Dates	3
	Durian	¼ cup
	Grapefruit, large	½ (11 ounces)
	Grapes, small	17 (3 ounces)
	Guava	1½ medium
	Jackfruit	½ cup
	Java plum	¾ cup
	Jujube	⅓ cup
	Kiwi	1 (3½ ounces)
	Korean melon	1 medium
	Korean pear (Asian pear)	1 medium
	Loquat	¾ cup
	Lychee	½ cup

(continued)

Type	Food	Portion Size
	Mango, cubed	½ cup
	Mangosteen	½ cup
	Mutsu apple	½ medium
	Nectarine, small	1 (5 ounces)
	Orange, small	1 (6½ ounces)
	Peach, medium	1 (6 ounces)
	Pear, large	½ (4 ounces)
	Persimmon	½ medium
	Pineapple, cubed	¾ cup
	Pitaya (dragon fruit)	1 medium
	Plums, small	2 (5 ounces)
	Rambutan	2 medium
	Raspberries	1 cup
	Strawberries	1¼ cup
	Tomatoes	¾ cup
	Watermelon, cubed	1¼ cups (13½ ounces)
Dried fruit		
	Apples	4 rings
	Apricots	8 halves
	Blueberries, cherries, cranberries, mixed fruit	2 tablespoons
	Figs	1½
	Prunes	3
	Raisins	2 tablespoons
Canned fruit, unsweetened		
	Applesauce, apricots, cherries, peaches, pears, pineapple, plums	½ cup
	Grapefruit, mandarin oranges	¾ cup
Fruit juice		
	Unsweetened apple, grapefruit, orange, pineapple	½ cup
	Fruit juice blends of 100% juice, grape, prune	⅓ cup

Vegetables

Your diet should include many types of nonstarchy vegetables. One-half of each meal should be comprised of nonstarchy vegetables. One-fourth should be comprised of a quality protein, and the remaining one-fourth a quality carbohydrate. Free foods are considered to be exempt from exchange rules and can be eaten in any quantity. Raw cabbage and spinach are two examples of "free foods." In general, the serving size for raw, nonstarchy vegetables is 1 cup; cooked is ½ cup. These items contain approximately 5 grams of carbohydrate or less.

TABLE A-3   Vegetables

Food	Portion Size
Asparagus	1 cup raw or ½ cup cooked
Bell peppers	1 cup raw or ½ cup cooked
Bamboo shoots, canned	½ cup
Bittermelon, raw	1½ cups
Broccoli	1 cup raw or ½ cup cooked
Brussels sprouts	1 cup raw or ½ cup cooked
Cabbage	1 cup raw or ½ cup cooked
Carrots	1 cup raw or ½ cup cooked
Cauliflower	1 cup raw or ½ cup cooked
Celery	1 cup raw or ½ cup cooked
Chayote, raw	1 cup
Chinese celery, raw	1 cup
Chinese eggplant, cooked	1 cup
Chinese mushroom, dried	2 medium
Cucumbers	1 cup raw or ½ cup cooked
Green beans	1 cup raw or ½ cup cooked
Leeks, cooked	½ cup
Kale	1 cup raw or ½ cup cooked
Peapods, cooked	½ cup

(continued)

Food	Portion Size
Spinach	1 cup raw or ½ cup cooked
Sprouts	½ cup
Straw mushrooms	½ cup
Taro, cooked	⅓ cup
Turnip, raw or cooked	1 cup
Water chestnuts, canned	½ cup
Water chestnuts, raw	4
Winter melon, cooked	1 cup
Zucchini	1 cup raw or ½ cup cooked

Milk

One milk exchange equals 12 grams of carbohydrate, and 8 grams of protein. Note that 2 percent or whole-milk products also count as one or two fat exchanges, so choose low-fat milk products more often. Table A-4 reflects different milk products.

TABLE A-4   **Milk**

Type	Food	Portion Size
Fat-free and low-fat milk and yogurt products		
	Buttermilk*	1 cup (8 ounces)
	Chocolate milk	1 cup (counts as 1 milk + 1 starch)
	Evaporated milk	½ cup
	Milk, skim or 1%	1 cup
	Yogurt, plain or flavored with a non-nutritive sweetener	⅔ cup (6 ounces)
	Yogurt, low-fat with fruit	⅔ cup (6 ounces) (counts as 1 milk + 1 fruit)

TABLE A-4 *(continued)*

Type	Food	Portion Size
Reduced-fat milk and yogurt products		
	Milk, 2%	1 cup (counts as 1 milk + 1 fat)
	Soy milk, light	1 cup (counts as 1 milk + 1 fat)
Whole milk and yogurt products		
	Buttermilk	1 cup
	Chocolate milk	1 cup
	Evaporated milk	½ cup
	Milk, whole	1 cup (counts as 1 milk + 2 fats)
	Soy milk	1 cup
	Yogurt, plain	1 cup
Other		
	Eggnog, whole milk	1 cup (counts as 1 milk + 2 fats)
	Rice drink, fat-free, plain	1 cup fat-free milk
	Rice drink, low-fat	1 cup milk + 1 fat

Meat and Meat Substitutes

A meat and meat substitute exchange is carbohydrate–free (negligible carbohydrate) and contains 7 grams of protein. The different exchange lists are based upon the fat and calories in a portion that gives you 7 grams of protein. Beans, peas, and lentils are an exception with respect to carbohydrate, where each portion also includes 15 grams carbohydrate and is considered a starch exchange, too (see Table A–1).

Lean and very lean meat, and meat substitutes

Very lean and lean meat and meat substitutes contain 0 carbohydrates, 7 grams protein, 1 gram or less fat, and 35 calories. Lean meat or meat substitutes contain 0 carbohydrate (except for beans, peas, and lentils), 7 grams of protein, 3 grams of fat, and 55 calories. Table A–5 lists the portion size containing 7 grams of protein for your best choices when you have diabetes.

TABLE A-5   **Lean and Very Lean Meat and Meat Substitutes**

Food	Portion size
Beef, select or choice, trimmed of fat: ground round, roast, round sirloin, tenderloin	1 ounce
Beef jerky*	½ ounce
Fish, fresh or frozen: catfish, cod, flounder, haddock, halibut, orange roughy, salmon, tilapia, trout, tuna	1 ounce
Herring, smoked*	1 ounce
Hot dog, 3 grams or less of fat per ounce (Note: May also contain carbohydrate)*	1
Lamb: roast, chop, leg	1 ounce
Lunch meat, 3 grams or less of fat per ounce: chipped beef, deli thin-sliced meats, turkey ham, turkey kielbasa, turkey pastrami*	1 ounce
Oysters, medium, fresh or frozen	6
Pork, lean: Canadian bacon,* chop, ham, tenderloin	1 ounce
Poultry without skin: chicken, Cornish hen, duck, goose, turkey	1 ounce
Sardines, canned*	2 medium
Shellfish: clams, crab, imitation shellfish, lobster, scallops, shrimp	1 ounce
Tuna, canned in water or oil, drained*	1 ounce
Veal: loin chop, roast	1 ounce
Cheese, 3 grams or less of fat per ounce*	1 ounce
Cottage cheese, fat-free, low-fat, or regular*	¼ cup
Egg substitute, plain	¼ cup
Egg whites	2
Baked beans	⅓ cup
Black, garbanzo, kidney, lima, navy, pinto, white (cooked)	½ cup
Lentils, cooked	½ cup
Black eyed, split, green peas (cooked)	½ cup
Refried beans, canned, fat-free	½ cup

Medium-fat meat and meat substitutes

Medium-fat meat or meat substitutes contain 0 carbohydrates, 7 grams of protein, 5 grams of fat, and 75 calories. Table A-6 lists the portion sizes for meat and meat substitutes containing 7 grams of protein and a notable amount of fat.

TABLE A-6   **Medium-Fat Meat and Meat Substitutes**

Food	Portion Size
Beef: corned beef, ground beef, meatloaf, prime rib, short ribs, tongue*	1 ounce
Cheese, 4 to 7 grams of fat per ounce: feta, mozzarella, pasteurized processed cheese spread, reduced-fat cheeses, string*	1 ounce
Eggs (limit to 3 a week)	1
Fish, fried	1 ounce
Lamb: ground, rib roast	1 ounce
Pork: cutlet, shoulder roast	1 ounce
Poultry: chicken with skin, dove, fried chicken, ground turkey, pheasant, wild duck or goose	1 ounce
Ricotta cheese*	¼ cup (2 ounces)

High-fat meat and meat substitutes

High-fat meat and meat substitutes contain 0 carbohydrates, 7 grams protein, 8 grams of fat, and 100 calories. These foods are high in saturated fat and calories. Table A-7 lists foods containing 7 grams of protein and this significant amount of fat. Your diet is healthier if you make these choices only rarely.

High-Fat Meats and Meat Substitutes

Food	Portion Size
Bacon, pork*	2 slices (1 ounce each before cooking)
Bacon, turkey*	3 slices (½ ounce each prior to cooking)
Cheese, regular: American, bleu, Brie, cheddar, hard goat, Monterey Jack, queso, Swiss*	1 ounce
Hot dog, regular: beef, chicken, pork, turkey or combination*	1 (counts as 1 fat and 1 meat exchange)
Lunch meat, 8 or more grams of fat per ounce: bologna, pastrami, hard salami*	1 ounce
Pork: ground, sausage, spareribs	1 ounce
Sausage, 8 or more grams of fat per ounce: bratwurst, chorizo, Italian, knockwurst, Polish, smoked, summer sausage*	1 ounce

Fats

One fat exchange equals 5 grams of fat and 45 calories. Table A-8 lists fats and a portion size according to whether they are predominantly monounsaturated, polyunsaturated, or saturated fat. The unsaturated fats are your best choice for heart health.

TABLE A-8 ## Monounsaturated, Polyunsaturated, and Saturated Fats

Type	Food	Portion Size
Monounsaturated fats		
	Almonds*	6
	Avocado	2 tablespoons (1 ounce)
	Brazil nuts*	2
	Cashews*	6
	Filberts (Hazelnuts)*	5
	Macadamia nuts	3
	Nut butters, trans-free: almond butter, cashew butter, peanut butter (smooth or crunchy)	1½ teaspoons

TABLE A-8 *(continued)*

Type	Food	Portion Size
	Oil: canola, olive, peanut	1 teaspoon
	Olives, black*	8 large
	Olives, green with pimento*	10 large
	Peanuts	10*
	Pecans*	4 halves
	Pistachios*	16
Polyunsaturated fats		
	Mayonnaise, reduced-fat	1 tablespoon
	Mayonnaise, regular	1 teaspoon
	Mayonnaise-style salad dressing, reduced-fat*	1 tablespoon
	Mayonnaise-style salad dressing, regular	2 teaspoons
	Oil: corn, cottonseed, flaxseed, grape seed, safflower, soybean, sunflower	1 teaspoon
	Pine nuts	1 tablespoon
	Salad dressing, reduced-fat	2 tablespoons
	Salad dressing, regular*	1 tablespoon
	Seeds: flaxseed, pumpkin, sesame, sunflower*	1 tablespoon
	Walnuts	4 halves
Saturated fats		
	Bacon, cooked, regular or turkey*	1 slice
	Butter, reduced-fat	1 tablespoon
	Butter, stick	1 teaspoon
	Butter, whipped	2 teaspoons
	Coconut, shredded	2 tablespoons
	Cream: half-and-half, whipped	2 tablespoons
	Cream, heavy	1 tablespoon
	Cream, light	1½ tablespoons
	Cream cheese, reduced-fat	1½ tablespoons
	Cream cheese, regular	1 tablespoon
	Oil: coconut, palm, palm kernel	1 teaspoon
	Shortening or lard	1 teaspoon
	Sour cream, reduced-fat	3 tablespoons
	Sour cream, regular	2 tablespoons

Free Foods

The specified portion sizes for free foods are less than 20 calories, and 5 grams carbohydrate or less. If you spread these throughout the day, up to three servings is often recommended for appetite control without affecting blood glucose levels. Remember that one exchange of a nonstarchy vegetable falls into this category, too. Table A-9 lists common free foods and a portion size fitting the free food definition. A portion size listed as *Unlimited* refers to the calorie and carbohydrate content of normal use. For instance, drinking a couple of glasses of "cooking wine" is outside of its normal use.

TABLE A-9   **Free Foods**

Type	Food	Portion Size
Beverages		
	Bouillon*, club soda, coffee (unsweetened or with sugar), flavored water (carbohydrate-free), tea (unsweetened or with sugar substitute), tonic water (sugar-free), water (plain, carbonated, mineral)	Unlimited
Condiments		
	Horseradish	Unlimited
	Lemon juice	Unlimited
	Mustard*	Unlimited
	Vinegar	Unlimited
Seasonings		
	Vegetable cooking spray	Unlimited
	Cooking wine	Unlimited
	Extracts (vanilla, peppermint, etc.)	Unlimited
	Garlic	Unlimited
	Herbs	Unlimited
	Hot sauce*	Unlimited
	Pimento	Unlimited

TABLE A-9 *(continued)*

Type	Food	Portion Size
	Spices without salt as an ingredient	Unlimited
	Worcestershire sauce*	Unlimited
Other		
	Gelatin, sugar free or unflavored	Unlimited
	Sugar-free gum	Unlimited
	Salad greens	Unlimited
Condiments with a limit		
	Barbeque sauce*	2 teaspoons
	Cream cheese, fat-free	1 tablespoon
	Creamer, liquid non-dairy	1 tablespoon
	Creamer, powdered non-dairy	2 teaspoons
	Pickle, dill*	1½ medium
	Gherkin pickles	¾ ounce
	Honey mustard*	1 tablespoon
	Jam or jelly, light or no sugar added	2 teaspoons
	Ketchup	1 tablespoon
	Margarine spread, fat-free	1 tablespoon
	Margarine spread, reduced fat	1 teaspoon
	Mayonnaise, fat-free	1 tablespoon
	Mayonnaise, reduced fat	1 teaspoon
	Mayonnaise-style salad dressing, fat-free	1 tablespoon
	Mayonnaise-style salad dressing, reduced fat	1 teaspoon
	Miso*	1½ teaspoons
	Parmesan cheese, freshly grated*	1 tablespoon

(continued)

Type	Food	Portion Size
	Pickle relish	1 tablespoon
	Salad dressing, fat-free Italian*	2 tablespoons
	Salad dressing, fat-free or low fat*	1 tablespoon
	Salsa	¼ cup
	Sour cream, fat-free or reduced fat	1 tablespoon
	Soy sauce, regular or Light*	1 tablespoon
	Sweet and sour sauce	2 teaspoons
	Sweet chili sauce	2 teaspoons
	Syrup, sugar-free	2 tablespoons
	Taco sauce	1 tablespoon
Other		
	Cocoa powder, unsweetened	1 tablespoon
	Hard candy, regular or sugar-free	1 piece
	Whipped topping, light or fat-free	2 tablespoons
	Whipped topping, Regular	1 tablespoon

Sweets and Desserts

Sweets and desserts are often very high in carbohydrates, fats, and calories, and should be eaten in moderation. This limited list of exchanges is provided for demonstration purposes, illustrating a few better choices for sweets and desserts, contrasted with a few choices that are going to be frustrating because of the portion size. Table A-10 gives the portion size containing 15 grams of carbohydrate for common sweets and desserts. Note than some of these foods also include more than 5 grams of fat for the serving size listed.

TABLE A-10 **Sweets and Desserts — Portions for 15-Grams Carbohydrate**

Food	Portion Size
Banana nut bread	½ ounce
Cake, unfrosted	1 ounce (+ 1 fat exchange)
Chocolate kisses	5 pieces (+ 1 fat exchange)
Frozen yogurt	½ cup
Gingersnap cookies	3 cookies
Glazed donut	½ donut (+ 1 fat exchange)
Hot chocolate, sugar-free or light	1 packet
Ice cream (fat-free)	⅓ cup
Large muffin	¼ muffin (+ 1½ fat exchanges)
Lemonade	¼ cup
Pan dulce	¼-x-4½-inches across
Pumpkin pie	½ pie (+ 1 fat exchange)
Soft drink, regular	5 ounces
Vanilla wafer	5 cookies (+ 1 fat exchange)

Appendix **B**

Glycemic Index and Glycemic Load Values

G lycemic index (GI) values represent the relative impact of a food on blood glucose levels compared to pure glucose (which has a GI of 100). Glycemic load (GL) takes into account both the GI value and the carbohydrate content of a food and provides a more comprehensive measure of a food's effect on blood glucose levels.

The values for the common carbohydrate foods listed in Table B-1 are approximate and can vary depending on preparation, ripeness, and cooking methods. Do not be surprised to see different values quoted in different sources. Many factors including other foods in a meal, insulin sensitivity, gut microbiome, and individual response can alter the way in which glucose rises after a meal, but having a general idea of the GI and GL value of a food can nevertheless provide a useful guide about the release of glucose when it is absorbed.

TABLE B-1   **GI and GL Values of Common Foods**

Food	Glycemic Index (GI)	Glycemic Load (GL)
Almonds	0	0
Apple	38	6
Apricot	34	2
Avocado	15	1
Banana	51	12
Black beans	30	7
Blueberries	53	6
Carrot	47	3
Cashews	25	3
Cherries	22	3
Chickpeas	28	9
Cornflakes	93	23
Dark chocolate (70%)	23	6
Grapes	59	11
Honey	58	17
Ice cream	61	9
Kidney beans	24	7
Kiwi	53	9
Lentils	28	5
Mango	51	12
Maple syrup	54	12
Milk (whole)	27	5
Oats	55	13
Orange	43	5
Papaya	58	8
Peach	42	5
Peanuts	14	1
Pear	38	4

TABLE B-1 *(continued)*

Food	Glycemic Index (GI)	Glycemic Load (GL)
Pineapple	59	8
Plum	39	3
Potato (boiled)	59	10
Quinoa	53	13
Rice, brown (boiled)	55	16
Rice, white (boiled)	73	17
Strawberries	40	1
Sweet potato	70	22
Walnuts	15	1
Watermelon	72	4
White Bread	71	10
Whole wheat bread	69	9
Yogurt (plain)	14	4

Appendix C

Examples of Bioactive Compounds in Foods

Literally thousands of bioactive compounds are found in common vegetables and fruits, including polyphenols, carotenoids, and glucosinolates. The anti-inflammatory and antioxidant effects of these chemicals may have a significant effect on reducing the risk of type 2 diabetes and its complications as well as many other chronic diseases. Diets like the Mediterranean diet are naturally rich in polyphenols and other bioactive compounds and have been shown to reduce markers of chronic inflammation.

Tables C-1, C-2, C-3, and C-4 list some of the most common bioactive compounds and the foods in which they occur in the highest quantity, although the amounts vary depending on various factors in the environment. This is just a sample of the many thousands of bioactive compounds that are being studied by chemists and nutrition scientists.

TABLE C-1   # Polyphenols in Foods and Possible Bioactivity

Polyphenol Class	Polyphenol Type	Example	Food Sources	Potential Health Benefits
Flavonoids	Flavonols	Quercetin	Onions, apples, berries, broccoli, green tea, capers, citrus fruits	Antioxidant, anti-inflammatory, cardiovascular health, allergy relief
Flavonoids	Flavonols	Kaempferol	Kale, spinach, broccoli, green tea, strawberries, fennel	Antioxidant, anti-inflammatory, cardiovascular health, anticancer properties
Flavonoids	Flavonols	Myricetin	Berries, grapes, red wine, pomegranate, walnuts, red onions	Antioxidant, anti-inflammatory, brain health, anticancer properties
Flavonoids	Flavanols (Catechins)	Epicatechin	Green tea, cocoa, red wine, apples, berries, cherries, pears	Antioxidant, cardiovascular health, blood sugar regulation
Flavonoids	Flavanols (Catechins)	Epigallocatechin gallate (EGCG)	Green tea, matcha, apples, berries, cocoa, dark chocolate	Antioxidant, metabolic health, brain health, weight management
Flavonoids	Flavanones	Hesperetin	Citrus fruits (oranges, lemons, grapefruits), tomatoes, parsley	Antioxidant, cardiovascular health, anti-inflammatory
Flavonoids	Flavanones	Naringenin	Grapefruit, tomatoes, oranges, lemons, grapefruit juice, hops	Antioxidant, cardiovascular health, metabolic health
Flavonoids	Flavones	Luteolin	Parsley, celery, chamomile tea, thyme, sage, peppermint	Antioxidant, anti-inflammatory, brain health, anticancer properties
Flavonoids	Flavones	Apigenin	Parsley, celery, chamomile tea, artichokes, basil, celery seed	Antioxidant, anti-inflammatory, brain health, anticancer properties
Flavonoids	Anthocyanins	Cyanidin	Blueberries, blackberries, cherries, grapes, cranberries, eggplant	Antioxidant, cardiovascular health, brain health, anti-aging

TABLE C-1 *(continued)*

Polyphenol Class	Polyphenol Type	Example	Food Sources	Potential Health Benefits
Flavonoids	Anthocyanins	Delphinidin	Blueberries, cranberries, raspberries, blackcurrants, red radishes	Antioxidant, cardiovascular health, brain health, anti-inflammatory
Phenolic acids	Hydroxybenzoic acids	Gallic acid	Coffee, tea, blueberries, blackberries, strawberries, red wine	Antioxidant, anti-inflammatory, cardiovascular health, anticancer properties
Phenolic acids	Hydroxybenzoic acids	Protocatechuic acid	Green tea, apples, pears, cinnamon, cocoa, cherry, vanilla	Antioxidant, anti-inflammatory, metabolic health, brain health
Phenolic acids	Hydroxycinnamic acids	Caffeic acid	Coffee, whole grains, apples, pears, artichokes, lettuce, parsnips	Antioxidant, anti-inflammatory, cardiovascular health, anticancer properties
Stilbenes	Resveratrol	Resveratrol	Red grapes, red wine, peanuts, mulberries, dark chocolate, pistachios	Antioxidant, anti-inflammatory, cardiovascular health, brain health
Other	Secoiridoides	Oleuropein, oleocanthal, Tyrosols	Extra-virgin olive oil	Anti-inflammatory, cardiovascular health including oxidation of LDL cholesterol, antioxidant properties
Other	Lignans	Secoisolariciresinol	Flaxseeds, sesame seeds, whole grains, berries, cruciferous vegetables	Antioxidant, hormonal balance, cardiovascular health, anticancer properties
Other	Lignans	Enterolactone	Flaxseeds, sesame seeds, whole grains, berries, cruciferous vegetables	Hormonal balance, anticancer properties, cardiovascular health

REMEMBER

Much more research is needed before we can fully explain whether, and how, antioxidant or other effects translate into effects that improve health. For some of the examples provided, the evidence is based on reliable experiments, but for others the data is less convincing. In most cases more evidence is needed to be able to say that studying a food containing a bioactive compound with possible anticancer effects will result in definite proof of its activity in the real world or provide the basis for manufacturing a new medicine. What is known is that diet plays an important role in preventing many chronic illnesses.

TABLE C-2

Carotenoids in Foods and Possible Bioactivity

Carotenoid Type	Food Sources	Potential Health Benefits
Alpha-carotene	Carrots, sweet potatoes, pumpkins, winter squash	Antioxidant, eye health, immune system support
Beta-carotene	Carrots, sweet potatoes, spinach, kale, apricots	Antioxidant, vision health, immune system support, skin health
Beta-cryptoxanthin	Oranges, papayas, peaches, mangoes	Antioxidant, immune system support, joint health
Lutein	Spinach, kale, collard greens, broccoli, avocado	Antioxidant, eye health, brain health, heart health
Lycopene	Tomatoes, watermelon, pink grapefruit, papaya	Antioxidant, heart health, prostate health, skin health
Zeaxanthin	Spinach, kale, collard greens, broccoli, eggs	Antioxidant, eye health, skin health, cognitive function, heart health

TABLE C-3

Glucosinolates in Foods and Possible Bioactivity

Glucosinolate	Food Sources	Potential Health Benefits
Gluconasturtiin	Watercress, garden cress, nasturtium flowers	Antioxidant, anticancer properties, respiratory health
Glucoraphanin	Broccoli, cauliflower, brussels sprouts, cabbage	Anticancer properties, detoxification, anti-inflammatory
Glucotropaeolin	Radishes, cabbage, watercress, mustard greens	Antioxidant, anti-inflammatory, anticancer properties
Progoitrin	Brussels sprouts, mustard greens, kale	Anticancer properties, thyroid health, anti-inflammatory
Sinapine	Broccoli, brussels sprouts, mustard seeds	Antioxidant, anti-inflammatory, cardiovascular health
Sinigrin	Mustard seeds, horseradish, wasabi, arugula	Anticancer properties, anti-inflammatory, digestive health

TIP

Bioactive compounds influence the taste of many foods (see Chapter 8). Some of the polyphenols in extra-virgin olive oil have been studied to establish how they affect its flavor. Some bitterness and pungency is considered a positive taste attribute for a high-quality extra-virgin olive oil and indicates that it is healthy, too, because of these polyphenols.

TABLE C-4 Phenolic Compounds in Extra-Virgin Olive Oil

Phenolic Compound	Taste Profile
Hydroxytyrosol	Bitter, pungent, slightly sweet
Tyrosol	Mildly bitter, slightly sweet
Oleuropein	Bitter, pungent, robust, herbal
Ligstroside	Bitter, pungent, slightly sweet
Oleocanthal	Peppery, slightly spicy, tingling sensation
Oleacein	Bitter, pungent, complex, slightly fruity
Verbascoside	Bitter, astringent, slightly sweet
Lignans (such as pinoresinol)	Woody, herbal, slightly bitter
Flavonoids (such as luteolin)	Bitter, astringent, slightly citrusy, herbal

Index

Numerics

15-gram snacks, 286

30-gram snacks, 286–287

A

A1C (hemoglobin A1C) measurement, 31, 46–47, 69–70

AACE (American Association of Clinical Endocrinologists), 46

ABC salad, 359

Academy of Nutrition and Dietetics, 54

ACCE (American College of Clinical Endocrinologists), 69

active transport, 41

acute inflammation, 37

ADA (American Diabetes Association), 30, 46, 69, 155, 188, 218

adenosine triphosphate (ATP), 40, 85

adipocytes, 71, 97

age factors, 33

alcohol

  calories and carbohydrates, 278–279

  hypoglycemia and, 279

  moderate consumption, 277–278

  public health guidelines, 276–277

  red wine, 277

  restaurant drinks, 269

allicin, 134

alpha cells, 42, 67

alternative sweeteners, 287

alums, 204

American Association of Clinical Endocrinologists (AACE), 46

American Association of Diabetes Educators, 54

American College of Clinical Endocrinologists (ACCE), 69

American Diabetes Association (ADA), 30, 46, 69, 155, 188, 218

amino acids, 101–102, 222, 249

amylin analog, 50

anthocyanins, 136

antibody proteins, 101

anti-inflammatory properties. *See also* bioactive compounds

  defined, 37

  extra-virgin olive oil, 242

  flavonoids, 136–137

  garlic, 364

  polyphenols, 136, 139

  sofrito, 132–133

  spices, 231, 366

antioxidants, 37, 129–130, 348, 350

antithrombotic properties, 136, 242–243

appetizers, 174, 270

apples, 357

arginine, 359

aromatics, 148, 364–365

artificial sweeteners, 287

Asian Noodle and Seven-Vegetable Salad with Sweet and Tangy Ginger Sauce, 316

Asparagus, Red Pepper, and Tempeh Stir-Fry with Soba Noodles and Sesame Seeds, 335

aspartame, 197, 287

Assorted Seafood Tartines with Microgreen, Red Cabbage, Carrot, and Corn Slaw, 334

athletes, 78, 281

Atkins, Robert, 252

Atkins diet, 252

ATP (adenosine triphosphate), 40, 85

autoimmune disorders, 27

autonomic neuropathy, 79

B

B vitamin complex, 106–108

Baba Ghanouj with Crudités and Roasted Chickpeas, 321–322

bacteria, gut microbiome, 120–121

bananas, 115, 358

bar snacks, 269

barley, 354

base recipes, 336–341

beans and legumes. *See also* Mediterranean diet

as budget-friendly option, 356

personalized meal planning, 226

as power foods, 349

shopping for, 203–204

stocking pantry with, 148

beets, 359

beta carotene, 134

beta cells, 41, 67, 85

beta-glucans, 354

beverages

alcohol, 276–279

coffee and tea, 279–280

energy drinks, 282

flavored waters, 280–281

soft drinks, 280–281

sports drinks, 281

water, 276

bioactive compounds

antioxidants, 129–130

carotenoids, 126, 133–135, 394

flavonoids, 136–137

garlic, 135

glucosinolates, 127, 135, 394

inflammation and, 130–133

non-flavonoid polyphenols, 137–140

oxidation, 129–130

phenolic compounds, 395

polyphenols, 127, 136, 392–393

recognizing foods with, 141–142

role in health, 127–129

taste, 140–141

BistroMD, 256

blender, 146

blood glucose

adenosine triphosphate, 40

carbohydrates, 40–41, 223

disaccharides, 40

fasting, 44

fiber and, 40

glucagon, 42–43

glycogen, 42

hemoglobin A1C test, 46–47

homeostasis, 10–11

insulin and, 41–42

measuring standards, 43–44

mitochondria, 40

oral glucose tolerance test, 44

overview, 3

polysaccharides, 40, 41

starches, 40

storing, 42–43

testing, 45–47

blood pressure

DASH diet and, 73–74, 245

diastolic pressure, 73, 245

hypertension, 20, 73, 116

Mediterranean diet, 74

potassium-to-sodium ratio, 74

systolic pressure, 73, 245

blood sugar. *See* blood glucose

Blue Zones project, 244

Blueberry-Almond Yogurt Bowls with Honey, Cinnamon, and Chia Seeds, 305

body mass index (BMI), 32, 70–71, 215, 217

bolus, 52

bread

diabetic exchanges, 157

eating out, 270

vitamin fortified, 203

white vs. whole grain, 96

breakfast

importance of, 302

personalized meal planning, 231–232

recipes, 303–308

Broccoli and Pecorino Cheese Soup with Stuffed Baby Portobello Mushrooms, 317–318

brown rice, 224

budget-friendly foods, 355–359

buffets, 272–273

butter, 205, 233

C

C reactive protein (CRP), 130

cabbage soup diet, 257

caffeic acid, 140

calcium, 111–112, 247, 249–250

calories
  calorie counting, 71
  nutrition labels, 150–151
  personalized meal planning and, 215

canned and jarred products, 200, 367

carb choice. *See also* exchange lists
  brown rice, 224
  comparing, 92–93
  defined, 215
  15-gram, 91, 144, 286
  fruit, 224
  personalized meal planning and, 219–221
  portion sizes, 153
  starchy vegetables, 224
  30-gram, 286–287

carbohydrates, 40–41
  choosing, 94–95
  complex carbohydrates, 88–91
  counting, 91–94
  exchange lists, 370–377
  fiber, 95–96
  fruit, 202
  glycemic index, 84
  glycemic load, 84
  Mediterranean diet, 241
  overview, 18–20, 84–86
  personalized meal planning and, 215, 223–224
  starchy vegetables, 202
  sugar, 86–88
  whole grains, 202–203

carcinogenic meat, 103

Cardamom-Scented Kefir, Pineapple, and Kiwi Smoothie, 310

cardiovascular health
  metabolic syndrome, 31, 75, 109
  nutrition and, 72–76

carotenes, 133

carotenoids, 106, 126, 133–135, 394

carrots, 358–359

catechins, 137

celiac disease, 78–79

cell membrane, 25–26

certified diabetes educator, 48

certified nutrition specialists (CNSs), 48, 214

Chicken Simmered in Tomatoes, Olives, and Capers with Sautéed Dandelion Greens and Salad, 327

Chicken Stock recipe, 341

children, diabetes management for, 76–77

chips and dips, 365

chocolate, 284–285, 351–352, 366–367

cholesterol
  atherosclerosis, 74–75
  fat and, 99–100
  high-density lipoproteins, 74–75, 99
  lipoproteins, 74–75
  low-density lipoproteins, 74–75, 99
  nuts and, 204

chromium, 112

chromium picolinate, 112

chronic inflammation, 131–132

Citrus-Marinated Salmon with Fiery Potatoes and Kale, 324

Clostridium botulinum, 200

CNSs (certified nutrition specialists), 48, 214

coffee, 279–280

community, sense of, 61

comorbidities with diabetes, 18

complete meals, 230–231

complete protein foods, 102

complex carbohydrates, 88–91

complications of diabetes
  COVID-19 and, 38
  defined, 11
  diabetic foot disease, 36
  heart attack and stroke, 35–36
  hyperglycemia, 35
  hypoglycemia, 35
  infections, 38
  inflammation and diabetes, 36–37
  kidney disease, 36
  long-term, 35–36
  neuropathy, 36
  overview, 34–35
  short-term, 35
  vision problems, 36

condiments, 207, 232–234

conditioned response, 162–163

conscious eating, 180–181

Continuing Survey of Food Intake by Individuals (CSFII), 165

continuous glucose monitors, 45

coumaric acid, 140

COVID-19, 38

cravings, 15–17, 166–167. *See also* emotional eating

CRP (C reactive protein), 130

CSFII (Continuing Survey of Food Intake by Individuals), 165

Cucumber and Smoked Salmon Pinwheels with Mixed Green Salad, 320

culinary medicine, 166

culinary therapy. *See also* diabetes management; holistic approach

  carbohydrates, 18–20

  common comorbidities with diabetes, 18

  diabetes management, 11–12

  healthy lifestyle, 55–62

  heart-healthy diet, 20–21

  homeostasis, 10–11

  investing in yourself, 21–22

  mind-body connection, 13–17

  overview, 9–10

cultural connection with food, 167–168

D

dairy products

  DASH diet, 245–246

  exchange lists, 376–377

  personalized meal planning, 226–227

  shopping, 207–208

  stocking pantry with, 148

dark chocolate, 284–285, 351–352, 366–367

DASH (dietary approaches to stop hypertension) diet

  blood pressure and, 73–74, 245

  calcium, 247

  dairy products, 245–246

  defined, 20

  fruit, 245–246

  grains, 245–246

  magnesium, 247

  overview, 244–245

  potassium, 247

  sodium, 247–248

dentist, 49

desserts, 270, 384–385

detours, 185

Diabetes Attitudes, Wishes, and Needs (DAWN) study, 47, 49

Diabetes Control and Complications Trial (DCCT), 46–47, 69

diabetes management. *See also* blood glucose

  choosing medical team, 47–49

  insulin therapy, 51–52

  medical nutrition therapy, 52–54, 214

  medications, 49–50

  overview, 11–12, 39–40

diabetes mellitus

  defined, 24

  gestational diabetes, 34

  glucose, 25–26

  insulin, 26

  Type 1 diabetes, 27–30

  Type 2 diabetes, 30–34

Diabetes Prevention Program (DPP), 31

Diabetic Exchange System, 156–157

diabetic foot disease, 36

diabetic ketoacidosis (DKA), 28

diabetologist, 48

diastolic pressure, 73

diet plans

  BistroMD, 256

  DASH diet, 244–248

  fad diets, 257–258

  Hello Fresh, 256

  Heritage diets, 243–244

  low-carb diets, 251–253

  Mediterranean diet, 238–243

  Noom, 256

  Nutrisystem, 255–256

  overview, 237–238

  vegetarian diets, 248–251

  Weight Watchers, 253–255

dietary approaches to stop hypertension diet. *See* DASH diet

dietary fat. *See* fats and oils

Dietary Inflammatory Index (DII), 132–133

dinner recipes, 323–333

disaccharides, 40, 87

DKA (diabetic ketoacidosis), 28

dopamine, 169–170

DPP (Diabetes Prevention Program), 31

DPP-4 enzyme, 50

Dried Beans recipe, 337

dysbiosis, 121

E

eating at home, 183

eating out

  analyzing menu items, 264–265

  appetizers, 270

  asking ahead, 266–267

  bread, 270

  bringing your own food, 267

  buffets, 272–273

  checking ahead, 262–263

  dessert, 270

  drinks and bar snacks, 269

  hors d'oeuvres, 270

  overview, 259–260

  portion distortion, 268

  remembering your meal plan, 261–262

  salad bar, 271

  sticking to plan, 263

  taking some home, 267–268

Eatwell Plate (U.K.), 217, 219

eggs, 207, 359

Egyptian Fuul Medammes with Extra-Virgin Olive Oil, Tomato, and Eggs, 309

elderly, nutrition and, 77–78

electrolytes, 114–116, 247

emotional eating

  cultural connection with food, 167–168

  emotional patterns that interfere with self-care, 14–15

  impulsive eating, 15–17

  mindless eating, 171–172

  overview, 166–167

  pleasure response, 168–170

  social connection with food, 168

  stress and, 170–171

empty calories, 151

endocrinologist, 48

endorphins, 169

endothelial function, 352

energy drinks, 282

energy production, 97

enzymes, 101

epicatechin, 137

essential amino acids, 102, 222

ethnicity and diabetes, 33

European Prospective Investigation into Cancer, 140

exchange lists

  carbohydrates, 370–377

  fats and oils, 380–381

  free foods, 382–384

  meat, 377–380

  overview, 369–370

  sweets and desserts, 384–385

extra-virgin olive oil. *See also* Mediterranean Diet

  anti-inflammatory properties, 242

  antithrombotic properties, 242–243

  overview, 204–207

  phenolic compounds in, 395

  polyphenols in, 139–140

  as power food, 348

  as substitute for salad dressing, 362–363

F

fad diets, 257–258

fasting blood glucose, 44

fats and oils. *See also* extra-virgin olive oil

  adipocytes, 97

  cholesterol and, 99–100

  energy production, 97

  exchange lists, 380–381

  hormones and, 97

  ketones, 97

  nuts and seeds, 282–283

  overview, 96–100

  saturated, 96, 99

  shopping, 205–207

  triglycerides, 96

  unsaturated, 96, 97–98

fat-soluble vitamins, 109, 134
fiber
  blood glucose and, 40
  insoluble, 95
  Mediterranean diet, 240
  overview, 95–96
  pectin, 350
  soluble, 20, 95
15-gram snacks, 286
fish and seafood
  choosing, 208–209
  omega-3 fatty acids, 75
  swapping meat for, 241–242
  vitamin D, 109
flavonoids, 136–137
flavor, enhancing, 185
flavored waters, 280–281
food as medicine, 1–2. *See also* culinary therapy
food cravings, 15–17, 166–167. *See also* emotional
  eating
food environment, 162–166
food grater, 146
Food Guide Pyramid, 217
food processor, 146
food storage, 163
food swaps
  aromatics, 364–365
  canned and jarred products, 367
  chips and dips, 365
  chocolate, 366–367
  overview, 361–362
  processed and packaged foods, 368
  red meat, 368
  salad dressings, 362
  sour cream, 363–364
  spices, 366
  tomato sauce, 362–363
food thermometer, 146
free foods, exchange list, 382–384
free radicals, 37, 129–130
French paradox, 138
Fresh Fruit Salad with Homemade Vanilla and Flax
  Seed Granola, 306

Fresh Herb and Parmigiano Crusted Fish with
  Apple, Beet, and Carrot Salad with Citrus
  Vinaigrette, 330
frozen food, 199, 367
fructose, 25
fruit
  carbohydrates, 224
  DASH diet, 245–246
  exchange lists, 373–374
  Mediterranean diet, 240–241
  as snack, 284
  stocking pantry, 147
  whole fruit, 94–95

G

garlic, 135, 364
gastroparesis, 79
genetics, Type 2 diabetes and, 32
genistein, 137
GFR (glomerular filtration rate), 79
ghrelin, 169
GI. *See* glycemic index
GL. *See* glycemic load
glomerular filtration rate (GFR), 79
GLP-1 hormone, 50, 129
glucagon, 42–43
glucose. *See* blood glucose
glucose tolerance factor, 112
glucosinolates, 127, 135, 394
gluten sensitivity, 78–79
glycemic index (GI)
  of common foods, 387–388
  defined, 84
  evaluating, 88–90
  Nutrisystem plan, 255
  tropical fruit, 202
glycemic load (GL)
  acid and, 350
  of common foods, 387–388
  defined, 84
  evaluating, 90
glycerol (glycerin), 96
glycogen, 19, 42, 85

glycolipids, 85

grains. *See* whole grains

grams and milligrams, 151–152

Greek yogurt, 227, 353, 363–364

gut microbiome, 120–123

H

HbA1C (hemoglobin A1C) measurement, 31, 46–47, 69–70

HCAs (heterocyclic amines), 104

HCG (human chorionic gonadotropin) diet, 257

HDL (high-density lipoproteins), 99

healthy eating and lifestyle

  asking for help with, 175

  commitment to, 61

  creating right environment for, 173–175

  making time for, 179–180

  meal planning and, 175–176

  overview, 55, 161–162

  physical activity, 56–58

  sense of community and, 61

  smoking cessation, 59

  spending time outdoors, 61–62

  stress management, 59–60

  valuing prevention, 62

healthy fats. *See also* extra-virgin olive oil; fats and oils

healthy halo effect, 201

heart attack and stroke, 35–36

heart-healthy diet, 20–21

Hearty Farro and Five-Vegetable Minestrone, 319

heirloom recipes, 234–235

Hello Fresh, 256

hemoglobin A1C (HbA1C) measurement, 31, 46–47, 69–70

herbs, 204, 365

Heritage diets, 243–244

hesperidin, 137, 350

heterocyclic amines (HCAs), 104

high-density lipoproteins (HDL), 99

holistic approach

  complications of diabetes, 34–38

  diabetes mellitus defined, 24–26

  gestational diabetes, 34

  overview, 23–24

  Type 1 diabetes, 27–30

  Type 2 diabetes, 30–34

Homemade Hummus and Whole Wheat Pita with Fresh Vegetables, 312

homeostasis, 10–11, 39. *See also* diabetes management

hormones, 26. *See also* insulin

  fat and, 97

  ghrelin, 169

  leptin, 169

hors d'oeuvres, 270

human chorionic gonadotropin (HCG) diet, 257

hydration, 292

hydrogenated fats, 99, 198

hydrogenation, 198

hydroxytyrosol, 139

hyperglycemia, 35, 78

hyperlipidemia, 100

hyperosmolar syndrome, 35

hypertension, 20, 73, 116. *See also* blood pressure

hypoglycemia, 26, 35, 78

hyponatremia, 115

I

I:C ratio (insulin to carbohydrate ratio), 51, 68

IL-6 (interleukin 6), 130

immunity, 38

impaired glucose tolerance, 44

impulsive eating, 15–17

incomplete protein foods, 102

infections, 38

inflammation

  biomarkers, 130

  C reactive protein, 130

  chronic inflammation, 131–132

  Dietary Inflammatory Index, 132–133

  interleukin 6, 130

  linking diabetes and, 36–37

  overview, 130–131

  proinflammatory foods, 131

  tumor necrosis factor alpha, 130

insoluble fiber, 95

insulin
  defined, 10–11
  hexamer, 117
  insulin bolus dosing, 93–94
  losing capacity to produce, 27–28
  monomer, 117
  overview, 41–42
  Type 1 diabetes, 10–11
  Type 2 diabetes, 10–11
insulin pumps, 52
insulin resistance, 30
insulin therapy, 51–52
insulin to carbohydrate ratio (I:C ratio), 51, 68
interleukin 6 (IL-6), 130
intermediate insulin formulations, 51–52
investing in yourself, 21–22
iodine, 209
isoflavones (phytoestrogens), 352

J

joules, 150

K

kale, as power food, 351
ketchup, 233
keto diet, 253
ketoacidosis, 97
ketones, 28, 97
kidney disease, 36
kidney failure, 79–80
King, Martin Luther, Jr., 6
kitchen scale, 144–145
knives, 145

L

labels, nutrition. See nutrition labels
lactose, 41, 85, 208
lada (latent autoimmune diabetes of adults), 29
lamb, 210
latent autoimmune diabetes of adults (lada), 29
LDL (low-density lipoproteins), 74–75, 99
leafy greens, as power food, 351

lean meats, 103
Lebanese Fattoush Salad with Citrus-Infused
    Chicken, 315
legumes. See beans and legumes
lemons, 350
lentils, 338, 356
leptin, 169
lifestyle changes
  achieving goals, 188–189
  adopting healthy habits, 182–184
  committing to future, 178–182
  detours, 185
  fads and quick fixes, 187–188
  overview, 177–178
  reasonable expectations, 186
  recordkeeping, 189
lignans, 139
limiting amino acids, 102
lipids, 96. See also fats and oils
liver cells, 42
long-acting insulin formulations, 52
long-term complications of diabetes, 35–36
low-carb diets
  Atkins diet, 252
  keto diet, 253
  overview, 251–252
  paleo diet, 253
low-carb snacks
  15-gram, 286
  overview, 285–286
  30-gram, 286–287
low-density lipoproteins (LDL), 74–75, 99
lunch
  Asian Noodle and Seven-Vegetable Salad with
      Sweet and Tangy Ginger Sauce, 316
  Baba Ghanouj with Crudités and Roasted
      Chickpeas, 321–322
  Broccoli and Pecorino Cheese Soup with Stuffed
      Baby Portobello Mushrooms, 317–318
  Cucumber and Smoked Salmon Pinwheels with
      Mixed Green Salad, 320
  Hearty Farro and Five-Vegetable Minestrone, 319
  Homemade Hummus and Whole Wheat Pita with
      Fresh Vegetables, 312
  Lebanese Fattoush Salad with Citrus-Infused
      Chicken, 315

Moroccan Rice, Lamb, Vegetable, and Lentil Soup, 313

overview, 311

personalized meal planning, 231–232

Roasted Sweet Potato, Avocado, and Quinoa Bowls with Honey- Lime Dressing and Cashews, 314

lycopene, 134–135

M

macronutrients. *See also* carbohydrates

building complete meals, 83–84

fat, 96–100

overview, 81–83

protein, 100–104

quality of food, 195–196

magnesium, 113–114, 247

mass-produced food, 164–166

mayonnaise, 233

meal planning. *See* personalized meal planning

meal skipping, 184

measuring cups, scoops, and spoons, 145

meat and meat substitutes

carcinogenic meat, 103

exchange lists, 377–380

red meat, 209–210, 368

medical nutrition therapy, 52–54, 214. *See also* culinary therapy

medical team

certified diabetes educator, 48

certified nutrition specialist, 48

dentist, 49

diabetologist, 48

endocrinologist, 48

mental health professional, 49

pharmacist, 48

podiatrist, 48

primary physician, 48

registered dietitians, 48

medications. *See also* insulin therapy

amylin analog, 50

compliance with, 49

GLP-1 hormone, 50

matching food and, 67–68

metformin, 50

side effects, 50

sodium glucose co-transporter 2 inhibitors, 50

thiazolidinediones, 50

Mediterranean diet

beans and legumes, 240

blood pressure and, 74

carbohydrates, 241

cost, 162

COVID-19 and, 38

dietary fiber, 240

Dietary Inflammatory Index and, 132

fruits and vegetables, 240–241

health benefits, 239

insulin resistance, 21

mortality and, 240

overview, 238

polyphenols, 129

protein and fat, 241–243

mental health professional, 49

menu-planning

avoiding temptation, 195

money-saving tips, 194–195

overview, 192–193

shopping list, 193

metabolic syndrome, 31, 75, 109

metabolism, 106

metformin, 50

mg/dl (milligrams per deciliter), 43–44

microflora, 353

micronutrients

gut microbiome, 120–123

minerals, 110–117

overview, 105

supplements, 117–120

vitamins, 106–110

Middle Eastern–Style Breakfast Platter, 308

milligrams per deciliter (mg/dl), 43–44

millimoles per liter (mmol/l), 43–44

mind-body connection

emotions and eating, 14–15

impulsive eating, 15–17

mind-body therapy, 14

overview, 13–14

mindless eating, 171–172
minerals
  calcium, 111–112
  chromium, 112
  magnesium, 113–114
  overview, 110
  potassium, 114–115
  sodium, 115–116
  zinc, 117
mitochondria, 40
mixed dishes and casseroles, 227–229
mmol/l (millimoles per liter), 43–44
money-saving shopping tips, 194–195
monosaccharides, 87
Monterey Bay Aquarium Seafood Watch list, 209, 349
morbidly obese BMI, 71
Moroccan Rice, Lamb, Vegetable, and Lentil
  Soup, 313
motor proteins, 101
muscle loss, 33–34
MyPlate, 217–219

N

National Mustard Museum, 233
National Weight Control Registry, 184
nephrologist, 79
nephropathy, 79
neuropathy, 36
neurotransmitters, 169–170
non-flavonoid polyphenols, 137–140
nonstarchy vegetables, 88, 92, 147, 201–202, 225
Noom, 256
nori, 107
Nurses' Health Study, 33, 132
nutrient-dense calories, 151
Nutrisystem, 255–256
Nutrisystem D plan, 255
nutrition
  A1C levels, 69–70
  athletes, 78
  cardiovascular health, 72–76
  celiac and gluten sensitivity, 78–79
  children, 76–77
  elderly, 77–78
  gastroparesis, 79
  kidney failure, 79–80
  matching medication and food, 67–68
  overview, 65–66
  weight loss, 70–72
nutrition apps, 155
nutrition labels
  calories, 150–151
  grams and milligrams, 151–152
  overview, 148–150
  serving sizes, 152
nuts and seeds
  as power food, 350
  shopping, 204
  as snack, 282–283

O

oats, as power food, 354
OGTT (oral glucose tolerance test), 44
oils. *See* fats and oils
oleic acid, 243
oleocanthal, 139
oleuropein, 139
oligomeric procyanidins, 138
oligosaccharides, 87–88
omega-3 fatty acids, 75, 97–98, 208, 243, 349
omega-6 fatty acids, 98, 206, 243
online resources
  Academy of Nutrition and Dietetics, 54
  American Association of Diabetes Educators, 54
  Cheat Sheet, 5
  Monterey Bay Aquarium Seafood Watch list,
    209, 349
  nutrition information, 155
  supplements, 120
oral glucose tolerance test (OGTT), 44
oranges, as power food, 350
organic food, 200–201
outdoor activities, 61–62
overweight BMI, 71
ovo-lacto vegetarians, 249–250
oxidation, 37, 99, 129–130, 348

oxidative stress, 37, 127, 130
Ozempic (semaglutide), 187

P

paleo diet, 253
pantry essentials
  beans and legumes, 148
  dairy, 148
  fruit, 147
  grains and starchy vegetables, 147
  healthy fats, 148
  healthy protein, 147
  nonstarchy vegetables, 147
  overview, 146
  spices and seasonings, 148
Pasta with Pistachio Pesto, Fresh Tuna, and Yellow
    Tomato Sauce, 331
Pavlov, Ivan, 162
peanut butter, 359
pectin, 350
personalized meal planning
  beans, 226
  breakfast and lunch, 231–232
  calorie requirements, 215
  carb portions, 219–221
  carbohydrates, 223–224
  complete meals, 230–231
  condiments, 232–234
  converting MyPlate into, 217–219
  dairy products, 226–227
  heirloom recipes, 234–235
  medical nutrition therapy and, 214
  mixed dishes and casseroles, 227–229
  overview, 213
  portion sizes, 216
  protein, 222–223
  recommended carbohydrate consumption, 215
  simple recipe formulas, 229–230
  snacks, 234
  starting simple, 221–222
  sugar-free foods, 227
  vegetables, 224–225
pharmacists, 48

phenolic compounds
  in extra-virgin olive oil, 395
  phenolic acids, 140
  phenolic alcohols, 139
phosphatidylcholine, 243
physical activity, 56–58
phytoestrogens (isoflavones), 352
phytonutrients, 126. *See also* bioactive compounds
pico de gallo, 233
plant proteins, 104
pleasure response, 168–170
Poached Egg and Avocado Toast with Warm Cherry
    Tomatoes and Sea Salt, 303–304
podiatrist, 48
Pollan, Michael, 197
pollo-pescetarian vegetarian, 248–249
polyphenols, 21, 127, 136, 367, 392–393
polysaccharides, 40, 41
portion distortion, 144, 268
portion sizes
  carb choice and, 153–155
  personalized meal planning and, 216
postprandial time frame, 45, 68
potassium, 114–115, 209, 247
potassium-to-sodium ratio, 74
potatoes, 358
poultry, 209, 241–242
power foods
  barley, 354
  beans and legumes, 349
  dark chocolate, 351–352
  extra-virgin olive oil, 348
  Greek yogurt, 353
  kale, 351
  leafy greens, 351
  lemons, 350
  nuts, 350
  oats, 354
  oranges, 350
  overview, 347
  salmon, 349
  soy, 352–353
  tuna, 349
  whole grains, 353–354

prebiotics, 122
prediabetes, 12, 30–31, 86
prevention, valuing, 62
primary physicians, 48
prioritizing health. *See* lifestyle changes
probiotics, 122–123
processed and packaged foods, 164–165, 196–199, 368
produce, 201–202. *See also* fruit; vegetables
pro-inflammatory foods, 37, 131
protein
  amino acids, 101–102
  animal sources of, 102–104
  beans and legumes, 203–204
  dairy products, 207–208
  eggs, 207
  Mediterranean diet, 241–243
  nuts and seeds, 204
  overview, 100–101
  personalized meal planning, 222–223
  plant proteins, 104
  stocking pantry, 147
protein digestibility corrected amino acid score, 222

Q

quercetin, 137

R

rapid insulin formulations, 51
reasonable expectations, 186
recipes. *See also* lunch
  base recipes, 337–341
  breakfast, 303–308
  collecting, 156
  converting, 156
  dinner, 323–333
recordkeeping, 189
Red Lentil Croquettes over Baby Spinach with Tzatziki Sauce, 325–326
red meat, 209–210, 368. *See also* meat and meat substitutes
reduction (redox), 130
registered dietitians, 48
resistance exercises, 58

resveratrol, 138
rheumatoid arthritis, 27
Roasted Sweet Potato, Avocado, and Quinoa Bowls with Honey- Lime Dressing and Cashews, 314
rosemarinic acid, 140

S

saccharin, 287
salad bar, 271
salad dressings, 234, 362
salad spinner, 145
salmon, 349
salsa, 233
saturated fat, 99, 205
scarcity, 163–164
scurvy, 106
Seafood Stock recipe, 340
secoiridoids, 139
secondary metabolites, 127
selenium, 209
self-care, 14–15, 21–22. *See also* culinary therapy
semaglutide (Ozempic), 187
serotonin, 169
serving size, nutrition labels, 152
Seven-Day Menu, 291–299
SGLT2 inhibitors (sodium glucose co-transporter 2 inhibitors), 50
shopping
  beans and legumes, 203–204
  canned foods, 200
  condiments, 207
  dairy products, 207–208
  eggs, 207
  extra-virgin olive oil, 204–205
  fats and oils, 205–207
  fish and seafood, 208–209
  frozen foods, 199
  identifying high-quality food, 195–196
  menu-planning, 192–195
  nuts and seeds, 204
  organic food, 200–201
  overview, 191
  poultry, 209
  prepackaged food, 196–198
  processed food, 198–199

produce, 201–202

red meat, 209–210

spices, herbs, and alums, 204

whole grains, 202–203

short-acting insulin formulations, 51

short-term complications of diabetes, 35

simple recipe formulas, 229–230

Sizzling Rosemary Shrimp over Cannellini Bean Puree and Sautéed Greens with Mixed Peppers, 332–333

smoking cessation, 59

snacks

dark chocolate, 284–285

fruit, 284

low-carb, 285–287

nuts and seeds, 282–283

personalized meal planning, 234

Seven-Day Menu, 299

veggies and dips, 284

yogurt, 283–284

social connection with food, 168

sodium, 74, 115–116, 232–233, 247–248

sodium glucose co-transporter 2 inhibitors (SGLT2 inhibitors), 50

soft drinks, 280–281

soluble fiber, 20, 95

sour cream, 233, 363–364

soy, 104, 107, 202, 223, 226, 352–353

soy sauce, 232–233

sphygmomanometer, 73

spices and seasonings, 148, 204, 366

sports drinks, 281

starches, 40, 370–372

starchy vegetables, 147, 202, 224. *See also* vegetables

steamer baskets, 146

sterol, 99. *See also* cholesterol

stilbenes, 138

stocking kitchen, 143–148

stress management

chronic stress, 171

cortisol, 171

emotional eating, 170–171

fight or flight response, 170

overview, 59–60

sleep quality and, 171

sucralose, 287

sugar

disaccharides, 87

fruit sugars vs. refined sugars, 20

monosaccharides, 87

oligosaccharides, 87–88

overview, 86–87

sugar alcohols, 93

sugar beets, 359

sugar substitutes, 287

sugar-free foods, 227

supplements, 117–120

sweets and desserts, 270, 384–385

systolic pressure, 73

T

table beets, 359

tea, 279–280

tempeh, 107, 353

thiamine (vitamin B1), 21

thiazolidinediones, 50

30-gram snacks, 286–287

timing meals and snacks, 183–184

TNF- alpha (tumor necrosis factor alpha), 130

tofu, 104, 353

Tomato Sauce recipe, 343

tomato sauce substitutes, 362–363

tools and gadgets

blender, 146

food grater, 146

food processor, 146

food thermometer, 146

kitchen scale, 144–145

knives, 145

measuring cups, scoops, and spoons, 145

salad spinner, 145

steamer baskets, 146

vegetable peelers, 146

trans fats, 99, 198

TRIGR study, 30

tropical fruit, 202

tumor necrosis factor alpha (TNF- alpha), 130

tuna, 349

Turkish-Style Eggplant and Chickpea Stew with Brown Basmati Rice Pilaf, 328–329

Type 1 diabetes
  causes of, 29–30
  defined, 10–11
  latent autoimmune diabetes of adults vs., 29
  losing capacity to produce insulin, 27–28

Type 2 diabetes
  age and, 33
  body mass index and, 32
  defined, 10–11
  ethnicity and, 33
  genetics and, 32
  muscle loss and, 33–34
  prediabetes and, 30–31
  visceral fat, 32

U

unconditioned response, 162
United Kingdom Prospective Diabetes Study (UKPDS), 46–47, 69
unsaturated fat, 97–98, 205
U.S. Department of Agriculture (USDA), 217

V

vanillic acid, 140
vegan diet, 250–251
vegetable peelers, 146
Vegetable Stock recipe, 339
vegetables. *See also* nonstarchy vegetables
  choosing, 95
  exchange lists, 375
  personalized meal planning, 224–225
  starchy, 147, 202, 224
  as substitute for chips and dip, 365

vegetarian diets
  overview, 248–249
  ovo-lacto vegetarians, 249–250
  vegan, 250–251
Vegetarian Society, 248
veggies and dips, 284
villi, 41
visceral fat, 32, 72
vision problems, 36

vitamins
  B complex, 106–108
  fat-soluable, 134
  overview, 106
  vitamin A, 209
  vitamin B1, 21
  vitamin B12, 250
  vitamin D, 108–110, 209, 250

W

Wansink, Brian, 171
Warm Raspberry and Cocoa Quinoa with Almond Milk and Sesame Seeds, 307
water, importance of, 276
weight loss
  fads and quick fixes, 187–188
  food swaps for, 361–368
  keys to success, 186
  nutrition and, 70–72
Weight Watchers, 253–255
whole grains
  DASH diet, 245–246
  defined, 94
  as power food, 353–354
  shopping, 202–203
  stocking pantry, 147
World Health Organization (WHO), 99

X

xanthophylls, 133

Y

yogurt
  as budget-friendly option, 357
  Greek yogurt, 227
  inulin, 284
  microflora, 283, 353
  as snack, 283–284

Z

zinc, 117, 208–209

About the Authors

Dr. Simon Poole, MBBS, DRCOG, FBMA, MIANE, is a primary care physician in Cambridge, England, with a particular interest in lifestyle medicine and nutrition as well as the management of long-term medical conditions. He has taught and undertaken research with Cambridge University and is a founding member of the British and European Associations of Lifestyle Medicine. Simon is a council member of The True Health Initiative and an International Senior Collaborator with the Global Centre for Nutrition and Health in Cambridge. He was awarded Fellowship of the British Medical Association for services to the profession in 2018, which included longstanding membership of Council of the Royal College of General Practitioners and Public Health Medicine Committee. Simon is a recognized international authority and speaker on lifestyle medicine, chairing the Food Values Conference series at the Pontifical Academy of Science of the Vatican, and the author of the award-winning book *The Olive Oil Diet* (Hachette) and *The Real Mediterranean Diet* (Cambridge Academic), and coauthor of *Diabetes For Dummies*, 6th Edition (Wiley).

Amy Riolo is a bestselling author and an award-winning chef, television host, and Mediterranean lifestyle ambassador. The author of 15 books on the Mediterranean diet and cuisine, diabetes-friendly cuisine, and the Mediterranean lifestyle, Amy has been named "The Ambassador of Italian Cuisine in the United States" by the Italian International Agency for Foreign Press, and the "Ambassador of the Italian Mediterranean Diet 2022–2024" by the International Academy of the Italian Mediterranean Diet in her ancestral homeland of Calabria, Italy. Amy is the brand ambassador for the Maryland University of Integrative Health and the Pizza University and Culinary Arts Center in Maryland. In 2019, she launched her own private label collection of premium Italian imported culinary ingredients called Amy Riolo Selections, which includes extra-virgin olive oil, balsamic vinegar, organic pasta, and pesto sauce from award-winning artisan companies. She is also coauthor of *Diabetes For Dummies*, 6th Edition (Wiley).

Dedication

From Simon: I dedicate this book to my sons, Adam and Tom, who are a constant inspiration to me for the way in which they are forging their lives with purpose and passion.

From Amy: I dedicate this book to my mother, Faith Riolo, for always inspiring me to learn, cook, and do my best, and to my Nonna Angela for teaching me everything I needed to know.

Authors' Acknowledgments

The authors would like to thank Dr. Alan Rubin and Toby Smithson for their excellent contributions to the previous edition of this book and all those at Wiley, especially Tracy Boggier, who have been so supportive of our commitment to bringing a holistic and positive approach to the prevention and treatment of diabetes and for being such a pleasure to work with. Katharine Dvorak, thank you for your amazing editing skills. We are also grateful to Kristie Pyles for her support and to Rachel Nix for her nutritional analysis support and careful recipe testing. Many thanks to Elizabeth Lipski, PhD, CNS, for her excellent technical review.

From Simon: I am, as ever, grateful to my wife, Roslyn, and family, friends, and colleagues acknowledged in the first book in the series, *Diabetes For Dummies,* who continue to provide generous support, invaluable feedback, and unwavering inspiration.

As I write this final section of our book, the National Health Service celebrates 75 years of providing universal healthcare to the people of the United Kingdom. During my 30 years of service in the NHS, I consider myself fortunate to work in a system that, despite its many challenges, aspires to care comprehensively for people "from cradle to grave," reduce health inequalities, and align its priorities with public health and lifestyle medicine organizations committed to prevention of illness and promotion of good health. The ethos of the organization always depends on those working in it, and I have been privileged to spend my career with professionals who show so much skill, dedication, and compassion in their care of patients. Those friends and colleagues have been my teachers and my inspiration as I have looked after patients through illness and worked to support those who wish to add years to life and life to years through enjoyable and beneficial lifestyle changes.

I am grateful to my coauthor of this book and of *Diabetes for Dummies,* 6th Edition, Amy Riolo, without whose wise, holistic, and creative partnership none of this would be possible.

From Amy: I owe my ability to write, cook, and promote the Mediterranean lifestyle strictly to destiny. Had I been born into another family or culture, and not had the opportunity to live, work, and travel throughout the Mediterranean region, it would never have been possible. After decades of witnessing not only my own family, but also people throughout the region live and eat with both pleasure and health, I am convinced, now more than ever, that this is a goal we can all achieve. For all of you who have shared a kitchen or a meal with me, I thank you.

My nonna, Angela Magnone Foti, taught me to cook and bake, as well as valuable lessons that served me outside of the kitchen. Because of her and our heritage, my first tastes of "Italian food" were Calabrian. Those edible time capsules formed a culinary bloodline between us and our relatives in southern Italy. Because of her, I am able to prepare many of the same dishes that my Italian relatives do, even though I am a fourth generation American. Nonna Angela gave me my first cookbook and showed me how cooking was not a mundane chore, but a form of magic that could unite people across distances and time.

My Yia Yia, Mary Michos Riolo, shared her beloved Greek traditions with me, and I am happy to say that they have become woven into my culinary fabric as well — especially because many Italian regions were Greek colonies in antiquity. My earliest memories of cooking were with my mother, Faith Riolo, who would sit me on the counter and roll more meatballs and cookies than I could count. She taught me that food was not just something we eat to nourish ourselves, but an edible gift that could be given to express love. I owe my love of food history and anthropology to my father, Rick Riolo, for planting the desire to answer the question, "I wonder how they eat" in my mind since childhood. It's a type of culinary curiosity that is never completely satisfied and gives me the motivation to continue my work each day. To my beloved little brother, Jeremy, you are my why, and I am grateful to be able to pass our family's knowledge down to you.

I would probably never have published a cookbook if it weren't for my mentor, Sheilah Kaufman, who patiently taught me much more than I ever planned on learning. I am proud to pass her knowledge on to others. I am very thankful to Chef Luigi Diotaiuti for his influence and for always believing in me, inspiring me, encouraging me to foster my culinary medicine interests, and much more. I am also very grateful for the presence of Dr. Sam Pappas in my career. To my current writing partner, Dr. Simon Poole, you are a pleasure to collaborate with, and I am always grateful for the passion, knowledge, and commitment that you bring to our work.

In Italy, I thank my fantastic, generous, and hospitable cousins Franco Riolo, his lovely wife, Pina, and Tonia Riolo; my beautiful cousin Serena Riolo, who I love cooking and spending time with; Serena's brother Vincenzo Riolo for the bond and memories we share; as well as to my dear cousin Angela Riolo for always clearing her schedule for me. To my Italian business partners Antonio Iuliano and Francesco Giovanelli, thank you for making my culinary dreams come true. I am also very grateful to Stefano Ferrari, owner of LIFeSTYLE and Cibo Divino, for importing and distributing my private-label products along with Vince Di Piazza of DITALIA for distributing them. Additional thanks go to all the retailers who carry my products.

There is not a day that passes that I don't thank my close friend and business partner Alex Safos of Indigo Gazelle Tours for his support and collaborations. Throughout recent years I have been fortunate to be able to call upon the assistance of many dear friends who I love like family. I am truly grateful to Francesco

Marra and the entire Marra family for naming me an Ambassador of Pizza University and Culinary Arts Center and for the gift of friendship. Thank you to my dear friend and marketing diva Gail Broeckel, the great Chef Paul Kolze, my favorite molecular gastronomist Edward Donnelly, the multi-talented Stuart Hershey, Chef Sedrick Crawley, and Certified Executive Chef Jeff Fritz. I would also like to thank Dr. John Rosa for recognizing my contributions to the field of culinary medicine and for all of the wonderful avenues of collaboration. To Marc Levin, President and CEO of the Maryland University of Integrative Health, thank you very much for the opportunity to represent you as an Ambassador. I am also very appreciative of my Alma Mater, Cornell University and Montgomery College for recognizing my achievements.

I am forever indebted to Dr. Norton Fishman for diagnosing me and creating a team of doctors to enable me to heal. To my late dear friend and sister, Kathleen Ammalee Rogers, I would not be here if it weren't for your care, support, and friendship, and I am always thankful to you for my health, career, and overall wellbeing. I am also forever grateful to Dr. Beth Tedesco and Dr. Mary Lee Esty for enabling me to overcome my own illness and fulfill my dreams. To my trusted friends like family, Jonathan Bardzik, Ann Hotung, Sharon Wolpoff, and Pina Dubbio, thank you for helping me create joy daily. And finally, I would like to thank you, the reader, for joining me on this journey into an enjoyable and rewarding way of life.

Publisher's Acknowledgments

Senior Acquisitions Editor: Tracy Boggier
Senior Managing Editor: Kristie Pyles
Project Editor: Katharine Dvorak
Technical Editor: Liz Lipski, PhD, CNS
Recipe Tester: Rachel Nix

Production Editor: Tamilmani Varadharaj
Cover Image: © fcafotodigital/Getty Images